Monographs in Oral Science

Vol. 25

Series Editors

A. Lussi Bern

M.C.D.N.J.M. Huysmans Nijmegen

H.-P. Weber Boston, Mass.

Erosive Tooth Wear

From Diagnosis to Therapy

2nd, revised and extended edition of
'Dental Erosion – From Diagnosis to Therapy', Vol. 20

Volume Editors

Adrian Lussi Bern
Carolina Ganss Giessen

61 figures, 41 in color, and 29 tables, 2014

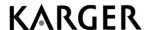

Basel · Freiburg · Paris · London · New York · Chennai · New Delhi ·
Bangkok · Beijing · Shanghai · Tokyo · Kuala Lumpur · Singapore · Sydney

Adrian Lussi
Department of Preventive, Restorative and
Pediatric Dentistry
University of Bern
Freiburgstrasse 7
CH–3010 Bern (Switzerland)

Carolina Ganss
Department of Conservative and Preventive
Dentistry, Dental Clinic
Justus Liebig University Giessen
Schlangenzahl 14
DE–35392 Giessen (Germany)

Library of Congress Cataloging-in-Publication Data

Dental erosion (Lussi)
  Erosive tooth wear : from diagnosis to therapy / volume editors, Adrian Lussi, Carolina Ganss. --
2nd, revised and extended edition.
      p. ; cm. -- (Monographs in oral science, ISSN 0077-0892 ; vol. 25)
  Preceded by Dental erosion / volume editor Adrian Lussi. c2006.
  Includes bibliographical references and indexes.
  ISBN 978-3-318-02552-1 (hard cover : alk. paper) -- ISBN 978-3-318-02553-8 (electronic version)
  I. Lussi, Adrian, editor. II. Ganss, Carolina, editor. III. Title. IV.
Series: Monographs in oral science ; v. 25. 0077-0892
  [DNLM: 1. Tooth Erosion. W1 MO568E v.25 2014 / WU 140]
  RK340
  617.6′3--dc23
                                                                    2014012875

Bibliographic Indices. This publication is listed in bibliographic services, including Current Contents® and Index Medicus.

© Copyright 2014 by S. Karger AG, P.O. Box, CH–4009 Basel (Switzerland)
www.karger.com
Printed in Germany on acid-free and non-aging paper (ISO 9706) by Kraft Druck GmbH, Ettlingen
ISSN 0077–0892
e-ISSN 1662–3843
ISBN 978–3–318–02552–1
e-ISBN 978–3–318–02553–8

Contents

List of Contributors

Martin Addy
School of Oral and Dental Sciences
University of Bristol
Lower Maudlin Street
Bristol BS1 2LY (UK)
E-Mail martin.addy@bristol.ac.uk

Thomas Attin
Center for Dental Medicine
Clinic for Preventive Dentistry, Periodontology
and Cariology
University of Zurich
Plattenstrasse 11
CH–8032 Zurich (Switzerland)
E-Mail thomas.attin@zzm.uzh.ch

Michele E. Barbour
School of Oral and Dental Sciences
University of Bristol
Lower Maudlin Street
Bristol BS1 2LY (UK)
E-Mail m.e.barbour@bristol.ac.uk

David Bartlett
Department of Prosthodontics
King's College London Dental Institute
Floor 25, Guy's Tower, St. Thomas' Street
London Bridge, London SE1 9RT (UK)
E-Mail david.bartlett@kcl.ac.uk

Marília Alfonso Rabelo Buzalaf
Department of Biological Sciences
Bauru Dental School
University of São Paulo
Al. Octávio Pinheiro Brisolla, 9-75
Bauru, SP 17012-901 (Brazil)
E-Mail mbuzalaf@fob.usp.br

Thiago Saads Carvalho
Department of Preventive, Restorative and
Pediatric Dentistry
School of Dental Medicine
University of Bern
Freiburgstrasse 7
CH–3010 Bern (Switzerland)
E-Mail thiago.saads@zmk.unibe.ch

Maria Davies
Periodontology
Clinical Trials Unit
Bristol Dental School
Lower Maudlin Street
Bristol BS1 2LY (UK)
E-Mail maria.davies@bristol.ac.uk

John D.B. Featherstone
Department of Preventive, Restorative and
Pediatric Dentistry Dental Sciences
University of California at San Francisco
Room 0603, Box 0758
707 Parnassus Avenue
San Francisco, CA 94143 (USA)
E-Mail jdbf@ucsf.edu

Dien L. Gambon
Department of Oral Biochemistry
Academic Centre for Dentistry Amsterdam (ACTA)
Louwesweg 1
NL–1066 EA Amsterdam (The Netherlands)
E-Mail dien.gambon@kpnmail.nl

Carolina Ganss
Department of Conservative and Preventive Dentistry
Dental Clinic
Justus Liebig University Giessen
Schlangenzahl 14
DE–35392 Giessen (Germany)
E-Mail carolina.ganss@dentist.med.uni-giessen.de

Matthias Hannig
Clinic of Operative Dentistry, Periodontology and
Preventive Dentistry
Saarland University, Building 73
DE–66421 Homburg (Germany)
E-Mail matthias.hannig@uks.eu

Christian Hannig
Clinic of Operative Dentistry
Medical Faculty Carl Gustav Carus, TU Dresden
Fetscherstraße 74
DE–01307 Dresden (Germany)
E-Mail christian.hannig@uniklinikum-dresden.de

Anderson T. Hara
Department of Preventive and Community Dentistry
Oral Health Research Institute
Indiana University School of Dentistry
415 North Lansing Street
Indianapolis, IN 46202-2876 (USA)
E-Mail ahara@iu.edu

Elmar Hellwig
Department of Operative Dentistry and
Periodontology
Center of Dental Medicine, University of Freiburg
Hugstetter Strasse 55
DE–79106 Freiburg (Germany)
E-Mail elmar.hellwig@uniklinik-freiburg.de

Marie-Charlotte Huysmans
College of Dental Sciences
Radboud University Medical Center
Radboud University Nijmegen, PO Box 9101
NL–6500 HB Nijmegen (The Netherlands)
E-Mail marie-charlotte.huysmans@radboudumc.nl

Thomas Jaeggi
Department of Preventive, Restorative and
Pediatric Dentistry
School of Dental Medicine
University of Bern
Freiburgstrasse 7
CH–3010 Bern (Switzerland)
E-Mail thomasjaeggi@bluewin.ch

Adrian Lussi
Department of Preventive, Restorative and
Pediatric Dentistry
School of Dental Medicine
University of Bern
Freiburgstrasse 7
CH–3010 Bern (Switzerland)
E-Mail adrian.lussi@zmk.unibe.ch

Ana Carolina Magalhães
Department of Biological Sciences
Bauru Dental School
University of São Paulo
Al. Octávio Pinheiro Brisolla, 9-75
Bauru, SP 17012-901 (Brazil)
E-Mail acm@usp.br

Vasileios Margaritis
College of Health Sciences
Walden University
100 Washington Ave. South, Suite 900
Minneapolis, MN 55401 (USA)
E-Mail vasileios.margaritis@waldenu.edu

Rebecca Moazzez
Department of Prosthodontics
King's College London Dental Institute
Floor 25, Guy's Tower, St. Thomas' Street
London Bridge, London SE1 9RT (UK)
E-Mail rebecca.v.moazzez@kcl.ac.uk

June Nunn
Department of Special Care Dentistry
Dublin Dental University Hospital
Lincoln Place
Dublin 2 (Ireland)
E-Mail june.nunn@dental.tcd.ie

Anne Peutzfeldt
Department of Preventive, Restorative and
Pediatric Dentistry
School of Dental Medicine
University of Bern
Freiburgstrasse 7
CH–3010 Bern (Switzerland)
E-Mail anne.peutzfeldt@zmk.unibe.ch

Joon Seong
Periodontology
Clinical Trials Unit
Bristol Dental School
Lower Maudlin Street
Bristol BS1 2LY (UK)
E-Mail j.seong@bristol.ac.uk

R. Peter Shellis
Department of Preventive, Restorative and
Pediatric Dentistry
School of Dental Medicine
University of Bern
Freiburgstrasse 7
CH–3010 Bern (Switzerland)
E-Mail peter.shellis@btinternet.com

Nadine Schlueter
Department of Conservative and Preventive Dentistry
Dental Clinic
Justus Liebig University Giessen
Schlangenzahl 14
DE–35392 Giessen (Germany)
E-Mail nadine.schlueter@dentist.med.uni-giessen.de

Anne Bjørg Tveit
Department of Cariology and Gerodontology
Institute of Clinical Dentistry
Faculty of Dentistry University of Oslo
NO–0317 Oslo (Norway)
E-Mail annebtv@odont.uio.no

Florian Just Wegehaupt
Center for Dental Medicine
Clinic for Preventive Dentistry, Periodontology
and Cariology
University of Zurich
Plattenstrasse 11
CH–8032 Zurich (Switzerland)
E-Mail florian.wegehaupt@zzm.uzh.ch

Nicola West
Periodontology
Clinical Trials Unit
Bristol Dental School
Lower Maudlin Street
Bristol BS1 2LY (UK)
E-Mail n.x.west@bristol.ac.uk

Annette Wiegand
Department of Preventive Dentistry, Periodontology
and Cariology
Georg August University Göttingen
Robert-Koch-Strasse 40
DE–35075 Göttingen (Germany)
E-Mail annette.wiegand@med.uni-goettingen.de

Alix Young
Department of Cariology and Gerodontology
Institute of Clinical Dentistry
Faculty of Dentistry University of Oslo
NO–0317 Oslo (Norway)
E-Mail a.y.vik@odont.uio.no

Domenick Zero
Department of Preventive and Community Dentistry
Oral Health Research Institute
Indiana University School of Dentistry
415 North Lansing Street
Indianapolis, IN 46202-2876 (USA)
E-Mail dzero@iupui.edu

Acknowledgements

The 2nd, revised and extended edition of the present book dealing with all aspects of erosive tooth wear was generously sponsored by the following bodies:

Platinum Sponsor

- GlaxoSmithKline, Weybridge, UK

Gold Sponsor

- Colgate Europe, Therwil, Switzerland

Silver Sponsors

- Procter & Gamble, Geneva, Switzerland
- Unilever Oral Care, London, UK
- Wrigley Oral Healthcare Program, Unterhaching, Germany

Sincere thanks goes to the experts who reviewed all chapters. Their commitment has ensured a high standard of the book.

The support of the University of Bern, Department of Preventive, Restorative and Pediatric Dentistry, is acknowledged. In particular, we wish to thank Ines Badertscher, Isabel Hug, Brigit Megert, Bernadette Rawyler and Hermann Stich for their outstanding contribution.

Adrian Lussi, Bern

Foreword to the First Edition

Dental Erosion: A challenge for the 21st century! This monograph offers a guide towards better oral health in the future. Erosive tooth wear is a multifactorial condition of growing concern to the clinician and the subject of extensive research – a view supported by the literature and impressions from many international conferences over recent decades. However, until now, no attempt has been made to collect and organize the available information in a single book. This volume of *Monographs in Oral Science* is the first book dealing solely with erosive tooth wear.

The thirteen chapters of the book present a broad spectrum of views on dental erosion, from the molecular level to behavioral aspects and trends in society. The multifactorial etiological pattern of erosive tooth wear is emphasized and is a strand connecting the different chapters of the book. It starts with the definition of erosion and describes the interaction of attrition, abrasion and erosion in tooth wear. The chapters on diagnosis of erosion and prevalence, incidence and distribution of the condition are followed by a chapter on the chemistry of erosion. Under the heading of extrinsic causes of erosion, several factors are analyzed and illustrated, amongst which are the consequences of our changing lifestyles and the effects of oral hygiene products and acidic medicines. The chapter on intrinsic causes of erosion focuses on gastroesophageal reflux disease and related issues. A separate chapter is devoted to dental erosion in children. Methods of assessment of dental erosion are presented and critically evaluated, concluding that the complex nature of erosive mineral loss and dissolution might not readily be encompassed by a single technique: a more comprehensive approach combining several different methods is recommended. The last three chapters cover dentinal hypersensitivity, risk assessment and preventive measures, and, finally, restorative options for erosive lesions.

Each chapter has a comprehensive list of references, encouraging the reader to consult the original articles for more details. Instructive intraoral photographs illustrate the text and guide the reader. An unusual step is that every chapter was reviewed not only by the editor but also by two external reviewers, ensuring the highest of standards.

This monograph describes current concepts of dental erosion and presents an overview of the literature, with special reference to clinically relevant implications. It is not only suitable for faculty members and researchers, but may also be recommended for dental students, practitioners and other dental professionals who are committed to preventing and treating dental erosion.

Birgit Angmar-Månsson, Stockholm

Preface

Eight years ago the first edition of the monograph *Dental Erosion – from Diagnosis to Therapy* appeared and was then the first of its kind to deal with all aspects of this important subject. Since then, new knowledge has been gathered which makes a better understanding of this multifactorial process possible. The more detailed knowledge resulted in this second edition which has now a slightly modified title, *Erosive Tooth Wear – from Diagnosis to Therapy*. The title as well as new chapters and their increased number mirror the extended knowledge. This second extended edition deals with all aspects of erosive tooth wear. The issues concerning epidemiology, histopathology, aetiology, preventive therapy as well as special problems concerning children are now covered more extensively.

A book is only up to date when the process from writing to publishing is very fast. We would like to thank all the authors for their timely writing of the chapters, the reviewers for correcting the chapters so quickly and the publisher for producing this monograph.

Finally, we thank the different bodies for their generous support of this book. It makes wide dissemination at a reasonable price possible.

Adrian Lussi, Bern
Carolina Ganss, Giessen

Lussi A, Ganss C (eds): Erosive Tooth Wear. Monogr Oral Sci. Basel, Karger, 2014, vol 25, pp 1–15
DOI: 10.1159/000360380

Erosive Tooth Wear: A Multifactorial Condition of Growing Concern and Increasing Knowledge

Adrian Lussi · Thiago S. Carvalho

Department of Preventive, Restorative and Pediatric Dentistry, School of Dental Medicine, University of Bern, Bern, Switzerland

Abstract

Dental erosion is often described solely as a surface phenomenon, unlike caries where it has been established that the destructive effects involve both the surface and the subsurface region. However, besides removal of the surface, erosion shows dissolution of mineral within the softened layer – beneath the surface. In order to distinguish this process from the carious process it is now called 'near surface demineralization'. Erosion occurs in low pH, but there is no fixed critical pH value concerning dental erosion. The critical pH value for enamel concerning caries (pH 5.5–5.7) has to be calculated from calcium and phosphate concentrations of plaque fluid. In the context of dental erosion, the critical pH value is calculated from the calcium and phosphate concentrations in the erosive solution itself. Thus, critical pH for enamel with regard to erosion will vary according to the erosive solution. Erosive tooth wear is becoming increasingly significant in the management of the long-term health of the dentition. What is considered as an acceptable amount of wear is dependent on the anticipated lifespan of the dentition and is, therefore, different for deciduous compared to permanent teeth. However, erosive damage to the teeth may compromise the patient's dentition for their entire lifetime and may require repeated and increasingly complex and expensive restorations. Therefore, it is important that diagnosis of the tooth wear process in children and adults is made early and that adequate preventive measures are undertaken. These measures can only be initiated when the risk factors are known and interactions between them are present.

© 2014 S. Karger AG, Basel

Change of Perception

Erosive tooth wear was for many years a condition of little interest to clinical dental practice, dental public health or dental research. Diagnosis was seldom made, especially in the early stages, and there was little, if anything, that could be done to intervene at this stage. However, perceptions have now changed. Problems and questions concerning erosive tooth wear now cover an ample area of research in dentistry, and it is a daily concern in the clinical practice. This will undoubtedly expand in the future, similarly to what has been occurring in the last decades.

A literature search in PubMed was carried out using the term 'tooth erosion' (MeSH terms) for the number of publications throughout the years. A steady increase can be observed in the number of publications, where less than 5 papers were published in 1970 and the number of studies increased to just over 10 in 1980. In 2000, the number of studies had increased considerably to almost 60 studies, whereas more recently, in 2012, the number had reached 100. Such an increase in the number of publications was also observed when the search on PubMed included all non-carious dental hard tissue defects, where terms related to abrasion and attrition were also incorporated in the search: ['tooth wear' (MeSH terms) OR 'tooth attrition' (MeSH terms) OR 'tooth erosion' (MeSH terms) OR 'tooth abrasion' (MeSH terms)]. A total of almost 40 studies were published in 1970 and this number increased to almost 50 in 1980. However, the number of studies doubled in 2000, when more than 100 studies were published on tooth wear, and more recently, in 2012, almost 250 studies appeared on PubMed. This goes to show that dental erosion and erosive tooth wear are becoming increasingly more significant both in research and in the clinic.

(Erosive) tooth wear is also of increasing importance in the long-term health of the dentition and the overall well-being of those who suffer its effects. Following the decline in tooth loss in the 20th century, the increasing longevity of teeth in the 21st century will render the clinically deleterious effect of wear more demanding on the preventive and restorative skills of the dental professional [1]. Awareness of dental erosion is still not widespread in the public, although in some countries there is knowledge and awareness concerning acidic foods and beverages [2–5]. In its early stages, and for the vast majority of the population, the changes seen in tooth erosion are of only cosmetic significance. In a survey in England, 34% of the children were aware of tooth erosion but only 8% could recall their dentist mentioning the condition [6]; 40% of children believed incorrectly that the best way to avoid erosion was regular toothbrushing, which shows some misunderstanding or lack of information. In addition, the awareness of dentists was considered low [6]. A recent study carried out with young adults from Norway (aged 19–20 years) showed that, although a great majority of the participants were aware of erosion, had knowledge about the causes of the condition (93.5%) and believed that the condition can be prevented (84.9%), a reasonable number of them still drank sugary soft drinks (17.5%) and juices (34.1%). This indicates the need for effective intervention strategies to reduce the level of consumption [2].

Change of Knowledge

Dental caries is a well-known phenomenon, where the destructive effects occur both on the surface as well as within the subsurface region. Unlike caries, dental erosion is more often defined as a purely surface phenomenon. Although most of the demineralization does occur on the tooth's surface, the pathophysiology of dental erosion is more complex than previously described. Initially, when a solution comes into the oral cavity, it first has to diffuse through the acquired enamel pellicle before it can interact with the enamel itself [see chapters by Shellis et al., this vol., pp. 163–179 and Hannig and Hannig, this vol., pp. 206–214]. The pellicle is a thin acellular biofilm, free of bacteria, that covers both hard and soft oral tissues and functions as a perm-selective barrier. It is mainly composed of proteins (mostly mucins) and peptides derived from saliva, but it can also include enzymes, glycoproteins, carbohydrates and lipids [7, 8]. Once the acid diffuses through the acquired enamel pellicle, it reaches the surface of enamel, where hydrogen ions (H^+) will start to dissolve the enamel crystals. The effect of the H^+ ions first triggers the dissolution of the prism sheath, and later of the prism core, thus leaving the well-known honeycomb appearance [9]. However, much emphasis has been placed solely on the effect of the H^+ ions on the interface between solution and enamel; nevertheless, Gray [10] in the 1960s and Featherstone and Rodgers [11] in the 1980s also argued for the importance of the undissociated (non-ionized) form of organic acids in the carious process.

When organic acids are present in solution such as saliva, part of acid molecules will remain in its undissociated form, whereas another part will dissociate [R-COOH (aq) $\rightleftarrows$ R-COO$^-$ (aq) + H$^+$ (aq)]. Gray [10] and Featherstone and Rodgers [11] suggested that, during the formation of the subsurface lesion in the early caries process, the undissociated form of the acid could penetrate the enamel pores faster than the dissociated form because of its lack of charge. Once within the enamel, these molecules then dissociate, thus acting as carriers of H$^+$ into the enamel mineral [10, 11]. These H$^+$ ions present within the enamel pores would then dissolve the mineral crystals. In the first issue of this book, this mechanism was also proposed to be valid for the development of erosive lesions [12, 13]. More recently, Shellis et al. [14] were able to prove experimentally that these processes are also valid for erosion, and erosive dissolution occurs not only at the interface between solution and enamel but also within the thin, partly demineralized softened enamel layer. For this process, they suggested the term 'near-surface demineralization'. Hence, near-surface demineralization describes the softening process during dental erosion, emphasizing the fact that dental erosion is not exclusively a surface phenomenon but also occurs within the limited extent of the softened layer (a few micrometres) due to the effect of the undissociated form of the organic acids [14]. Furthermore, the authors also concluded that this process depends primarily on the concentration of the undissociated form of the organic acids within the enamel pores rather than on the buffering properties of the acid itself [14].

During the superficial and near-surface demineralization processes, the outflow of ions from the dental hard tissues will subsequently lead to a local rise of pH and ions in the liquid layer adjacent to the tooth mineral [15]. This semi-static layer of solution (the 'Nernst layer') will then have an increased concentration of ions,

eventually becoming saturated and not demineralizing enamel further. However, an increase in agitation (e.g. when a patient is swishing the drink in the mouth) may produce a constant replacement of the Nernst layer, which will not reach saturation level, and thus enhance the dissolution process [16]. This process is of particular importance when a substance is only slightly undersaturated with respect to tooth mineral. With such substances, only agitation will lead to a distinct dissolution of dental hard tissue. In any case, the continuous outflow of ions from the dental hard tissues will lead to the formation of a softened layer, which is vulnerable to outside mechanical forces (e.g. toothbrushing) and subsequent irreversible tooth substance loss.

With regard to dentine, the events occurring during erosion are, in principle, the same but the presence of the organic dentine matrix adds more complexity to the condition. The organic dentine matrix reduces the diffusion of the demineralizing agent (i.e. acid) deeper into the region as well as the outward flux of minerals from the dental hard tissues [17]. It has been assumed that the organic dentine matrix has a sufficient buffering capacity to retard further demineralization and that chemical or mechanical degradation of the dentine matrix promotes demineralization [18, 19]. These erosive processes are halted when no new acids are provided. Further, the amount of drink in the mouth in relation to the amount and flow of saliva present will modify the process of dissolution [1].

In addition to the few factors already mentioned in this chapter (pellicle, type of organic acid and its undissociated form, organic dentine matrix, etc.), many others are involved in erosive tooth wear. Figure 1 attempts to reveal the multifactorial predisposing factors and aetiologies of the erosive condition. Over time, many patient-related and nutritional factors will interact with the tooth surface, and they will either wear the surface away or indeed protect it, depending upon their fine balance. The interplay of all these

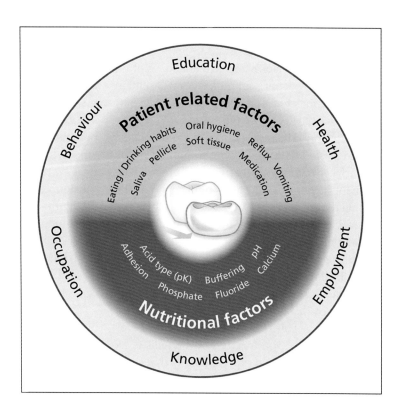

Fig. 1. Interactions of the different factors for the development of erosive tooth wear.

factors is crucial and helps explain why some individuals exhibit more erosion than others. The interaction of many factors listed in the inner circles of figure 1 will determine the onset and severity of dental erosion. However, even if individuals are exposed to exactly the same acid challenge in their diets, their individual biological factors will also play a substantial role in the development of the erosive lesions. Similar to the carious process [20], the factors listed in the outer circle will influence the whole process of erosion too, either in the development or the defence of the condition. In any case, dentists can only initiate adequate preventive (non-interventive) and successful therapeutic (interventive) measures when all these issues are taken into consideration.

It is often observed that people who show signs and symptoms of erosive lesions are usually not aware of, and may easily be confused by, the different causative factors and erosive potential of the drinks and foodstuffs affecting their oral health. So, on the one hand it is a prerequisite that dentists have a comprehensive knowledge of the different risk and protective factors in patients, which will only be revealed when a comprehensive case history is undertaken. On the other hand, dentists must bear in mind that some causative factors, such as reflux, are not readily apparent to patients but should still be investigated. When dealing with dental erosion, the main focus is strongly placed on the consumption of acidic soft drinks, whereas silent gastroesophageal reflux can be easily overseen. Different studies have shown that about 35% of patients who had not reported symptoms of gastroesophageal reflux, nor had treatment for it, presented actual pathological reflux when assessed with 24-hour oesophageal pH measurements [21–24]. This silent gastroesophageal reflux must also be taken into account when examining patients presenting erosive tooth wear.

In this same context, cases of eating disorders can go undetected, leading to an underestimation of the role of intrinsic causes in the development of dental erosion.

It is also important to understand that there is no fixed 'critical pH' value for a solution to cause dental erosion. Generally, in relation to erosive solutions, the main focus is overly concentrated on the hydrogen ion concentration (pH). Although pH is a crucial factor, it alone does not explain the erosive potential of erosive drinks and foodstuffs. In addition to other patient-related biological factors [25], titratable acidity, calcium, phosphate and fluoride levels in the erosive solution will all play a considerable role in the erosive potential of drinks and foodstuffs [26, 27].

Change of Concepts

It is often observed that several points that have either been studied mostly in the laboratory or are generally true for dental caries have been extrapolated to dental erosion. Dental erosion is, however, considerably different to dental caries, and these concepts should be revised. Below we debate two main points that should be reconsidered in relation to dental erosion.

There Is No Fixed Critical pH Value concerning Dental Erosion

The 'critical pH' is a pH value at which a solution is just saturated with respect to a specific solid, e.g. enamel mineral. This means that if a specific solution has a pH below the critical pH value, the solution is considered undersaturated with respect to the solid and is capable of causing dissolution of this solid. On the other hand, if the pH of the solution is above the critical pH value, the solution is then supersaturated with respect to the solid and precipitation of minerals will tend to occur [28]. The critical pH value depends on both the solubility of the solid of interest and on the concentrations (or more correctly on the activi-

ties) of the relevant mineral constituents of the solution. In the case of tooth mineral, the principal relevant constituents are calcium, phosphate and, to a lesser extent, fluoride activity. These minerals determine the degree of saturation of the solution, which is the driving force for either dissolution or precipitation [15, 27].

In relation to caries, the plaque fluid is the relevant 'solution' from which the critical pH value is calculated. In the resting plaque fluid, the calcium and phosphate concentrations are around 3.5 and 13.2 mmol/l, respectively, whereas fermenting plaque fluid contains 8.2 mmol/l of calcium and 13.5 mmol/l of phosphate [29]. On the basis of these average concentrations, the critical pH for enamel was calculated to be between pH 5.5 and 5.7. Although the concentrations of calcium and phosphate are rather constant for a given person, they will vary between different people and hence will influence the critical pH, thus partly explaining the inter-individual differences in critical pH values [15].

By definition, dental erosion is the dissolution of tooth mineral in the absence of plaque. Therefore, the critical pH value mentioned above – determined from the composition of plaque fluid – cannot be considered as a guide to whether dental erosion will occur. In the context of dental erosion, the relevant 'solution' from which the critical pH value is calculated is actually the erosive solution itself. More exactly, the critical pH value for dental erosion will depend on the concentration of the relevant mineral constituents in each erosive solution. In this case, the concentration of calcium is the most important factor determining the critical pH, but fluoride and phosphate concentrations, among other components, will also play a role. Considering that these concentrations will vary from solution to solution, and they will be different to those found in plaque fluid, the critical pH for enamel will also vary in the case of erosion. In cases where the mineral concentrations are higher than the values found in plaque fluid, the solution will not be able to dissolve

Table 1. pH of different beverages and foodstuffs (in part from Lussi et al. [27]) and the calculated critical pH (pHc) with respect to hydroxyapatite

Tested Agents	pH	pH_c[1]		Tested Agents	pH	pH_c[1]
Soft drinks				*Teas and coffee*		
Carpe Diem Kombucha fresh	3.0	5.6		Black tea	6.6	5.6
Coca-Cola	2.5	5.1		Peppermint	7.5	5.4
Coca-Cola light	2.6	5.2		Rosehip	3.2	5.3
Fanta regular	2.7	6.1		Wild berries	6.8	5.6
Ice tea classic	2.9	6.2		Espresso	5.8	5.6
Ice tea lemon	3.0	6.3				
Ice tea peach	2.9	6.4		*Salad dressing*		
Pepsi Cola	2.4	5.5		French classic	4.0	4.8
Pepsi Cola light	2.8	5.5		French light	3.9	4.5
Rivella blue	3.3	4.9				
Rivella green	3.2	4.9				
Rivella red	3.3	4.9				
Sinalco	3.1	5.8				
Sprite	2.5	6.5				
Sports drinks						
Gatorade	3.2	5.8				
Isostar	3.9	4.6				
Fruit juices						
Apple juice	3.4	5.1				
Carrot juice	4.2	5.0				
Grapefruit juice	3.2	5.0				
Orange juice 1	3.7	5.0				
Orange juice 2	3.6	5.0				
Apricot	3.3	5.1				
Kiwi	3.3	4.8				
Orange	3.6	5.2				
Alcoholic drinks						
Bacardi Breezer	3.2	6.2				
Beer (Carlsberg)	4.2	5.2				
Beer (Eichhof)	4.1	5.0				
Champagne	3.0	5.1				
Red wine 1	3.4	5.1				
Red wine 2	3.7	5.1				
Smirnoff Ice vodka	3.1	5.6				
White wine	3.6	5.1				
Medicinal						
Alca-C fizzy tablet	4.2	5.6				
Alka-Seltzer fizzy tablet	6.2	5.9				
Neocitran	2.9	4.9				
Siccoral	5.4	6.3				
Vitamin C fizzy tablet 1	3.9	5.9				
Vitamin C fizzy tablet 2	3.6	5.1				
Yoghurt (natural)	3.9	3.9				
Mineral water						
Flavored mineral water (Valser)	3.3	5.3				

For the [Ca], [P_i], [F] values and change of enamel surface hardness, see table 3 in chapter by Lussi and Hellwig [this vol., pp. 220–229]. pH_c = Critical pH.
[1] pH_c values were calculated by R.P. Shellis (Department of Preventive, Restorative and Pediatric Dentistry, University of Bern, Bern, Switzerland, and School of Oral and Dental Sciences, University of Bristol, Bristol, UK).

tooth mineral even if its pH is below 5.5 (lower than the critical pH concerning dental caries). For example, sour milk has a calcium concentration of 69 mmol/l and a phosphate content of 39.2 mmol/l. This solution is, therefore, considered supersaturated with respect to enamel and, even with a pH of 4.2, it has no erosive impact on enamel [see table 3 in the chapter by Lussi and Hellwig, this vol., pp. 220–229]. Similarly, in spite of presenting a pH of 4.0, orange juice supplemented with calcium (42.9 mmol/l) and phosphate (31.2 mmol/l) did not erode enamel, even after enamel was immersed in the juice for 7 days, while the non-supplemented orange juice caused deep erosive lesions [30]. Jensdottir et al. [31] calculated the critical pH of different drinks and obtained values ranging from 4.3 to 6.4. In the present chapter, we also present values of critical pH with respect to hydroxyapatite for drinks and medicaments used in the study by Lussi et al. [27] (table 1). In our case, critical pH values ranged from 3.9 to 6.5. However, it is important to bear in mind that when the pH is below approximately 3.9, the solution will be undersaturated with respect to the enamel mineral. In other words, the solution will most probably dissolve the tooth mineral independently of its fluoride, phosphate or calcium concentration, although the latter will, nonetheless, modulate the rate of dissolution. Consequently, we can observe that there is no fixed critical pH value concerning dental erosion.

After an Erosive Challenge, There Is No Specific Waiting Period before Brushing the Teeth
Toothbrushing has long been related to erosive tooth wear. When the acid comes into contact with the tooth surface, the superficial and near-surface demineralization processes lead to a softening of the enamel. Once the enamel surface is softened, it is more prone to suffer from the detrimental effects of the toothbrush, which can actually remove the softened layer and cause enamel substance loss.

Several studies have shown that fluoride toothpastes have a certain beneficial effect against dental erosion, but the prevalence of dental erosion is still increasing despite the general use of fluoride toothpaste [32]. Several studies have analysed the effect of different waiting periods after an erosive challenge before toothbrushing. This concept relies on the possible remineralizing effect of saliva to allow enough time for the softened enamel surface to 're-harden' before applying abrasive forces with a toothbrush. The interaction of erosion and abrasion will have different impacts on enamel and dentine, and the effectiveness of the waiting periods is still a matter of debate [see chapter by Wiegand and Schlueter, this vol., pp. 215–219].

In the in vitro study by Attin et al. [33], the authors evaluated the period of remineralization necessary for eroded enamel to resist the effect of toothbrushing, where they used bovine enamel in a cyclic erosion model consisting of 1 min exposure to soft drink, incubation in artificial saliva for different time periods, and later toothbrushing. The authors observed that the longer the remineralization time, the greater the resistance

against abrasion [33]. This study was carried out using artificial saliva, which has a greater remineralization potential than human saliva since it does not contain many of the proteins that actually inhibit mineral deposition on the tooth surface.

The effect of human saliva was observed in the results from in situ studies. Jaeggi and Lussi [34] analysed the effect of different waiting periods prior to performing toothbrushing. Human enamel specimens were prepared and eroded in citric acid for 3 min. These specimens were then maintained in situ for either 0 (toothbrushing immediately after intraoral exposure), 30 or 60 min. The authors observed less enamel abrasion after 60 min of intraoral exposure, and this effect was associated with the resting saliva secretion [34]. A similar result was also observed by Attin et al. [35], where they suggested a waiting period of 60 min before performing toothbrushing after an erosive challenge. Interestingly, despite the fact that these in vitro and in situ studies showed a statistically significant effect of waiting period prior to toothbrushing, they have all observed substantial enamel substance loss even after the 60-min waiting period. In other words, although a statistically significant effect has been observed with a waiting period of 60 min, saliva was not able to re-harden the softened enamel layer to prevent substance loss and hence a clinically significant effect was not present. This is reflected in the in situ study by Ganss et al. [36], where the authors observed that even after a waiting period of 2 h, no protective effect against enamel abrasion was detected. Figure 2 shows the effect of the waiting period on eroded enamel. When an eroded enamel surface (6 min incubation in 1% citric acid, pH = 3.6) is examined with a scanning electron microscope immediately after the erosive challenge, the typical honeycomb appearance of dental erosion is clearly observed (fig. 2a). This typical appearance was also still observed even after 2 h of in situ exposure to human saliva (fig. 2b).

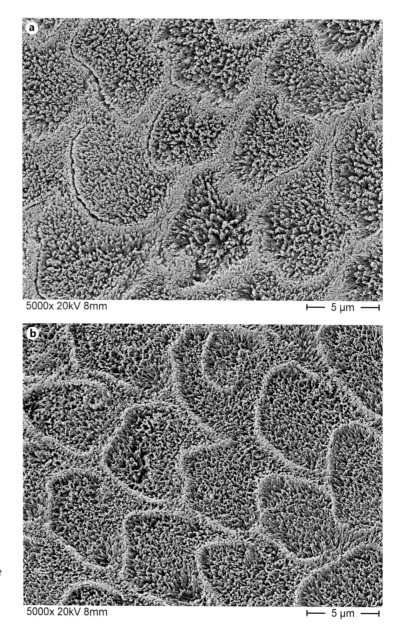

Fig. 2. Typical honeycomb appearance of eroded (6 min; 1% citric acid; pH = 3.6) enamel surface immediately after the erosive challenge (**a**) and after 2 h in situ exposure to human saliva (**b**).

From a different point of view, Wiegand et al. [37] observed in their in situ study that tooth substance loss was significantly lower when toothbrushing was applied before an erosive challenge rather than after 5 min of intraoral exposure. In any case, we must bear in mind that in vivo circumstances are considerably different to those observed in in situ (and in vitro) studies, and it is difficult to extrapolate and generalize these results to the clinical situation. This is shown in the recent epidemiological study by Bartlett et al. [38] with 3,187 adults from seven European countries, which throws light on this issue. The authors observed that there was no as-

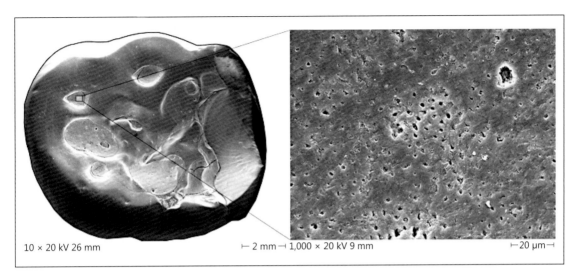

10 × 20 kV 26 mm   ⊢ 2 mm ⊣ 1,000 × 20 kV 9 mm   ⊢20 μm⊣

Fig. 3. Eroded tooth with involvement of dentine with open dentine tubules.

sociation between erosive tooth wear and the waiting period for toothbrushing after breakfast, but they found that the type of toothbrush and brushing movement were significantly associated with erosive tooth wear [38]. So, changing detrimental brushing habits is substantially more important to prevent dental erosion rather than asking erosion patients to wait before brushing their teeth. Furthermore, if there was clinically significant remineralization during the short waiting period before toothbrushing, the open dentine tubules related to dentine hypersensitivity would close, leading to less hypersensitivity pain symptoms. However, even in erosive lesions with involvement of dentine, where the dentine is exposed to the oral environment, open tubules can still be visualized (fig. 3), which may explain the cases of hypersensitivity. This is reflected in the recent population-based study by West et al. [39], who measured dentine hypersensitivity in 3,187 patients (18–35 years) from seven European countries, and observed no association between dentine hypersensitivity and the interval to toothbrushing. Consequently, advice on specific toothbrushing periods should not be generalized to all patients, but should be provided punctually to specific groups of high-risk patients (see chapter by Wiegand and Schlueter, this vol., pp. 215–219). Also, patients who frequently vomit, or who suffer from frequent episodes of reflux, could benefit from the use of mouth rinsing.

Another important point to bear in mind is that, despite the well-known fact that remineralization can take place in initial subsurface caries lesions in the presence of saliva, the mineral uptake concerning dental erosion is confined only to the surface and near-surface demineralized (softened) enamel layer. Therefore, the term 'remineralization', in the manner that is commonly understood and accepted in the field of cariology, should be reconsidered with regards to dental erosion [15]. In that case, the benefits of any waiting period before toothbrushing are still questionable and may not be the best preventive approach for all erosion patients. Nevertheless, controlled clinical trials are still necessary to better understand the extent of mineral gain of erosion lesions in in vivo situations, and further enlighten this debate.

Change of Definitions

The terms 'erosion', 'dental erosion' and 'erosive tooth wear' are often used interchangeably when referring to the effects of acids on the surfaces of teeth. When the surface of the tooth is first attacked by acids, the resulting loss of structural integrity leaves a softened layer on the tooth's surface, which renders it vulnerable to abrasive forces [40]. These abrasive forces will remove the softened layer on enamel, causing tooth hard substance loss, but they have no significant effect on a sound tooth surface, where hardly any abrasion can be measured when the surface is not softened [41]. Tooth hard substance loss can also occur without significant involvement of abrasion, and some cases of prolonged repeated erosive challenges (e.g. vomiting) can result in dental erosion. On the other hand, available evidence suggests that erosive challenges in vivo are brief; hence erosion alone is perhaps not likely to be a major direct cause of surface loss in real life. For this reason, Shellis et al. [40] suggested that the term 'dental erosion' should include only the cases of initial partial demineralization ('softening') and any surface loss caused solely by extended exposure to acids, whereas the term 'erosive tooth wear' should include the effects of any mechanical abrasive forces. Therefore, the terms 'dental erosion' and 'erosive tooth wear' should be used to refer to the chemical and chemical-mechanical processes, respectively. In any case, early diagnosis of dental erosion/erosive tooth wear is definitely important.

In some cases, dental professionals may dismiss very minor tooth surface loss as a normal and inevitable occurrence of daily living. When these signs of wear are 'within normal limits', no specific intervention is necessary. Although a certain degree of erosive tooth wear may be considered physiological, which depends on the patient's age, it is nevertheless important to correctly diagnose early stages of the erosive process. Since there is no device available for the specific detection of dental erosion in routine dental practice, the clinical appearance is the most important feature for dental professionals to diagnose dental erosion. However, erosive tooth wear only becomes evident at routine examination at its later stages, when the appearance and shape of the teeth are altered due to the condition and dentine has become exposed, possibly causing sensitivity. These changes are of particular significance because a smooth silky-glazed sometimes dull appearance, intact enamel along the gingival margin and change in colour, as well as cupping and grooving on occlusal surfaces, are considered as some of the clinically typical signs of 'early' erosive tooth wear. However, these signs are only clinically visible when there is already some kind of tooth hard substance loss. Furthermore, it is not only difficult to diagnose the erosive process at an early stage; it is also difficult to determine whether dentine is exposed or not at a later stage of tooth wear [42]. Still, even if dentists are able to correctly diagnose tooth wear, they must face the challenge of the differential diagnosis of the main factor/cause, e.g. erosion, abrasion or attrition; this is mainly because of the lack of awareness of the multifactorial and overlying aetiologies [43]. Nonetheless, timely and adequate preventive measures can only be provided to the patients when the dentists correctly diagnose the condition.

Change of Consumption of Acidic Foods and Beverages

As life styles have changed through the decades, the total amount and frequency of consumption of acidic foods and drinks have also changed. Soft drink consumption in the USA increased by 300% in 20 years [44], and serving sizes increased from 185 g (6.6 oz) in the 1950s to 340 g (12 oz) in the 1960s and 570 g (20 oz) in the late 1990s. Around the year 1995, between 56 and 85% of children at school in the USA consumed at least one soft drink daily, with the highest amounts ingested by adolescent males. From this group, 20% consumed four or more servings daily [45]. In a recent publication [46], it was reported that between 2003 and 2009 soft drink consumption increased by more than 60% in Hungary, India, Turkey, Venezuela and Vietnam (65.2, 95.2, 82.8, 66.8 and 99.5%, respectively). In contrast, a decrease of more than 10% in soft drink consumption was reported in Germany, Italy, Portugal and Sweden (10.8, 11.5, 12.6 and 11.1%, respectively). The report also showed that the greatest consumer of soft drinks was the USA, with over 27 million litres sold in the year 2009 [46]. In 2007, the worldwide annual consumption of soft drinks reached 552 billion litres, the equivalent of just under 83 litres per person per year. An increase was projected for the year 2012, when the value would reach 95 litres per person per year [47]. However, the annual consumption per person in 2012 has reached 165 litres in the USA and 146 litres in Mexico [48]. In the UK, the annual consumption of carbonates per person also increased from 94.4 litres in 2007 to 102.6 litres in 2012 [49]. Canada and Finland lead the annual fruit juice consumption with 60 litres and 48 litres per capita, respectively, in 2012. Sports drinks and energy drinks are consumed less than soft drinks, but their annual consumption per person is also increasing. The USA is the leading consumer of sports drinks, with an annual consumption of 18 litres per person, whereas Europe is the leading consumer of energy drinks; in the UK, consumption increased from 4.4 litres in 2007 to 7.6 litres in 2012 [49], and in Austria, the home market and headquarters of Red Bull, the annual consumption of energy drinks per person reached nearly 8 litres in 2012. Recently, the European Food and Safety Authority commissioned a study on the consumption of energy drinks in adults, adolescents and children in the EU, in which over 52,000 participants from 16 different EU countries were included [50]. The prevalence of consumption was highest in the adolescent group, with an average of 68% of teenagers having consumed energy drinks at least once

in the last year, and the prevalence of consumption was 30% in adults, 19% in children aged 6–10 and even 2% in the younger children aged 3–5 years. Strikingly, 16% of children were considered high chronic consumers, who stated to have been drinking energy drinks 3 times a week or more during the last months before the survey. This added up to an average consumption volume of 0.95 litres per week per child. In addition, the high consumption of energy drinks can lead to a high caffeine exposure of a calculated average of 42.9 mg/day (1.98 mg/kg b.w./day) [50].

Studies in children and adults have shown that four or more servings per day are associated with the presence and progression of erosion when other risk factors are present [51, 52]. With such an increase in the popularity of soft drinks, sports drinks and energy drinks, the consumption of other nutritive products (e.g. milk) may decrease in children and adolescents. This could result in more serious health issues other than dental erosion, such as calcium deficiency, thus jeopardizing the accrual of maximal peak bone mass at a critical time in life [53].

Change of Prevalence

National dental surveys are not routinely undertaken and when conducted they seldom have included measures of tooth wear, specifically erosive tooth wear. The prevalence of erosion in the UK dental health survey increased from the year 1993 to 1996/1997 [54]. There was a trend towards a higher prevalence of erosion in children aged between 3.5 and 4.5 years, and in those who consumed carbonated drinks on most days, compared with toddlers consuming these drinks less often. In another UK study, 1,308 children were examined at the age of 12 years and 2 years later; 5% of the subjects aged 12 years and 13% 2 years later had deep erosive enamel lesions. Dentinal lesions were found in 2% of the examined subjects at the age of 12 years and rose to 9% 2 years later. The incidence of new cases also increased; 12% of 12-year-old children who demonstrated no evidence of erosion developed the condition over the subsequent 2 years. New and more advanced lesions were seen in 27% of the children over the study period [55]. A longitudinal study of 12-year-old adolescents showed an increased incidence of 24% over 18 months. From those who already presented erosive lesions at baseline, 60% presented a progression in terms of lesion depth and/or number [56]. Figures 4–6 show the progression of erosive lesions on incisors and molars after different time periods. Active erosive lesions will progress when no adequate preventive measures are implemented or if the patients do not comply with the measures proposed by the dentist. To determine the progression of erosive defects, 55 adults were examined on two separate occasions 6 years apart [52]. All persons were informed about the risk of erosive tooth wear but no active preventive care during the study period was performed. A distinct progression of erosion on occlusal and facial surfaces was found. The occurrence of occlusal erosive lesions with involvement of dentine rose from 3 to 8% (26–30 years old at the first examination) and from 8 to 26% (46–50 years old at the first examination). The increase in facial erosions was smaller but again more marked for the older group. In this longitudinal study, the subjective evaluation of dentine hypersensitivity remained unchanged despite the marked increase of erosive and wedge-shaped defects.

Dentine hypersensitivity is a relatively common phenomenon and erosive tooth wear has been implicated as a predisposing factor [57]. In the population-based study by West et al. [39], 3,187 patients were clinically assessed for dentine hypersensitivity and they completed a questionnaire on the risk factors for this condition, including questions on lifestyle, diet and oral health, among other factors. The authors observed that although only 26.8% of the participants declared experiencing dentine hypersensitivity, overall more than 40% of the patients actually experienced dentine hypersensitivity on at least one tooth during cold air stimulation. Also, a strong, progressive relationship was observed between dentine hypersensitivity and erosive tooth wear [39], and hypersensitivity was strongly associated with patients reporting frequent heartburn, gastric reflux and, to a lesser extent, vomiting. So, it is important to recognize this association, especially regarding patient preventive therapies and the clinical management of pain.

Conclusion

The overall increase in the worldwide consumption of acidic foods and beverages in the last few years and the increased prevalence of erosive tooth wear observed in some studies may reflect the changes in perception of dental erosion. During the last decades, an increasingly greater interest in dental erosion has been observed in the clinical dental practice, in dental public health and in dental research. Originally thought as a solely superficial event, the pathophysiology of dental erosion is now considered to implicate demineralization both at the interface between solution and enamel and within the thin, partly demineralized softened enamel layer (near-surface demineralization). Although the condition has been referred to by different terms ('erosion', 'dental erosion' or 'erosive tooth wear') and there is still a need for the standardization of nomenclature, timely and adequate preventive measures are nonetheless only possible when the dentists correctly diagnose the condition. For that, dentists should explore the numerous factors that play a role in the onset and severity of dental erosion.

In order to provide the best preventive and therapeutic measures for patients, dentists must primarily investigate all risk factors related to the patient, bearing in mind concealed factors (like silent gastroesophageal reflux) as well as the many aspects associated with the erosive poten-

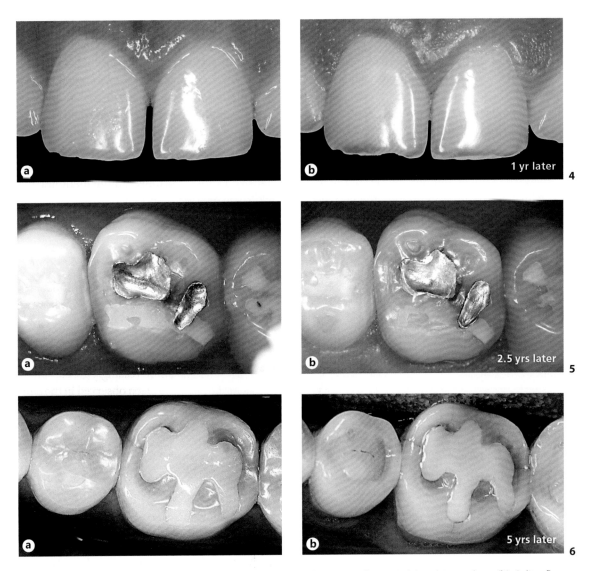

Fig. 4. Erosive tooth wear on the incisors of a 14-year-old adolescent at first visit (**a**) and 1 year later (**b**). Saliva flow rate 2.4 ml/min with high buffer capacity; known risk factors: pathological gastroesophageal reflux.

Fig. 5. Erosive tooth wear on occlusal surfaces of a 14-year-old adolescent at first visit (**a**) and 2.5 years later (**b**). The patient suffered from dentine hypersensitivity; known risk factors: gastroesophageal reflux and consumption of ice tea and acidic beverages.

Fig. 6. Erosive tooth wear on occlusal surfaces of a 30-year-old patient at first visit (**a**) and 5 years later (**b**). Involvement of dentine is clearly observed, with a composite filling rising above the level of the adjacent tooth surface; known risk factors: soft drinks (sip-wise) and silent reflux (only later discovered).

tial of drinks and foodstuff such as the concentration of relevant mineral constituents (calcium and phosphates) that lead to the lack of a unique 'critical pH' value concerning dental erosion. These risk factors should then be coupled with the evident signs of erosive tooth wear observed during the clinical examination. In addition, dentists must take into consideration the reported symptoms (thermal or tactile sensitivity) as well as the wishes, hopes and possibilities of the individual patient in order to provide the best available treatment. In cases where restorative treatment becomes inevitable, all preparations must follow the principles of minimally invasive treatment. Furthermore, it is of foremost importance to bear in mind that any restorative procedure can only be beneficial to patients if they thoroughly comply with adequate preventive measures. Consequently, preventive measures should be initiated as early as possible to reduce the erosive challenge and to increase the protective and defensive factors, thus bringing the equilibrium back to the oral environment.

References

1 Zero DT, Lussi A: Erosion – chemical and biological factors of importance to the dental practitioner. Int Dent J 2005; 55:285–290.

2 Asmyhr O, Grytten J, Holst D: Occurrence of risk factors for dental erosion in the population of young adults in Norway. Community Dent Oral Epidemiol 2012;40:425–431.

3 Harpenau LA, Noble WH, Kao RT: Diagnosis and management of dental wear. J Calif Dent Assoc 2011;39:225–231.

4 Hermont AP, Oliveira PA, Auad SM: Tooth erosion awareness in a Brazilian dental school. J Dent Educ 2011;75: 1620–1626.

5 Stewart KF, Fairchild RM, Jones RJ, Hunter L, Harris C, Morgan MZ: Children's understandings and motivations surrounding novelty sweets: a qualitative study. Int J Paediatr Dent 2013;23: 424–434.

6 Dugmore CR, Rock WP: Awareness of tooth erosion in 12-year-old children and primary care dental practitioners. Community Dent Health 2003;20:223–227.

7 Hannig C, Hannig M, Attin T: Enzymes in the acquired enamel pellicle. Eur J Oral Sci 2005;113:2–13.

8 Zimmerman JN, Custodio W, Hatibovic-Kofman S, Lee YH, Xiao Y, Siqueira WL: Proteome and peptidome of human acquired enamel pellicle on deciduous teeth. Int J Mol Sci 2013;14:920–934.

9 Meurman JH, Frank RM: Scanning electron microscopic study of the effect of salivary pellicle on enamel erosion. Caries Res 1991;25:1–6.

10 Gray JA: Kinetics of the dissolution of human dental enamel in acid. J Dent Res 1962;41:633–645.

11 Featherstone JD, Rodgers BE: Effect of acetic, lactic and other organic acids on the formation of artificial carious lesions. Caries Res 1981;15:377–385.

12 Lussi A: Erosive tooth wear – a multifactorial condition of growing concern and increasing knowledge. Monogr Oral Sci 2006;20:1–8.

13 Featherstone JD, Lussi A: Understanding the chemistry of dental erosion. Monogr Oral Sci 2006;20:66–76.

14 Shellis RP, Barbour ME, Jesani A, Lussi A: Effects of buffering properties and undissociated acid concentration on dissolution of dental enamel in relation to pH and acid type. Caries Res 2013;47: 601–611.

15 Lussi A, Schlueter N, Rakhmatullina E, Ganss C: Dental erosion – an overview with emphasis on chemical and histopathological aspects. Caries Res 2011; 45(suppl 1):2–12.

16 Shellis RP, Finke M, Eisenburger M, Parker DM, Addy M: Relationship between enamel erosion and liquid flow rate. Eur J Oral Sci 2005;113:232–238.

17 Hara AT, Ando M, Cury JA, Serra MC, Gonzalez-Cabezas C, Zero DT: Influence of the organic matrix on root dentine erosion by citric acid. Caries Res 2005; 39:134–138.

18 Ganss C, Klimek J, Starck C: Quantitative analysis of the impact of the organic matrix on the fluoride effect on erosion progression in human dentine using longitudinal microradiography. Arch Oral Biol 2004;49:931–935.

19 Kleter GA, Damen JJ, Everts V, Niehof J, Ten Cate JM: The influence of the organic matrix on demineralization of bovine root dentin in vitro. J Dent Res 1994;73:1523–1529.

20 Fejerskov O: Changing paradigms in concepts on dental caries: consequences for oral health care. Caries Res 2004;38: 182–191.

21 Ronkainen J, Aro P, Storskrubb T, et al: High prevalence of gastroesophageal reflux symptoms and esophagitis with or without symptoms in the general adult Swedish population: a Kalixanda study report. Scand J Gastroenterol 2005;40:275–285.

22 Ohara S, Kouzu T, Kawano T, Kusano M: Nationwide epidemiological survey regarding heartburn and reflux esophagitis (in Japanese). Nihon Shokakibyo Gakkai Zasshi 2005;102:1010–1024.

23 Wang FW, Tu MS, Chuang HY, Yu HC, Cheng LC, Hsu PI: Erosive esophagitis in asymptomatic subjects: risk factors. Dig Dis Sci 2010;55:1320–1324.

24 Cho JH, Kim HM, Ko GJ, et al: Old age and male sex are associated with increased risk of asymptomatic erosive esophagitis: analysis of data from local health examinations by the Korean National Health Insurance Corporation. J Gastroenterol Hepatol 2011;26:1034–1038.

25 Lussi A, von Salis-Marincek M, Ganss C, Hellwig E, Cheaib Z, Jaeggi T: Clinical study monitoring the pH on tooth surfaces in patients with and without erosion. Caries Res 2012;46:507–512.

26 Lussi A, Jaeggi T: Chemical factors. Monogr Oral Sci 2006;20:77–87.

27 Lussi A, Megert B, Shellis RP, Wang X: Analysis of the erosive effect of different dietary substances and medications. Br J Nutr 2012;107:252–262.

28 Dawes C: What is the critical pH and why does a tooth dissolve in acid? J Can Dent Assoc 2003;69:722–724.

29 Ten Cate JM, Larsen MJ, Pearse EIF, Fejerskov O: Chemical interactions between the tooth and oral fluids; in Fejerskov O, Kidd E (eds): Dental Caries – The Disease and Its Clinical Management, ed 2. Oxford, Blackwell Munksgaard, 2008, pp 209–231.

30 Larsen MJ, Nyvad B: Enamel erosion by some soft drinks and orange juices relative to their pH, buffering effect and contents of calcium phosphate. Caries Res 1999;33:81–87.

31 Jensdottir T, Bardow A, Holbrook P: Properties and modification of soft drinks in relation to their erosive potential in vitro. J Dent 2005;33:569–575.

32 Ganss C, Schulze K, Schlueter N: Toothpaste and erosion. Monogr Oral Sci 2013;23:88–99.

33 Attin T, Buchalla W, Gollner M, Hellwig E: Use of variable remineralization periods to improve the abrasion resistance of previously eroded enamel. Caries Res 2000;34:48–52.

34 Jaeggi T, Lussi A: Toothbrush abrasion of erosively altered enamel after intraoral exposure to saliva: an in situ study. Caries Res 1999;33:455–461.

35 Attin T, Knöfel S, Buchalla W, Tütüncü R: In situ evaluation of different remineralization periods to decrease brushing abrasion of demineralized enamel. Caries Res 2001;35:216–222.

36 Ganss C, Schlueter N, Friedrich D, Klimek J: Efficacy of waiting periods and topical fluoride treatment on toothbrush abrasion of eroded enamel in situ. Caries Res 2007;41:146–151.

37 Wiegand A, Egert S, Attin T: Toothbrushing before or after an acidic challenge to minimize tooth wear? An in situ/ex vivo study. Am J Dent 2008;21:13–16.

38 Bartlett DW, Lussi A, West NX, Bouchard P, Sanz M, Bourgeois D: Prevalence of tooth wear on buccal and lingual surfaces and possible risk factors in young European adults. J Dent 2013;41:1007–1013.

39 West NX, Sanz M, Lussi A, Bartlett D, Bouchard P, Bourgeois D: Prevalence of dentine hypersensitivity and study of associated factors: a European population-based cross-sectional study. J Dent 2013;41:841–851.

40 Shellis RP, Ganss C, Ren Y, Zero DT, Lussi A: Methodology and models in erosion research: discussion and conclusions. Caries Res 2011;45(suppl 1):69–77.

41 Voronets J, Lussi A: Thickness of softened human enamel removed by toothbrush abrasion: an in vitro study. Clin Oral Investig 2010;14:251–256.

42 Ganss C, Klimek J, Lussi A: Accuracy and consistency of the visual diagnosis of exposed dentine on worn occlusal/incisal surfaces. Caries Res 2006;40:208–212.

43 Bartlett D: The implication of laboratory research on tooth wear and erosion. Oral Dis 2005;11:3–6.

44 Cavadini C, Siega-Riz AM, Popkin BM: US adolescent food intake trends from 1965 to 1996. West J Med 2000;173:378–383.

45 Gleason P, Suitor C: Food for thought: children's diets in the 1990s. Princeton, Mathematica Policy Research, 2001.

46 Euromonitor International: Who Drinks What: Identifying International Drinks Consumption Trends, ed 2. 2011. http://www.euromonitor.com.

47 Packer CD: Cola-induced hypokalaemia: a super-sized problem. Int J Clin Pract 2009;63:833–835.

48 Which Countries Consume the Most Soft Drinks? http://ladyofthecakes.wordpress.com/2013/04/09/which-countries-consume-the-most-soft-drinks/2013.

49 BSDA: The 2013 UK Soft Drinks Report: Refreshing the Nation. http://www.britishsoftdrinks.com/PDF/2013UKsoftdrinksreport.pdf 2013:20.

50 Zucconi S, Volpato C, Adinolfi F, et al: Gathering consumption data on specific consumer groups of energy drinks. European Food Safety Authority, 2013. http://www.efsa.europa.eu/publications.

51 O'Sullivan EA, Curzon ME: A comparison of acidic dietary factors in children with and without dental erosion. ASDC J Dent Child 2000;67:186–192.

52 Lussi A, Schaffner M: Progression of and risk factors for dental erosion and wedge-shaped defects over a 6-year period. Caries Res 2000;34:182–187.

53 American Academy of Pediatrics Committee on School Health: Soft drinks in schools. Pediatrics 2004;113:152–154.

54 Nunn JH, Gordon PH, Morris AJ, Pine CM, Walker A: Dental erosion – changing prevalence? A review of British National children's surveys. Int J Paediatr Dent 2003;13:98–105.

55 Dugmore CR, Rock WP: The progression of tooth erosion in a cohort of adolescents of mixed ethnicity. Int J Paediatr Dent 2003;13:295–303.

56 El Aidi H, Bronkhorst EM, Truin GJ: A longitudinal study of tooth erosion in adolescents. J Dent Res 2008;87:731–735.

57 Addy M: Tooth brushing, tooth wear and dentine hypersensitivity – are they associated? Int Dent J 2005;55:261–267.

Prof. A. Lussi
Department of Preventive, Restorative and Pediatric Dentistry
School of Dental Medicine, University of Bern
Freiburgstrasse 7
CH–3010 Bern (Switzerland)
E-Mail adrian.lussi@zmk.unibe.ch

Lussi A, Ganss C (eds): Erosive Tooth Wear. Monogr Oral Sci. Basel, Karger, 2014, vol 25, pp 16–21
DOI: 10.1159/000359931

Is Erosive Tooth Wear an Oral Disease?

Carolina Ganss

Department of Conservative and Preventive Dentistry, Dental Clinic, Justus Liebig University Giessen, Giessen, Germany

Abstract

Erosive tissue loss is part of the physiological wear of teeth. Clinical features are an initial loss of tooth shine or luster followed by flattening of convex structures; with continuing acid exposure, concavities form on smooth surfaces, or grooving and cupping occur on incisal/occlusal surfaces. Dental erosion must be distinguished from other forms of wear, but can also contribute to general tissue loss by surface softening, thus modifying physical wear processes. The determination of dental erosion as a condition or pathology is relatively easy in the case of pain or endodontic complications, but is ambiguous in initial stages and in terms of function or esthetics. The impact of dental erosion on oral health is discussed. However, it can be concluded that in most cases dental erosion is best described as a condition, with the acid being of nonpathological origin.

© 2014 S. Karger AG, Basel

Definition of Erosive Tooth Wear

During a lifetime, teeth are exposed to a number of physical and chemical insults, which to a various extent contribute to the wear and tear of dental hard tissues.

The variety of processes includes the following: (1) the friction of exogenous material (e.g. during mastication, toothbrushing, holding tools) forced over tooth substances (abrasion), (2) the effect of antagonistic teeth (attrition), (3) the impact of tensile and compressive forces during tooth flexure (abfraction) and (4) the chemical dissolution of tooth mineral (erosion; table 1). All of these factors to a greater or lesser extent occur in the dentition, and wear results from the simultaneous and/or synergistic action of these processes [see chapter by Shellis and Addy, this vol., pp. 32–45].

The morphology and severity of defects may substantially vary depending on the predominant etiological factor (fig. 1).

Dental erosion can be defined as dissolution of tooth by acids when the surrounding aqueous phase is undersaturated with respect to tooth mineral [1]. When the acidic challenge is acting for long enough, a clinically visible defect occurs. On smooth surfaces, the original luster of the tooth dulls. Later, the convex areas flatten or shallow concavities become present, which are mostly located coronal to the enamel-cementum junction. On occlusal surfaces, cusps become rounded

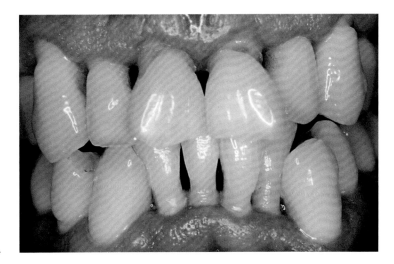

Fig. 1. A 50-year-old woman with multiple forms of wear: 11 and 21 cervical abrasions due to abusive flossing; 13 and 23 wedge-shaped defects; 32–42 toothbrush abrasion.

Table 1. Terminology, definition and etiology of various types of physical and chemical tooth wear

Terminology	Definition and etiology
Abrasion	Physical wear as a result of mechanical processes involving foreign substances or objects (three-body wear) Etiological factors are oral hygiene procedures (e.g. excessive brushing/flossing, effect of abrasives in toothpastes), habits (e.g. holding objects) or occupational exposure to abrasive particles The resulting morphology of defects can be diffuse or localized depending on the predominant impact Wedge-shaped defects are also attributed to abrasion A special form of abrasion is demastication, which means wear from chewing food, tissue loss is located on incisal and/or occlusal surfaces and depends on the abrasiveness of the individual diet
Attrition	Physical wear as a result of the action of antagonistic teeth with no foreign substances intervening (two-body wear) Characteristic features are antagonistic plane facets with sharp margins
Abfraction	Physical wear as a result of tensile or shear stress in the cemento-enamel region provoking microfractures in enamel and dentine (fatigue wear) Wedge-shaped defects are also attributed to abfraction
Erosion	Chemical wear as a result of extrinsic or intrinsic acids or chelators acting on plaque-free tooth surfaces Characteristic clinical features of (tribo) chemical wear are loss of surface structure, melted appearance, cupping or grooving on occlusal/incisal surfaces, and shallow concavities coronal from the cemento-enamel junction

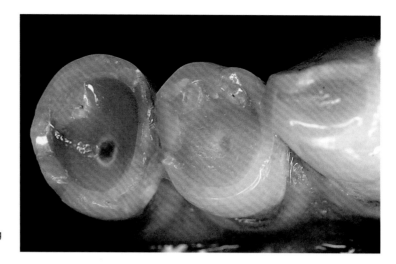

Fig. 2. Frank and near pulp exposure (45 and 44) in a 58-year-old male with advanced wear of unknown etiology. He complained about a sudden pinprick-like feeling when chewing.

or cupped and edges of restorations appear to rise above the level of the adjacent tooth surfaces. In severe cases, the whole tooth morphology disappears and the vertical crown height can be significantly reduced. For morphology of erosive wear, see chapter by Ganss and Lussi [this vol., pp. 22–31].

The result of continuing acid exposure, however, is not only a clinically visible defect but also a change in the physical properties of the remaining tooth surface. It is recognized that erosive demineralization results in a significant reduction in microhardness [2, 3], making the softened surface more prone to mechanical impacts [4]. Although independent in origin, erosion is therefore linked to other forms of wear not only because it contributes to the individual overall rate of tooth tissue loss, but also by modifying physical wear [see chapter by Shellis and Addy, this vol., pp. 32–45].

Although listed in the International Classification of Diseases [5], erosive tissue loss cannot be regarded as pathology per se. Unlike caries and periodontitis, which should not occur at all, erosive and physical wear contribute to the physiological loss of tooth tissue occurring throughout lifetime.

Is Erosive Tooth Wear an Oral Disease?

Attempts have been made to distinguish between pathological and physiological loss of tooth tissues [6]:

Tooth wear can be regarded as pathological if the teeth become so worn that they do not function effectively or seriously mar the appearance before they are lost due to other causes or the patient dies. The distinction of acceptable and pathological wear at a given age is based upon the prediction of whether the tooth will survive the rate of wear.

'Function' in a professional view means: (1) the interplay of the dental arches (occlusion); (2) the action of musculature and temporomandibular joint and (3) the biological integrity of teeth.

Regarding the latter, formation of reactionary and reparative dentine and obturation of dentinal tubules are responses that compensate for the loss of tissue occurring from continuing erosive demineralization and loss of enamel. In the case that the progression of erosive wear exceeds the reparative capacity of the dentinal-pulp complex (fig. 2), and when excessive (erosive) wear occurs, possible complications are

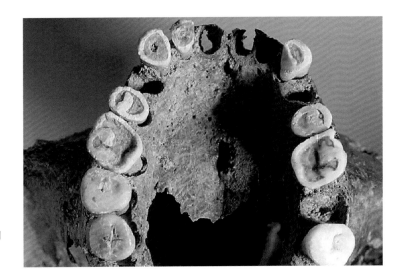

Fig. 3. Medieval subject (estimated age 50–70 years) with advanced generalized wear.

pain, pulpal inflammation, necrosis and periapical pathology.

The prevalence of endodontic sequelae has not been systematically studied but is estimated to occur in roughly 10% of patients with significant wear [7]. Pain, however, is not only induced by near or frank pulp exposure but can occur as soon as dentine is exposed. The etiology of dentinal hypersensitivity has been extensively described, and it appears that the absence of a smear layer and patent tubules are the relevant factors, which would favor the exposure to acids as the primary etiology [8]. However, even if not studied systematically, hypersensitivity from the clinical experience appears as only a minor problem in most subjects with erosive wear.

Continuing hypersensitivity, acute pain or pulp necrosis with periapical inflammation would doubtlessly represent a pathological condition. However, even severe (erosive) tooth wear can be localized to single teeth or generalized without any clinical symptoms, a condition which refers to considerations regarding the significance of the morphology of teeth for occlusion, musculature and joints.

The teeth of prehistoric hunter-gatherers are often characterized by extensive wear in both arches. Although a decrease in wear is seen on the dentition of premodern and recent people, its presence appears to be a constant feature [9]. Observations from anthropologists, therefore, led to substantially different concepts of occlusion than those generally accepted in dentistry. Begg [10] suggested that an 'attritional occlusion' rather than a nonattritional occlusion is the anatomically and functionally correct feature. 'Attritional occlusion' refers to a dentition that is affected by various wear processes which are present in heavy-wear environments (fig. 3). Edge-to-edge occlusion and working/nonworking contacts are the major features in this concept, whereas scissors occlusion and interlocking cusp relation appear as a retention in a juvenile condition which is 'unexpected' if the history of the human body is considered. Since his publication, a number of aspects regarding this theory have been investigated, which are extensively reviewed by Kaifu et al. [11]. They considered tooth wear in the context of evolutionary adaptation and conclude: 'Our synthesis of the available evidence suggests that the human dentition is "designed" on the premise that extensive wear will occur'. In this concept, even extensive wear can be regarded as a condition rather than a pathology, provided that the amount of loss is related to the expected life span. For assessment of progression, see Ganss and Lussi [this vol., pp. 22–31].

The concept of attritional occlusion is in stark contrast to theories generally accepted in dentistry. Most concepts of an ideal occlusion include a defined centric occlusion and a canine or group guidance without nonworking contacts. Probably the most inflexible concept of an ideal nonattritional occlusion was presented by Lee [12]. He suggested that a physiological occlusion should feature a 4-mm overbite and a 3-mm overjet and, on lateral excursions, canines cause the posterior teeth to disclude. But most importantly, he stated that teeth without any signs of wear were essential for a properly functioning dentition. The consequence of premise is that any wear of teeth, no matter how small, is regarded as pathological.

Based on the concept of a nonattritional occlusion, an enormous body of literature has been published regarding the role of occlusion in the etiology of temporomandibular disorders (TMD). Based on this concept, erosive tooth wear involving loss of occlusal morphology and resulting in a lack of canine or group guidance, nonworking contacts and loss of vertical height would increase the risk of developing TMD. However, clinical studies reveal none or weak associations between deviations from an ideal occlusion and TMD [13–16]. Correspondingly, there is no evidence that occlusal adjustment should be part of any recommended treatment for TMD [17]. Clinical studies investigating the association of TMD and generalized erosive tooth wear are absent, but several investigations on the morphology of the temporomandibular joint in prehistoric subjects with wear have been published. It has been demonstrated that structural changes to the fossa and condyle occur either as degenerative (i.e. bony erosion, proliferation or eburnation) [18, 19] or adaptive changes [20–22]. These studies, however, have obvious limitations, at least insofar as they cannot be correlated with the clinical situation.

The description of function by professionals might significantly differ from a patient's perspective and, accordingly, clinical judgments have only limited power in interpreting subjective oral health and psychosocial well-being [23]. Considering the emotional and social significance of food, the individual's need for function of the dentition would address masticatory ability, which comprises chewing capacity and chewing with comfort rather than the objective chewing efficiency. The finding that shortened dental arches with all molars missing was sufficient to satisfy the needs of most individuals [23] means the general relevance of wear for masticatory ability is difficult to assess. Esthetics, however, appears to be more important for many people than function [23]. Beauty has been closely associated with truth and goodness. Individuals endowed with physical beauty are seen as virtuous and trustful, and are given more social credit than subjects afflicted with ugliness. White teeth represent health and youth, and vice versa a worn and yellowish dentition is attributed to old age and loss of power. This notion is strongly supported by Rufenacht [24]. Even if it is assumed that there must be universal norms of esthetics, beauty ideals are the result of culture and related to time and fashion. Hence, the concepts and impacts of bodily beauty vary considerably between people [25]. Overall, (erosive) tooth wear potentially impacts the oral health-related quality of life [26] and it is often the individual who first recognizes his or her tooth wear as a pathological condition. But it is the dentist's responsibility to consider the complexity surrounding the concepts of beauty and the sequelae of bodily changes and, most importantly, to enhance the patients in making an informed decision, particularly if extensive and expensive restorations are considered.

Considering the various aspects addressed above, it appears that the difference between a condition and pathology is dependent on the concepts of health and disease. In any case, erosion might be considered to be pathological when occurring in combination with pain or acute endodontic complications. It is also reasonable to consider that minor-to-moderate tissue loss is a normal feature of the aging dentition. But in asymptomatic advanced erosive wear the differentiation between a physiological and pathological state becomes more difficult to distinguish. The question of whether, and in which cases, erosion is an oral disease is currently open for debate. In general terms, though, dental erosion is best described as a condition brought about by an acid insult, with the acid being of nonpathological origin.

Future research and discussion of the role of erosive tooth wear in oral health is needed, but the matter also appears to be stimulating for reflecting on concepts of health and disease in dentistry in general.

References

1 Larsen MJ: Chemical events during tooth dissolution. J Dent Res 1990;69: 575–580.
2 Lussi A, Jaeggi T, Jaeggi-Schärer S: Prediction of the erosive potential of some beverages. Caries Res 1995;29:349–354.
3 Lussi A, Portmann P, Burhop B: Erosion on abraded dental hard tissues by acid lozenges: an in situ study. Clin Oral Invest 1997;1:191–194.
4 Attin T, Koidl U, Buchalla W, Schaller HG, Kielbassa AM, Hellwig E: Correlation of microhardness and wear in differently eroded bovine dental enamel. Arch Oral Biol 1997;42:243–250.
5 World Health Organisation: ICD-10 Online Version. International Statistical Classification of Diseases and Related Health Problems. 2010.
6 Smith BG, Knight JK: An index for measuring the wear of teeth. Br Dent J 1984; 156:435–438.
7 Sivasithamparam K, Harbrow D, Vinczer E, Young WG: Endodontic sequelae of dental erosion. Aust Dent J 2003;48: 97–101.
8 Addy M, Pearce N: Aetiological, predisposing and environmental factors in dentine hypersensitivity. Arch Oral Biol 1994;39(suppl):33S–38S.
9 Kaifu Y: Changes in the pattern of tooth wear from prehistoric to recent periods in Japan. Am J Phys Anthropol 1999; 109:485–499.
10 Begg PR: Stone age man's dentition. Am J Orthod 1954;40:298–312, 373–383, 462–475, 517–531.
11 Kaifu Y, Kasai K, Townsend GC, Richards LC: Tooth wear and the 'design' of the human dentition: a perspective from evolutionary medicine. Am J Phys Anthropol 2003;37(suppl):47–61.
12 Lee R: Esthetics in relation to function; in Rufenacht CR (ed): Fundamentals in Esthetics. Chicago, Quintessence, 1990, pp 137–183.
13 Mohlin B, Axelsson S, Paulin G, Pietilä T, Bondemark L, Brattström V, Hansen K, Holm AK: TMD in relation to malocclusion and orthodontic treatment. Angle Orthod 2007;77:542–548.
14 Van´t Spijker A, Kreulen CM, Creugers NH: Attrition, occlusion, (dys)function, and intervention: a systematic review. Clin Oral Implants Res 2007;18:117–126.
15 Manfredini D, Castroflorio T, Perinetti G, Guarda-Nardini L: Dental occlusion, body posture and temporomandibular disorders: where we are now and where we are heading for. J Oral Rehabil 2012; 39:463–471.
16 Türp JC, Schindler H: The dental occlusion as a suspected cause for TMDs: epidemiological and etiological considerations. J Oral Rehabil 2012;39:502–512.
17 Koh H, Robinson PJ: Occlusal adjustment for treating and preventing temporomandibular joint disorders. Cochrane Database Syst Rev 2003;1: CD003812.
18 Richards LC: Degenerative changes in the temporomandibular joint in two Australian aboriginal populations. J Dent Res 1988;67:1529–1533.
19 Richards LC: Tooth wear and temporomandibular joint change in Australian aboriginal populations. Am J Phys Anthropol 1990;82:377–384.
20 Owen CP, Wilding RJ, Morris AG: Changes in mandibular condyle morphology related to tooth wear in a prehistoric human population. Arch Oral Biol 1991;36:799–804.
21 Owen CP, Wilding RJ, Adams LP: Dimensions of the temporal glenoid fossa and tooth wear in prehistoric human skeletons. Arch Oral Biol 1992;37:63–67.
22 Wedel A, Borrman H, Carlsson GE: Tooth wear and temporomandibular joint morphology in a skull material from the 17th century. Swed Dent J 1998;22:85–95.
23 Elias AC, Sheiham A: The relationship between satisfaction with mouth and number and position of teeth. J Oral Rehabil 1998;25:649–661.
24 Rufenacht CR: Fundamentals of Esthetics. Chicago, Quintessence, 1990.
25 Hilhorst M: Physical beauty: only skin deep? Med Health Care Philos 2002;5: 11–21.
26 Pagagianni CE, van der Meulen MJ, Naeije M, Lobbezoo F: Oral health-related quality of life in patients with tooth wear. J Oral Rehabil 2013;40:185–190.

Prof. C. Ganss
Department of Conservative and Preventive Dentistry
Dental Clinic, Justus Liebig University Giessen, Schlangenzahl 14
DE–35392 Giessen (Germany)
E-Mail carolina.ganss@dentist.med.uni-giessen.de

Lussi A, Ganss C (eds): Erosive Tooth Wear. Monogr Oral Sci. Basel, Karger, 2014, vol 25, pp 22–31
DOI: 10.1159/000359935

Diagnosis of Erosive Tooth Wear

Carolina Ganss[a] · Adrian Lussi[b]

[a]Department of Conservative and Preventive Dentistry, Dental Clinic, Justus Liebig University Giessen, Giessen, Germany; [b]Department of Preventive, Restorative and Pediatric Dentistry, School of Dental Medicine, University of Bern, Bern, Switzerland

Abstract

The clinical diagnosis 'erosion' is made from characteristic deviations from the original anatomical tooth morphology, thus distinguishing acid-induced tissue loss from other forms of wear. Primary pathognomonic features are shallow concavities on smooth surfaces occurring coronal from the enamel-cementum junction. Problems from diagnosing occlusal surfaces and exposed dentine are discussed. Indices for recording erosive wear include morphological as well as quantitative criteria. Currently, various indices are used, each having their virtues and flaws, making the comparison of prevalence studies difficult. The Basic Erosive Wear Examination (BEWE) is described, which is intended to provide an easy tool for research as well as for use in general dental practice. The cumulative score of this index is the sum of the most severe scores obtained from all sextants and is linked to suggestions for clinical management. In addition to recording erosive lesions, the assessment of progression is important as the indication of treatment measures depends on erosion activity. A number of evaluated and sensitive methods for in vitro and in situ approaches are available, but the fundamental problem for their clinical use is the lack of reidentifiable reference areas. Tools for clinical monitoring are described.

Current Approach to Erosive Tooth Wear

'Diagnosis is the intellectual course that integrates information obtained by clinical examination of the teeth, use of diagnostic aids, conversation with the patient and biological knowledge. A proper diagnosis cannot be performed without inspecting the teeth and their immediate surroundings' [1]. This definition, originally formulated for caries, is also true for erosive tooth wear. It means that a grid pattern of criteria is pelted over the patient and thereafter the signs and symptoms are first ordered and then classified in the second step. In the same process, the native tooth anatomy and morphology memorized engram-like is compared with the actual appearance.

The different chemical and physical insults on teeth cause loss of dental hard tissue with some characteristic patterns. The classification of wear is made from clinically observed morphological features described as the difference to an imagined ideal tooth morphology. Some indices do assume information as to the etiology such as attrition, abrasion and erosion. This approach is open to debate for two reasons: (1) an association between defect morphology and the respective etiological factors has not been validly estab-

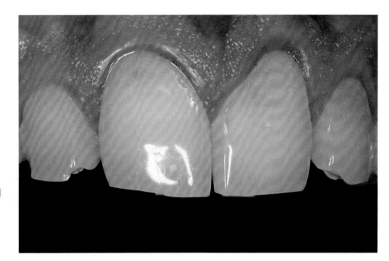

Fig. 1. Facial erosive tooth wear. Note the intact enamel along the gingival margin and the silky-glazed appearance of the tooth. Age of patient: 28 years. Known etiological factors: acidic drinks, gastroesophageal reflux.

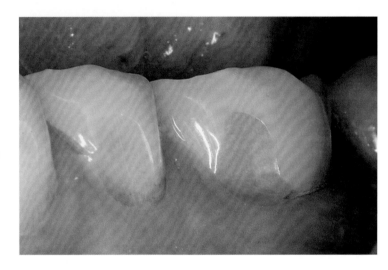

Fig. 2. Facial erosive tooth wear. No intact enamel along the gingival margin, but a silky-glazed appearance of the surface. Age of patient: 35 years. Known etiological factors: acidic fruits (lemon, orange) and fresh squeezed lemon and orange juice.

lished and (2) the presumed etiology predetermines scientific strategies and could introduce bias. It has therefore been argued that assessing wear as the super ordinate phenomenon disregarding the shape of lesions would overcome these disadvantages [2]. It is, however, important to note that the tissue loss ceases from progression when the cause is eliminated. Therefore, on a patient level it is a prerequisite to detect the condition early, to distinguish it from other defects and to search for the main cause in order to start the adequate preventive measures. From a clinical as well as from a scientific point of view, it would be necessary to have differentiating diagnostic criteria available.

Morphology and Differential Diagnosis of Erosive Tooth Wear

The early signs of erosive tooth wear appear as a smooth silky-shining sometimes dull surface. In the more advanced stages changes in the original morphology occur (fig. 1–10).

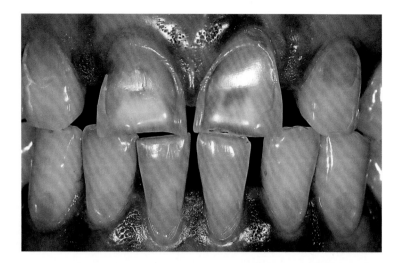

Fig. 3. Severe facial erosive tooth wear. Age of patient: 25 years. Known etiological factors: lemon slices under the lip, fruit juices.

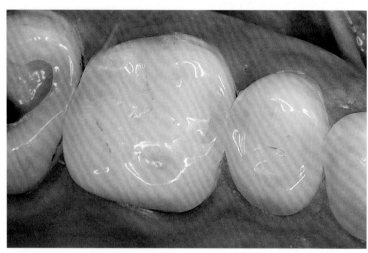

Fig. 4. Occlusal erosive tooth wear. Note rounding of the cusps and grooves. Age of patient: 29 years. Known etiological factors: soft drinks, sipping of 0.5 liters of acidic sports drinks per day.

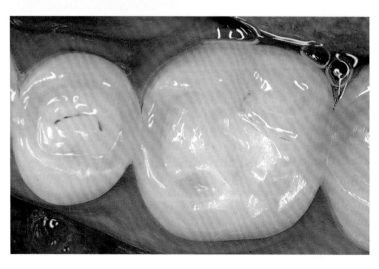

Fig. 5. Occlusal erosive tooth wear. Age of patient: 29 years (same patient as in fig. 4). The signs of erosive tooth wear are more pronounced. Known etiological factors: soft drinks, sipping of 0.5 liters of acidic sports drinks per day.

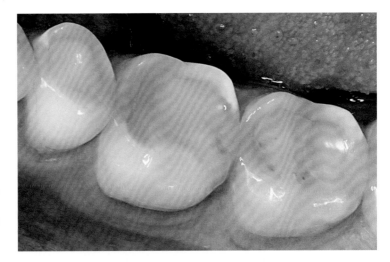

Fig. 6. Severe occlusal erosive tooth wear. Original morphological features not present. Age of patient: 29 years. Known etiological factor: gastroesophageal reflux.

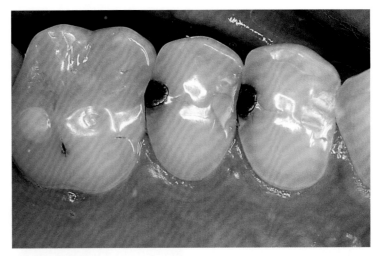

Fig. 7. Severe oral and occlusal erosive tooth wear. Note the worn oral cusps and the restorations rising above the level of the adjacent tooth surface. Age of patient: 29 years (same patient as in fig. 6). Known etiological factor: gastroesophageal reflux.

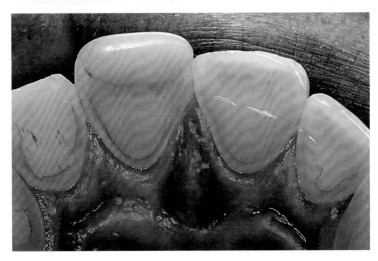

Fig. 8. Severe oral erosive tooth wear. Note the intact enamel along the gingival margin. Age of patient: 29 years (same patient as in figs. 6, 7). Known etiological factor: gastroesophageal reflux.

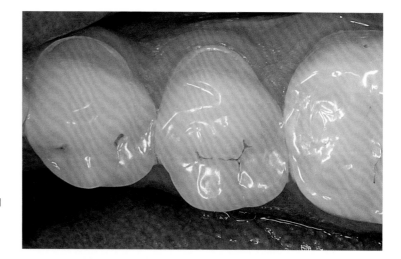

Fig. 9. Severe occlusal and buccal erosive tooth wear. Note the intact cervical enamel band on the buccal side. Age of patient: 25 years. Known etiological factor: gastroesophageal reflux.

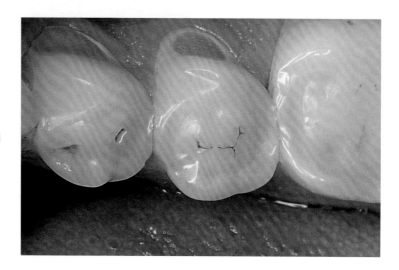

Fig. 10. Severe occlusal and buccal erosive tooth wear. Note the discoloured buccal surfaces indicating inactive erosive lesions after the cause was treated. A very small progression on the occlusal surfaces may be seen. Age of patient: 30 years (same patient as in fig. 9; 5 years later).

On smooth surfaces, the convex areas flatten or concavities become present, the width of which clearly exceed the depth. Undulating borders of the lesion are possible. Initial lesions are located coronal from the enamel-cementum junction with an intact border of enamel along the gingival margin. The reason for the preserved enamel band could be due to some plaque remnants, which act as a diffusion barrier for acids or due to an acid-neutralizing effect of the sulcular fluid, which is slightly alkaline [3]. Further acid attacks can lead to pseudo-chamfers at the margin of the eroded surface (fig. 1–3, 8, 9).

Erosion can be distinguished from wedge-shaped defects, which are located at or apical to the enamel-cementum junction. The coronal part of wedge-shaped defects ideally has a sharp margin and cuts at right angles into the enamel surface, whereas the apical part bottoms out to the root surface. The depth of the defect clearly exceeds its width.

The initial features of erosion on occlusal and incisal surfaces are the same as described above.

Further progression leads to a rounding of the cusps, grooves on the cusps and incisal edges, and restorations rising above the level of the adjacent tooth surfaces. In severe cases the whole occlusal morphology disappears (fig. 4–7). Erosive lesions have to be distinguished from attrition. The latter are often flat and have glossy areas with distinct margins and corresponding features at the antagonistic teeth. Much more difficult is the distinction between occlusal erosion and abrasion/demastication, which sometimes are of similar shape [4–6]. Indeed, erosion and abrasion appear most often as a combination of these processes. In other words: erosion involves two types of wear of enamel: mechanical wear of the thin softened layer (erosive tooth wear) and, in extreme cases, the direct removal of hard tissue by prolonged demineralization [see also chapter by Shellis and Addy, this vol., pp. 32–45].

Whenever possible, the clinical examination should be accomplished by a thorough history taking with respect to general health, diet and habits and by the assessment of saliva flow rates [see chapter by Lussi and Hellwig, this vol., pp. 220–229].

Clinical Assessment of Erosive Wear

Erosive tooth wear from a clinical viewpoint is a surface phenomenon, occurring on areas accessible to visual diagnosis. The diagnostic procedure is therefore a visual rather than an instrumental approach.

A number of indices for the clinical diagnosis of erosive tooth wear have been proposed [7], which more or less are modifications or combinations of the indices published by Eccles [8] and Smith and Knight [9] [see also chapter by Margaritis and Nunn, this vol., pp. 46–54]. All erosion indices include diagnostic criteria to differentiate erosions from other forms of tooth wear as well as criteria for the quantification of hard

tissue loss. The size of the area affected is often given as the proportion of the affected surface to the sound tooth surface. The depth of a defect is estimated by using the criterion of dentine exposition. Thereby, a relation between exposed dentine and the amount of substance loss is implicated. Most working groups have developed their own index modifications, which have not yet reached broader use.

Two items included in the erosion indices are currently under discussion:

(1) The morphological criteria for occlusal/incisal surfaces are not strongly associated with erosive tissue loss. A study including subjects with substantially different nutrition patterns (an abrasive, an acidic and an average western diet [5]) has clearly shown that the shape of occlusal/incisal lesions was similar in the abrasive and the acidic diet groups. During the process of breaking food, three-body abrasion can occur as a result of the food bolus being moved between antagonistic teeth. In the early stage of chewing, when the food bolus separates the occlusal/incisal surfaces, the important feature is that the teeth do not mate and that this process tends to abrade the softer regions of the tooth surface, resulting in a hollowing out of the dentine [11]. Significant occlusal tooth wear from mastication can occur either in the presence of high amounts of abrasives in the food bolus or in the case of acid softening of enamel and dentine. This three-body abrasion would result in rounding and cupping of the cusps and grooves on incisal edges, making a differentiation between abrasion and erosion on occlusal surfaces difficult.

In contrast to the occlusal morphology, shallow defects on facial surfaces localized coronally from the enamel-cementum junction were common in the acidic diet group but were not observed in the abrasive diet group [5]. Consequently, flat-shaped defects occurring on smooth surfaces could be appraised as pathognomonic rather than the defects on the occlusal surfaces.

Table 1. Criteria from the BEWE index for grading erosive wear [10]

Score	Criteria
0	No erosive tooth wear
1	Initial loss of surface texture
2	Distinct defect; hard tissue loss <50% of the surface area
3	Hard tissue loss ≥50% of the surface area

In scores 2 and 3 dentine is often involved.

(2) The visual diagnosis of exposed dentine is difficult. Since changes in anatomical form, color or luster appeared to be easy to observe, the validity of this criterion still is not fully established.

In a recent study, teeth with signs of occlusal/incisal tooth wear of various etiology and severity were visually and histologically investigated regarding the presence of exposed dentine [12]. The study revealed two interesting findings. The first was that the accuracy (closeness of the visual decision to histological findings) was poor. Only 65% of areas with exposed dentine, 88% of areas with enamel present and 67% of all areas examined were diagnosed correctly. The second finding was that exposed dentine was not related to significant amounts of tissue loss – a result that was also found in primary teeth [13]. Dentine was exposed in all cases of cupping or grooving even if only minor substance loss occurred. If cupping/grooving is assumed to be basically related to dentinal exposure, the present grading of initial and advanced occlusal lesions should be reassessed.

Diagnosing exposed dentine, however, could be important for the therapeutic approach in cases of erosion or as a prognostic factor with respect to the progression rate.

In view of these methodological considerations, a new index, the Basic Erosive Wear Examination (BEWE), was developed at a workshop held on current epidemiological approaches in the field of dental erosion entitled 'Current ero-

sion indices – flawed or valid' [14]. The BEWE was designed to avoid grading lesions according to whether and to what extent dentine is exposed. It is a simple scoring system quantifying the size of a given lesion as the percentage of the surface affected. All teeth (vestibular, occlusal and palatal surfaces) except third molars are graded. The dentition is divided into sextants; the most severe score in a sextant is recorded and a cumulative score from all sextants is calculated and represents the index value. The index is not only directed to epidemiological studies but is also intended to help clinicians with managing the condition (tables 1, 2).

First attempts to validate the BEWE have been published [15, 16] and it has also been used in epidemiological studies [17–19]. This new approach, however, surely warrants further validation and improvement.

Assessment of Progression Rate

The assessment of progression is important as it determines whether preventive measures are necessary, or whether interventions implemented were successful, and may help with decision making with respect to when and how to restore worn teeth (see table 2).

Progression can be estimated by depth [20–22], area [23] or volume [24]. Little information is available about clinical wear rates. They were estimated to be up to 40 μm annually [20, 21, 24–

Table 2. Recommendations for clinical management according to BEWE scores [10]

Cumulative score of all sextants	Criteria
≤2	Routine maintenance and observation; repeat at 3-year intervals
3–8	Oral hygiene and dietary assessment and advice; routine maintenance and observation; repeat at 2-year intervals
9–13	Oral hygiene and dietary assessment and advice; identify the main etiological factor(s) for tissue loss and develop strategies to eliminate respective impacts; consider fluoridation measures or other strategies to increase the resistance of tooth surfaces; ideally, avoid the placement of restorations and monitor erosive tooth wear with study casts, photographs or silicone impressions; repeat at 6- to 12-month intervals
≥14	Oral hygiene and dietary assessment and advice; identify the main etiological factor(s) for tissue loss and develop strategies to eliminate respective impacts; consider fluoridation measures or other strategies to increase the resistance of tooth surfaces; ideally, avoid restorations and monitor erosive tooth wear with study casts, photographs or silicone impressions; especially in cases of severe progression consider special care that may involve restorations; repeat at 6- to 12-month intervals

The cut-off values are based on the experience and studies of one of the authors (A.L.) and have to be reconsidered.

26], but in many subjects wear rates were well below 15 μm while in few others rampant wear is seen [26]. It has been assumed that erosive wear is not a steady condition but may occur in bursts depending on varying lifestyle or risk factors like episodes of reflux [25, 26]. It is further difficult to determine a 'physiological' wear rate, not only because there is currently no scientific concept for that. Referring to Smith and Knight [9], tooth wear rates need to be seen in view of whether 'the tooth will survive the rate of wear'; in other words, a given wear rate may need intervention at young, but not at older, age.

Clinical signs for progression are a frosty appearance and absence of extrinsic staining. However, the quantitative assessment of tissue loss is difficult as reference areas on the tooth surface might change over time. Monitoring erosive wear in individual patients by comparing consecutive good quality study casts or photos allows for a visual estimation of wear progression and in principle seems well suitable for decision making on treatment options, but may be difficult to establish in general dental practice [27]. Study casts have also been used for gathering incidence data in epidemiological studies [28, 29].

Various procedures have been suggested for exact quantification of tissue loss [30]. Optical methods use microscopic techniques generating consecutive images of dental casts, which are superimposed [31, 32]. Surface mapping strategies aim to generate computerized superimposed 3D digital images by scanning consecutive dental casts profilometrically or with an optical 3D sensor [21, 33] or by using electroconductive replicas [23]. Most of these methods require extensive equipment and are time consuming, which makes them less suitable for investigating larger groups. One study nonetheless managed to investigate a groups of 251 schoolchildren aged 11–13 years at baseline and at 9- and 18-month intervals. Impressions were taken and electroconductive replicas were scanned. The method was capable of identifying fluoride applications as a significant protecting factor against erosive tooth wear [25].

A relatively practicable procedure was suggested by Bartlett et al. [20], which was further modified by Schlueter et al. [22]. Metal markers were bonded on tooth surfaces serving as reference and identification areas for profilometric measurements. The procedure appears somewhat less sensitive compared to elaborate surface mapping, but is applicable without extensive equipment.

These methods use study models, which is time consuming and adds a source of imprecision. Therefore, methods for application in the oral cavity are desirable. One method potentially suitable for such purposes is optical coherence tomography. This is an interferometric technique, where light of various sources is applied to biological tissues and from the reflectivity profile of the sample a 3D scan is obtained. It has been successfully used to monitor the effect of esomeprazole versus placebo in a clinical trial with patients with gastroesophageal reflux disease [34]. Another method is applying ultrasound, but the reproducibility of this method is limited [35]. A major disadvantage of both methods is that they can only quantify enamel loss.

A more promising perspective might be to use intraoral scanning devices for digital impressions, but so far it seems as if these techniques have not been adapted/applied for monitoring erosive tooth wear. Further details on the methods for assessing erosive tooth wear can be found in the chapter by Attin and Wegehaupt [this vol., pp. 123–142].

Even if attempts have been made to introduce methods for the assessment of progression rates, there is still need for thoroughly evaluated, sensitive, practicable and preferably chairside procedures.

Future Perspectives

Four major points regarding the diagnosis of erosive tooth wear appear important for future activities:

- There is need for standardization of terminology and indices
- Items of currently used indices should be reconsidered with respect to the validity of diagnostic criteria (particularly for occlusal surfaces) and grading (the relevance and diagnosis of exposed dentine)
- It is necessary to consider the differentiation between pathological and physiological erosive tooth wear (on an individual level as well as in the frame of epidemiological research), which, inter alia, is a matter of age and progression rate
- The development of practicable and preferably chairside diagnostic tools for progression rate is needed

References

1 Kidd EAM, Mejàre I, Nyvad B: Clinical and radiographic diagnosis; in Fejerskov O, Kidd EAM (eds): Dental Caries. The Disease and Its Clinical Management. Copenhagen, Blackwell Munksgaard, 2003, pp 111–128.

2 Bartlett D: The implication of laboratory research on tooth wear and erosion. Oral Dis 2005;11:3–6.

3 Stephen KW, McCrossan J, Mackenzie D, MacFarlane CB, Speirs CF: Factors determining the passage of drugs from blood into saliva. Br J Clin Pharmacol 1980;9:51–55.

4 Bell EJ, Kaidonis J, Townsend G, Richards L: Comparison of exposed dentinal surfaces resulting from abrasion and erosion. Aust Dent J 1998;43:362–366.

5 Ganss C, Klimek J, Borkowski N: Characteristics of tooth wear in relation to different nutritional patterns including contemporary and medieval subjects. Eur J Oral Sci 2002;110:54–60.

6 Kaidonis J: Tooth wear: the view of the anthropologist. Clin Oral Investig 2008; 12(suppl 1):S21–S26.

7 Bardsley PF: The evolution of tooth wear indices. Clin Oral Investig 2008; 12(suppl 1):S15–S19.

8 Eccles JD: Dental erosion of nonindustrial origin. A clinical survey and classification. J Prosthet Dent 1979;42:649–653.

9 Smith BG, Knight JK: An index for measuring the wear of teeth. Br Dent J 1984;156:435–438.

10 Bartlett D, Ganss C, Lussi A: Basic Erosive Wear Examination (BEWE): a new scoring system for scientific and clinical needs. Clin Oral Invest 2008;12:S65–S68.

11 Mair LH· Wear in the mouth: the tribological dimension; in Addy M, Embery G, Edgar WM, Orchardson R (eds): Tooth Wear and Sensitivity. Clinical Advances in Restorative Dentistry. London, Martin Dunitz, 2000, pp 181–188.

12 Ganss C, Klimek J, Lussi A: Accuracy and consistency of the visual diagnosis of exposed dentine on worn occlusal/incisal surfaces. Caries Res 2006;40:208–212.

13 Al-Malik MI, Holt RD, Bedi R, Speight PM: Investigation of an index to measure tooth wear in primary teeth. J Dent 2001;29:103–107.

14 Ganss C, Lussi A: Current erosion indices – flawed or valid. Clin Oral Investig 2008;12(suppl 1):S1–S3.

15 Mulic A, Tveit AB, Wang NJ, Hove LH, Espelid I, Skaare AB: Reliability of two clinical scoring systems for dental erosive wear. Caries Res 2010;44:294–299.

16 Dixon B, Sharif MO, Ahmed F, Smith AB, Seymour D, Brunton PA: Evaluation of the basic erosive wear examination (BEWE) for use in general dental practice. Br Dent J 2012;213:E4.

17 Alves Mdo S, da Silva FA, Araújo SG, de Carvalho AC, Santo AM, de Carvalho AL: Tooth wear in patients submitted to bariatric surgery. Braz Dent J 2012;23:160–166.

18 Bartlett DW, Lussi A, West NX, Bouchard P, Sanz M, Bourgeois D: Prevalence of tooth wear on buccal and lingual surfaces and possible risk factors in young European adults. J Dent 2013;41:1007–1013.

19 Mantonanaki M, Koletsi-Kounari H, Mamai-Homata E, Papaioannou W: Dental erosion prevalence and associated risk indicators among preschool children in Athens, Greece. Clin Oral Investig 2013;17:585–593.

20 Bartlett DW, Blunt L, Smith BG: Measurement of tooth wear in patients with palatal erosion. Br Dent J 1997;182:179–184.

21 Pintado MR, Anderson GC, DeLong R, Douglas WH: Variation in tooth wear in young adults over a two-year period. J Prosthet Dent 1997;77:313–320.

22 Schlueter N, Ganss C, De Sanctis S, Klimek J: Evaluation of a profilometrical method for monitoring erosive tooth wear. Eur J Oral Sci 2005;113:505–511.

23 Chadwick RG, Mitchell HL: Conduct of an algorithm in quantifying simulated palatal surface tooth erosion. J Oral Rehabil 2001;28:450–456.

24 Lambrechts P, Braem M, Vuylsteke-Wauters M, Vanherle G: Quantitative in vivo wear of human enamel. J Dent Res 1989;68:1752–1754.

25 Chadwick RG, Mitchell HL, Manton SL, Ward S, Ogston S, Brown R: Maxillary incisor palatal erosion: no correlation with dietary variables? J Clin Pediatr Dent 2005;29:157–163.

26 Rodriguez JM, Austin RS, Bartlett DW: In vivo measurements of tooth wear over 12 months. Caries Res 2012;46:9–15.

27 Bartlett DW, Palmer I, Shah P: An audit of study casts used to monitor tooth wear in general practice. Br Dent J 2005;199:143–145.

28 Ganss C, Klimek J, Giese K: Dental erosion in children and adolescents – a cross-sectional and longitudinal investigation using study models. Community Dent Oral Epidemiol 2001;29:264–271.

29 Bartlett DW: Retrospective long-term monitoring of tooth wear using study models. Br J Clin Pharmacol 2003;194:211–213.

30 Huysmans MC, Chew HP, Ellwood RP: Clinical studies of dental erosion and erosive wear. Caries Res 2011;45:60–68.

31 Sorvari R, Kiviranta I: A semiquantitative method of recording experimental tooth erosion and estimation occlusal wear in the rat. Arch Oral Biol 1988;33:217–220.

32 Mistry M, Grenby TH: Erosion by soft drinks of rat molar teeth assessed by digital image analysis. Caries Res 1993;27:21–25.

33 Mehl A, Gloger W, Kunzelmann KH, Hickel R: A new optical 3-D device for the detection of wear. J Dent Res 1997;76:1799–1807.

34 Wilder-Smith CH, Wilder-smith P, Kaeakami-Wong H, Voronets J, Osann K, Lussi A: Quantification of dental erosions in patients with GERD using optical coherence tomography before and after double-blind, randomized treatment with esomeprazole or placebo. Am J Gastroenterol 2009;104:2788–2795.

35 Louwerse C, Kjaeldgaard M, Huysmans MC: The reproducibility of ultrasonic enamel thickness measurements: an in vitro study. J Dent 2004;32:83–89.

Prof. C. Ganss
Department of Conservative and Preventive Dentistry
Dental Clinic, Justus Liebig University Giessen
Schlangenzahl 14
DE–35392 Giessen (Germany)
E-Mail carolina.ganss@dentist.med.uni-giessen.de

Lussi A, Ganss C (eds): Erosive Tooth Wear. Monogr Oral Sci. Basel, Karger, 2014, vol 25, pp 32–45
DOI: 10.1159/000359936

The Interactions between Attrition, Abrasion and Erosion in Tooth Wear

R. Peter Shellis[a, b] • Martin Addy[a]

[a]School of Oral and Dental Sciences, University of Bristol, Bristol, UK; [b]Department of Preventive, Restorative and Pediatric Dentistry, School of Dental Medicine, University of Bern, Bern, Switzerland

Abstract

Tooth wear is the result of three processes: abrasion (wear produced by interaction between teeth and other materials), attrition (wear through tooth-tooth contact) and erosion (dissolution of hard tissue by acidic substances). A further process (abfraction) might potentiate wear by abrasion and/or erosion. Knowledge of these tooth wear processes and their interactions is reviewed. Both clinical and experimental observations show that individual wear mechanisms rarely act alone but interact with each other. The most important interaction is the potentiation of abrasion by erosive damage to the dental hard tissues. This interaction seems to be the major factor in occlusal and cervical wear. The available evidence is insufficient to establish whether abfraction is an important contributor to tooth wear in vivo. Saliva can modulate erosive/abrasive tooth wear, especially through formation of pellicle, but cannot prevent it.   © 2014 S. Karger AG, Basel

Tooth wear is the progressive loss of dental hard tissues through three processes. The first two are mechanical processes: abrasion (wear produced by interaction between teeth and other materials) and attrition (wear through tooth-tooth contact). These can contribute simultaneously to oc-clusal wear [1]. The third process – erosion – is caused primarily by demineralization of hard tissue by acidic substances. This can in itself result in tissue loss but usually erosive wear is an interactive process in which mechanical wear through attrition or abrasion is enhanced by the initial demineralization. It has been postulated that in a fourth wear-related process (abfraction) abnormal occlusal loading predisposes cervical enamel to mechanical and chemical wear [2]. All four processes are distinguished from the loss of dental hard tissues through dental caries or acute trauma.

The terms abrasion, attrition and erosion have been adapted from everyday usage and their meanings in the dental context diverge from those in other fields, especially tribology, the science of wear, friction and lubrication [3]. In tribological terms, attrition would be recognized as two-body abrasion, in which two moving surfaces contact each other directly and wear is produced by breaking away of asperities. Dental abrasion is a form of three-body wear, in which two moving surfaces are separated by an intervening slurry of abrasive particles, which remove material from both surfaces. Dental erosion would be described as tribochemical wear, in which attack by a chemical agent weakens the structure of the superficial region of the material and enhances its susceptibility to mechanical forces. Abfraction would be described as a form of fatigue. Clearly, the terminology of dental wear has limitations. The term erosion is used to describe either the effects of exposure to acid on dental hard tissue or the overall chemical-mechanical wear process. In this book, we will call the initial acid attack erosion, while recognizing that it should more precisely be termed corrosion [4], and refer to the overall chemical-mechanical wear process as erosive wear [5]. This is justified by the long-established use of the term erosion in dentistry, always with the recognition that, the mouth being a dynamic environment, both mechanical and chemical forces are at work. Retention of this terminology avoids the danger of a disconnect between dental research and clinical practice.

In preindustrial populations of humans, there was extensive wear of the dentition [1] – a natural consequence of the coarse diet, often admixed with abrasive particles such as millstone grit. The main wear processes in such populations were abrasion and attrition, and wear involved mainly the occlusal, incisal and approximal surfaces. Because of the constancy of the diet, wear increased linearly with age and this makes it possible to predict the extent of wear at a given age [6] or to estimate age from the extent of wear [7]. Since the Industrial Revolution the diet in the West has become softer and easier to masticate and this has resulted in a marked reduction in mechanical wear. Thus, while the rate of incisor wear has been estimated as 280–360 µm/year in prehistoric humans [8], teeth in modern humans wear at only 0–35 µm/year [9–11]. Because tooth wear in modern Western populations is ordinarily low, high levels of wear tend to be associated with pathological causes, and wear is not confined to the occlusal and incisal surfaces. The main forms of abnormal wear are cervical wear, heavy occlusal wear and erosive wear at many surfaces: all

three involve interactions of more than one wear process [3, 12, 13]. A major interaction is that between mechanical processes (abrasion and attrition) and erosion, since the latter both removes hard tissue directly and renders tooth surfaces more susceptible to mechanical wear, so that overall wear no longer increases linearly with time.

While much of our understanding of wear comes from in vitro studies which exclude the effects of the oral environment, it is clear from epidemiological surveys and from numerous experimental studies that individual oral and dental factors can modulate tooth wear in vivo [13–15]. Most of these are probably poorly understood at this time but there is evidence that saliva affects tooth wear in a number of ways.

In this review, we first discuss the three main tooth wear processes individually. We then discuss how these interact to produce clinical wear patterns, evaluate the significance of abfraction and consider the role of saliva in modulating wear.

Tooth Wear Mechanisms

Dental Attrition

Attrition creates flat facets with a smooth, shiny appearance and which microscopically present fine, parallel scratch marks [1]. Occlusal wear due to attrition is characterized by equal wear and matching facets on the opposing teeth [12]. Since attrition is created by tooth-to-tooth contact, it should in principle occur by two-body wear but mechanistically it cannot be differentiated sharply from three-body dental abrasion, since particles of enamel detached during attrition can act as abrasive particles [16, 17].

In vitro, the rate of enamel/enamel attrition under loads of 0.2–16 kg increases with time and load, and is strongly influenced by the presence and nature of lubricant [17–19]. In loads >10 kg, water-lubricated wear is greater than that between dry or saliva-lubricated surfaces but saliva-lubricated wear only exceeds wear of dry enamel at loads >14 kg [19]. Presumably, water or saline can keep detached particles of enamel in suspension and thus facilitate three-body abrasion, whereas mucins and other salivary macromolecules reduce frictional forces by coating both the wear surfaces and the particles. Burak et al. [20] observed that at loads of 6 and 10 kg, the rate of dentine/dentine attrition was greater than that of enamel/enamel attrition but at 14 kg the rates were the same. They suggested that dentine wear was greater at lower loads because of its relatively low mineral content, but that at high loads the fibrous organic matrix would help to reduce fracture, whereas the more highly mineralized enamel would lack this mechanism.

Experimental studies of attrition to date have used loads somewhat lower than those observed during the occlusal contact phase of chewing (approx. 27 kg [21]) and much lower than those which can occur in bruxism [22], so further experimentation using higher loads would be informative, as would studies of enamel/dentine attrition.

Wear on incisal edges is generally attributed to attrition. Attrition can also be involved in wear of buccal and lingual surfaces, particularly with certain malocclusions and also approximal surfaces. Pathological wear of occlusal surfaces, i.e. wear beyond the limited amount that can be considered as physiological, has generally been ascribed to parafunctional habits, notably bruxism. However, it often seems to have a multifactorial etiology and so is discussed later in the context of interactions of wear mechanisms.

Dental Abrasion

In the dental context, definitions sometimes assume that all abrasion is pathological [e.g. 23]. However, while abusive toothbrushing can produce pathological levels of abrasion, this view seems mistaken. It has been suggested that many dental health problems are caused or exacerbated by the almost complete lack of abrasive wear from the diet in modern Western populations [24]. Further, tooth cleaning, while being the most common cause of abrasion, is also indispensable to oral health.

As dentine is softer than enamel, it is more susceptible to abrasion, the difference between the tissues decreasing as the hardness of the abrasive particles increases [25]. On the teeth of people consuming abrasive diets, the dentine wears faster than enamel once the cuspal enamel has been removed, giving a 'cupped' or 'scooped' appearance [1]. The abraded dentine surface is covered by a smear layer and so is not associated with problems of sensitivity [1].

In Western populations, clinical data and studies in vitro show that the major abrasive agent is toothpaste [12, 26]. Brushing without paste has no effect on enamel and clinically minuscule effects on dentine [27] but features of the toothbrush, notably filament arrangement, density and texture, can modulate the abrasivity of the toothpaste [28, 29]. Toothbrushing wear is time dependent and appears to be influenced by many factors, including the frequency, duration and force of brushing [26]. The sites of predilection for dentine wear seem to be correlated with toothbrushing habits; the sides, teeth and sites at most risk are those known to receive most attention during brushing.

The major factor in dentine wear appears to be the relative dentine abrasivity (RDA) of the toothpaste, i.e. the abrasivity determined relative to a standard paste using an International Organization for Standardization (ISO) laboratory test. ISO stipulates that toothpastes should not exceed 2.5 times the standard paste (RDA = 100). This gives a range of 0–250 but the majority of toothpastes in developed countries have RDA ≤100. Difficulties arise in extrapolating RDA to clinical outcome. In vitro, wear increases with RDA [29, 30] but in situ the relationship is much less clear and there is often considerable variability in wear measurements [31–33].

Only dentifrices with high relative enamel abrasivity cause appreciable rates of enamel wear, usually because they use nonhydrated alumina, which is harder than enamel. Dentifrices with relative enamel abrasivity <10 produce very little wear of enamel in vitro or in situ [30, 32–35]. Wiegand et al. [36] reported that the abrasion of sound enamel was influenced by brushing force (1.5–4.5 N) over 20–200 brushing strokes but not thereafter up to 1,000 strokes. This might be a 'running-in' phenomenon [25] related to the initial removal of the smear layer, in which the enamel has been damaged by the specimen preparation process.

There seem to be no differences in susceptibility to abrasion between human deciduous and permanent dentine and enamel [37, 38].

It has been concluded that normal toothbrushing habits with toothpastes that conform with the ISO standard will, in a lifetime's use, cause virtually no wear of enamel and clinically insignificant abrasion of dentine: a wear rate of approximately 0.5 mm in 50 years has been cited [26].

Dental Erosion and Erosive Tooth Wear
The acids responsible for dental erosion may be intrinsic (regurgitated gastric acid) or extrinsic (acidic industrial vapors or dietary components such as soft drinks, pickles and acidic fruits). Epidemiological data, and studies in vitro and in situ, suggest that of the three individual wear processes erosion is the most common threat for tooth surface loss [14, 15]. Erosion of dentine appears to be an etiological factor in dentine hypersensitivity [39].

Enamel. Enamel exposed to acid loses mineral from a layer extending a few micrometers below the surface (fig. 1): a process known as softening [40], which renders the surface tissue highly vulnerable to mechanical wear. For histology of enamel erosion, see chapter by Ganss et al. [this vol., pp. 99–107]. With time, as softening progresses further into the enamel, dissolution in the most superficial enamel can reach the point where the outer enamel is lost completely [41, 42]. The pH fall at tooth surfaces following a single ingestion of an acidic drink seems to be fairly short-lived [43] and likely to produce only softening, but repeated intake of erosive drinks might favor some tissue loss by demineralization. In vivo, erosion can therefore involve two types of wear of enamel: mechanical wear of the thin softened layer (erosive tooth wear) and, in extreme cases, the direct removal of hard tissue by prolonged demineralization.

The mineral content of enamel from human deciduous teeth is lower than that from permanent teeth. The two often seem to be equally susceptible to erosion in vitro [37, 44–46] but greater erosion of deciduous tooth enamel has been reported in situ [47, 48].

Dentine. In vitro, the initial effect of exposing dentine to acid is dissolution at the junction between the peritubular and intertubular dentine, with subsequent loss of the peritubular dentine and widening of the tubule lumen [49]. This pattern of dissolution persists during subsurface demineralization (fig. 2) and results in the formation of a superficial layer of demineralized collagenous matrix which is very important in the process of dental erosion, since it mechanically protects the underlying residual dentine and also affects chemical reactions between the latter and the oral environment. For instance, it acts as a diffusion barrier which affects the rate and pattern of dentine erosion [50, 51]. The removal of this layer during wear in vivo probably involves both mechanical and chemical forces and is discussed later. In vivo, the dentinal tubules are filled with neutral, supersaturated tissue fluid. If the dentine surface is lost, e.g. by wear, this fluid will be able to flow out because of the pressure within the pulp. The extent to which these phenomena modify the process of dissolution described above remains to be evaluated.

The extent of dentine erosion is the depth to which mineral has been lost and the persistence of the demineralized layer interferes with the accuracy of measurement by some methods [52, 53]. Optical profilometry detects only the outer

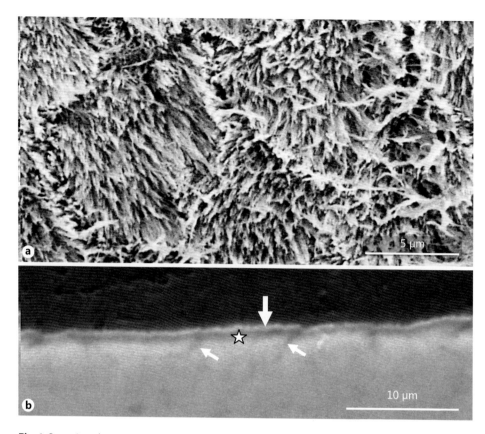

Fig. 1. Scanning electron microscope images of human enamel exposed to 14 mmol/l citric acid, pH 3.2 for 20 min. **a** Polished surface of enamel after citric acid erosion (secondary electron image). The prismatic structure can be seen (especially at left), as well as individual fine, partly-dissolved crystals. **b** Cross-section of specimen similar to (**a**), which has been highly polished and imaged using backscattered electron imaging. Contrast arises mainly from variations in average atomic number: lighter areas are more mineralized. The white line at the enamel surface (vertical broad arrow) is due to gold applied during preparation of the eroded surface, as in (**a**): its thickness arises from gold penetrating between the partly-dissolved crystals. Below this layer is a thin dark region (star) which has undergone initial demineralization. These two layers together represent the total thickness of the softened layer. Some advance demineralization extending obliquely down prism boundaries can also be seen (white arrows). See Shellis et al. [68] for SEM preparation details.

surface of the demineralized dentine and so cannot be used to measure erosion depth. The stylus of a mechanical profilometer can penetrate the demineralized layer but does not consistently reach the boundary with the unaffected dentine and so underestimates depth, although it probably provides information on relative depth. Accurate estimates of erosion depth can be obtained by using sections – by longitudinal micro-radiography, which provides integrated measurements of mineral content through the depth of a specimen, or by removal of the demineralized dentine to allow use of either optical or mechanical profilometry [52, 53]. A combination of either of the latter two methods with optical profilometry of the eroded/abraded surface allows the thickness of residual dentine to be estimated [54].

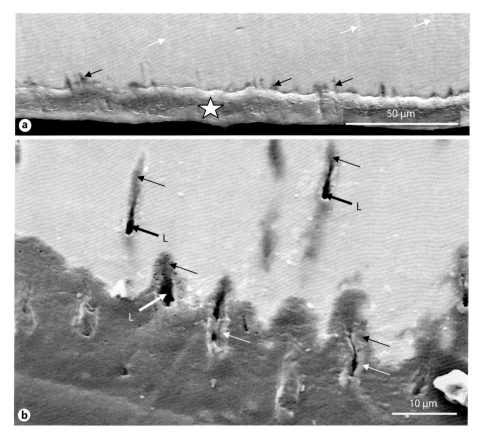

Fig. 2. Polished vertical sections of dentine exposed to 14 mmol/l citric acid, pH 3.2, for 20 min: backscattered electron imaging (see Shellis et al. [68] for details of specimen preparation). **a** Low-power image. Contrast in demineralized layer (marked by a star) is partly due to relief and partly to average atomic number. Top: sound dentine, with undemineralized tubules (white arrows) which are lighter than surrounding intertubular dentine. Demineralization front is irregular because of preferential demineralization along tubules (black arrows). **b** Higher power view of demineralization front, showing advance of demineralization along tubules, with loss of peritubular dentine and enlargement of tubules. Thin white arrows: partly-demineralized peritubular dentine. Thick arrows + L: lumina of dentinal tubules. Thin black arrows: Demineralization at interface between peritubular dentine and intertubular dentine.

In vitro, Hunter et al. [45] found no difference in susceptibility to erosion of dentine from deciduous and permanent teeth in vitro, whereas Wegehaupt et al. [38] found dentine from permanent teeth to be slightly more susceptible. The latter agrees with the results of in situ experiments at a high frequency of acid exposure (4×/day) [48]. All of these results were obtained by stylus profilometry and so are subject to some error.

Interactions between Tooth Wear Processes

It has been recognized for a long time that interactions between different mechanisms contribute strongly to the clinically observed pattern of wear. Attrition and abrasion can operate together in occlusal wear [1], but there is a consensus that interactions between erosion and mechanical wear processes are the most important in vivo. To this must be added a probable role of proteases in dentine wear. We describe the numerous experimental investigations on these interactions as a preliminary to considering clinical studies. It is appropriate also to discuss here the theory that abfraction might potentiate other wear mechanisms.

Dental Attrition and Erosion

Attrition of enamel after short exposure to citric acid increases the depth of tissue loss compared to specimens with erosion only [55]. Other experiments have compared wear of enamel by attrition at different loads and under neutral and acidic conditions. At loads up to 16 kg, enamel/enamel attrition in vitro is much higher in the presence of HCl (pH 1.2) than in water [19]. However, this extreme erosive challenge is likely to occur in vivo only in individuals who vomit frequently, e.g. bulimics [56]. Attrition is much lower in the presence of dilute acetic acid (pH 3.0) or citric acid (pH 3.2), which are much closer to more usual erosive stimuli, than in the presence of water or saline [17–19]. Enamel surfaces which had been rubbed together in citric acid solution at pH 3.2 were smooth, with only slight grooving, and it was suggested that acid softening would both reduce the friction between the surfaces and also dissolve potentially abrasive enamel particles fractured off the surfaces [17]. Studies of enamel surfaces worn by attrition under higher loads representative of chewing or bruxism, and in the presence and absence of acid, would be of interest.

In the only in vitro study of the effect of acidic pretreatment on dentine attrition, it was found that a 20-min treatment of dentine with 1% citric acid (pH 2.3) increased the volume of the wear scar produced by attrition against an enamel cusp by 60% [57].

The Role of Dental Abrasion and Other Forces in Erosive Wear

Enamel. It is well established that exposure of enamel to acid renders it more vulnerable to abrasion. Rats drinking an acidic drink instead of water showed occlusal and lingual wear of the molars, whether they were consuming soft or hard food [58]. In vitro, softened enamel is more susceptible to abrasion, not only by toothbrush and paste [31, 36, 37, 59–61] but even by milder challenges such as toothbrushing without paste [62] or friction from the human tongue [55, 63]. The thickness of tissue removed by erosion followed by abrasion is greater than the sum of the losses caused by erosion and abrasion separately [37]. Thus, whereas enamel is scarcely abraded by normal toothbrushing practices, it becomes vulnerable to abrasion after an erosive challenge; this is the reason for the large increase in wear under erosive conditions.

There is a gradient of mineral loss in softened enamel [64] and the outer extremities of the crystals are thinned and extremely vulnerable to mechanical forces (fig. 1) [64]. The thickness of enamel removed by abrasion depends on the thickness of the softened layer (and hence on the conditions of erosion); for instance, the thickness of softened enamel removed by ultrasonication increased with increasing erosion time [42]. After brief exposure to acid (simulating in vivo conditions), brushing with toothpaste removes about 250–500 nm of enamel [36, 65]. Removal of softened enamel also depends on the strength of the applied mechanical force. Ultrasonication removes only the outer, more demineralized part of the softened enamel [64, 66]. Brushing with water removes more softened enamel than ultrasonication but less than brushing with paste [66]. Increasing pressure enhances the removal of softened enamel by brushing [36], as does input of additional energy (power brushing or sonication [67]).

Brushing in the presence of acid enhances wear by about 50% compared with brushing after acid exposure [62], probably because increased fluid movement accelerates mineral dissolution [68]. This phenomenon might explain the increased risk of erosion associated with consumption of unusual quantities of acidic raw foods [69].

Dentine. Studies utilizing stylus profilometry suggested that eroded dentine is vulnerable to toothbrush abrasion [38, 59, 70–72] but it has become clear that the demineralized layer is remarkably resistant to abrasion [52, 53]. Although the amount of demineralized dentine increased with brushing force, about three quarters of the layer remained even after brushing under a load of 4 N [54]. As with sound dentine, abrasion of eroded dentine increases with RDA (range 10–100) [30].

In vivo, eroded dentine is exposed to a number of proteolytic enzymes. Some occur in saliva and may be of host or bacterial origin, while pepsin occurs in regurgitated gastric juice. These enzymes could attack demineralized dentine and hence augment the effects of abrasion. Saliva of bulimic patients showing clinical erosion has raised levels of pepsin and of proteolytic and collagenolytic activity compared to healthy controls [73]. When dentine was exposed to trypsin after erosion, pepsin simultaneously with erosion or both treatments, there were no clear differences from erosion-only controls until the 6th and last day, when tissue loss in the pepsin/ trypsin group became significantly greater than in the control group [74]. Brushing increased both total tissue loss and loss of the demineralized layer in dentine eroded with HCl containing pepsin and then treated with trypsin [75]. The load applied during brushing had no effect on dentine wear.

It has been speculated that matrix metalloproteinases (MMPs) located within dentine could be exposed and activated during the erosion process and hence could contribute to tissue breakdown [76]. The evidence for this hypothesis is indirect and consists of the finding that substances which inhibit MMPs also seem to reduce dentine erosion. However, there are problems with these data. Firstly, erosion and abrasion were analyzed using mechanical pro-

filometry, which is not completely reliable for these purposes. Secondly, other things being equal, inhibition of MMPs should not affect erosion but only the stability of the demineralized dentine. The fact that the agents tested have reduced or even prevented erosion [77–80] thus suggests that their primary effect is on the demineralization process and not on MMPs. Finally, it should be noted that Ganss et al. [52] and others produced erosive dentine lesions under conditions (alternating low pH erosive acid and artificial saliva at neutral pH) which are claimed to optimize MMP activity [76], and yet found that the demineralized dentine is resistant to abrasion.

From the foregoing, it is clear that much more work is required to elucidate the role of proteolytic enzymes in the erosive wear of dentine.

Abfraction

The principal idea in the theory of abfraction, which was put forward to account for the creation of wedge-shaped noncarious cervical lesions (NCCL), is that off-axis loading of tooth cusps would cause concentrations of tensile stress in the cervical region, leading to microcrack formation, particularly in the enamel, which resists tensile stress less well than dentine. It was hypothesized that the cervical region would consequently be susceptible to abrasive and erosive wear [2].

The evidence for abfraction as an important factor in tooth wear seems to be inconclusive [4, 81, 82]. In particular, there seems to be no firm clinical evidence for the phenomenon and some clinical observations seem to conflict with predictions of the hypothesis. For instance, NCCL are mostly located apical to the cement-enamel junction, suggesting that the initiating event is not breakdown of the cervical enamel [83]. A clinical study found that occlusal adjustment to remove abnormal stresses in the cervical region did not halt the progression of NCCL [84].

There are also problems with nonclinical studies. Most supporting evidence for abfraction comes from analyses of stress distributions in loaded teeth, but many of these studies have used unrealistic models of tooth structure [4, 82, 85] or have yielded results that conflict with the predictions of the abfraction hypothesis [82]. Experimental studies suggest that wedge-shaped cervical lesions can be created by toothbrushing in teeth that are either unloaded or under continuous axial load [86]. While axial loading reduced cervical toothbrushing wear, off-axis loading had no significant effect [86]. It is always possible that experiments on extracted teeth are influenced by pre-existing cracks in the cervical enamel but these results cast doubt on the validity of the abfraction hypothesis. Periodic off-axis stressing of whole tooth crowns increased the rate of erosion of cervical enamel in 1% lactic acid (pH 4.5) [87], but in this study only tissue loss on the crown surface subject to tensile stress was examined and examination of both surfaces is essential to test the abfraction hypothesis. Staninec et al. [88] found that tissue loss from beams of dentine subjected to bending stress was greater at pH 6 than at pH 7, but more wear occurred on the compression surface of the beam than on the tension surface and this is contradictory to the abfraction hypothesis.

Clinical Observations

At present, it is difficult to determine, in a given individual, the relative importance in tooth wear of the processes discussed above. However, much evidence on general interactions between wear processes in clinical tooth wear has accumulated from case reports and from clinical and epidemiological studies of tooth wear. The clinical evidence is supplemented by detailed examination of worn teeth and dentitions by microscopic and other techniques.

Occlusal Wear

Heavy wear of the occlusal surfaces was once generally assumed to be attributable to attrition during bruxism. However, several studies have found that occlusal wear may be related to a variety of factors, including occlusal variations, dusty environments, salivary variables and intake of acidic foods and drinks [89–92]. Such studies and observations on wear patterns suggest that erosion and abrasion, as well as attrition, contribute to occlusal wear [16, 93–95], although Khan et al. [93] identified attrition as the major cause of wear in maxillary anterior teeth of positively identified bruxers. In modern populations, wear patterns similar to those found in populations consuming an abrasive diet are mimicked in persons subsisting on a diet which has a relatively low abrasivity, provided that it is also erosive. An example is that of people living on a raw food diet which is both fibrous and has a high acid content [69].

Cervical Wear

The most common sites for abnormal tooth wear in modern populations are the buccal cervical regions and there has been considerable interest in the etiology of NCCL. Most researchers consider these lesions to have a multifactorial origin, with prominent contributions from erosion and abrasion [81, 85, 94–98]. A longitudinal study of wedge-shaped defects identified frequency of brushing as a significant risk factor [92]. In a case-control study [99], only variables considered to be related to abrasion were significant risk factors for cervical lesions in a subject-level model, while variables related to tooth flexure and erosion were also significant risk factors in a tooth-level model. In historical or aboriginal populations, in which the diet is abrasive but not erosive, NCCL are rare or absent [1, 69, 94, 96]; this indicates that the potentiation of abrasion by erosion is a key factor.

As noted above, it has been suggested that abfraction is a major factor in the creation of NCCL.

Studies [100, 101] which considered cervical lesion characteristics in relation to occlusal wear or malocclusion estimated that the proportion of lesions possibly due to abrasion was no more than 15–38%.

Saliva and Tooth Wear

There is clear variation in clinical tooth wear between people. One biological factor that could contribute strongly to this variability is saliva. Young and Khan [102] suggested that NCCL tended to occur at sites which were exposed to least clearance by saliva. Hellwig et al. [103] exposed enamel samples cyclically to acidified saliva and to natural saliva and found that erosion lesions developed in saliva from subjects with erosion progressed faster than in saliva from erosion-free subjects. There is considerable variation in the rate at which saliva recovers from undersaturation following an acid challenge [104]. However, identifying protective salivary factors has proved a problem, in that there is great inconsistency between studies. Some identified no differences in salivary properties between subjects with and without erosion [105, 106]. Other studies have identified a wide range of factors which differed between these groups. Unstimulated salivary flow rate was found to be lower in subjects with erosion than in subjects without erosion in four studies [56, 107–109] (in one study [107] this was the case only in 16- to 20-year-olds). Urea concentration has been found to be lower in subjects with erosion in two studies [107, 110] (in the former study [107] this was again the case only in 16- to 20-year-olds). Two studies [109, 111] found lower buffer capacity among subjects with erosion, while low buffer capacity was found to be more common in subjects at high risk of NCCL than in low-risk subjects [92]. Low flow rate and buffer capacity were also associated with an increased fall in salivary pH [109]. Other variables found to differ between these groups, but only in single studies, are concentrations of phosphate, calcium, sodium, potassium, chloride and protein [56, 107, 108, 112]. Among gastric reflux patients, some studies have identified low salivary flow rate [113] or low buffering capacity as risk factors for erosion in two studies [114, 115] but another study did not [116].

In most studies, test groups were selected on the basis of whether they showed clinical signs of erosive wear. However, there are many reasons why some persons show more erosive wear than others, e.g. total intake of acidic products. A better approach to determining the role of saliva might be first to test the rate at which in situ erosion occurs in volunteers under controlled conditions and then to correlate erosion with salivary variables in volunteers who show high and low erosion rates.

Salivary pellicle reduces the amount of mineral lost during an erosive challenge, having a greater effect on the erosion of enamel than on that of dentine [117]. It has been suggested that the thickness and protective properties of the pellicle influence site variations in erosion [118] but this hypothesis does not seem to be supported experimentally [119]. However, surprisingly large variations in the protective effect between individuals have been detected in vitro [120, 121]. The protective effect of pellicle lasts only for a short time as, during acid exposure, the pellicle is removed except for the dense basal layer and its protective effect is lost [119, 122]. In vitro tests indicate that to achieve a significant protective effect, exposure to saliva for 2 min for dentine and 1 h for enamel would be required [123]. During the time when pellicle is still forming, the denuded tooth surface would remain vulnerable to erosion.

The pellicle seems to show some resistance to brushing, since Hannig [124] found that the basal pellicle layer was still intact after 10 s of brushing with saliva alone. After brushing for 10 s with saliva/silica slurry, the basal pellicle layer was still not completely removed and Hannig [124] suggested that this layer could modify wear. However, brushing with silica pastes for 10 s would cause no significant wear of sound enamel and this hypothesis needs to be tested using softened enamel. Moreover, the finding that brushing removes the outer pellicle substantiates the suggestion [125] that brushing immediately before eating or drinking might degrade the protective effect of the pellicle against erosion.

It has been known for a long time that softened enamel exposed to a remineralizing solution or to saliva for an adequate time can regain mineral and thus reacquire mechanical strength [40]. Numerous studies aimed at determining the time required for this process to repair softened dental tissues have been carried out and are reviewed in the chapters by Shellis et al., Lussi et al., Hara et al. [this vol., pp. 163–179, pp. 1–15, pp. 197–205].

References

1 Kaidonis JA: Tooth wear: the view of the anthropologist. Clin Oral Invest 2008; 12(suppl):54–58.

2 Grippo JO: Abfractions: a new classification of hard tissue lesions of teeth. J Esthet Dent 1991;3:14–19.

3 Mair LH: Wear in the mouth: the tribological dimension; in Addy M, Embery G, Edgar WM, Orchardson R (eds): Tooth Wear and Sensitivity. London, Martin Dunitz, 2000, pp 181–188.

4 Michael JA, Townsend GC, Greenwood LF, Kaidonis JA: Abfraction: separating fact from fiction. Aust Dent J 2009;54: 2–8.

5 Shellis RP, Ganss C, Ren Y, Zero D, Lussi A: Methodology and models in erosion research: discussion and conclusions. Caries Res 2011;45(suppl 1): 69–77.

6 Richards LC, Kaidonis JA, Townsend GC: A model for the prediction of tooth wear in individuals. Aust Dent J 2003; 48:259–262.

7 Miles AEW: The Miles method of assessing age from tooth wear revisited. J Archaeol Sci 2001;28:973–982.

8 Bermúdez de Castro JM, Martinón-Torres M, Sarmiento S, Lozano M, Arsuaga JL, Carbonell E: Rates of anterior tooth wear in Middle Pleistocene hominins from Sima de los Huesos (Sierra de Atapuerca, Spain). Proc Natl Acad Sci USA 2003;100:11992–11996.

9 Lambrechts P, Braem M, Vuylsteke-Wauters M, Vanherle G: Quantitative in vivo wear of human enamel. J Dent Res 1989;68:1752–1754.

10 Pintado MR, Anderson GC, DeLong R, Douglas WH: Variation in tooth wear in young adults over a two-year period. J Prosthet Dent 1997;77:313–320.

11 Rodriguez JM, Austin RS, Bartlett DW: In vivo measurements of tooth wear over 12 months. Caries Res 2012;46: 9–15.

12 Bartlett DW, Smith BGN: Definition, classification, and clinical assessment of attrition, erosion and abrasion of enamel and dentine; in Addy M, Embery G, Edgar WM, Orchardson R (eds): Tooth Wear and Sensitivity. London, Martin Dunitz, 2000, pp 87–92.

13 Meurman JH, Sorvari R: Interplay of erosion attrition and abrasion in tooth wear and possible approaches to prevention; in Addy M, Embery G, Edgar WM, Orchardson R (eds): Tooth Wear and Sensitivity. London, Martin Dunitz, 2000, pp 171–180.

14 Nunn JH: Prevalence and distribution of tooth wear; in Addy M, Embery G, Edgar WM, Orchardson R (eds): Tooth Wear and Sensitivity. London, Martin Dunitz, 2000, pp 93–104.

15 Zero DT, Lussi AS: Etiology of enamel erosion: intrinsic and extrinsic factors; in Addy M, Embery G, Edgar WM, Orchardson R (eds): Tooth Wear and Sensitivity. London, Martin Dunitz, 2000, pp 121–140.

16 Xhonga FA: Bruxism and its effect on the teeth. J Oral Rehabil 1977;4:65–76.

17 Eisenburger M, Addy M: Erosion and attrition of human enamel in vitro. Part I. Interaction effects. J Dent 2002;30: 341–347.

18 Eisenburger M, Addy M: Erosion and attrition of human enamel in vitro. Part II. Influence of time and loading. J Dent 2002;30:349–352.

19 Kaidonis JA, Richards LC, Townsend GC, Tansley GD: Wear of human enamel: a quantitative assessment. J Dent Res 1998;77:1983–1990.

20 Burak N, Kaidonis JA, Richards LC, Townsend GC: Experimental studies of human dentine wear. Arch Oral Biol 1999;44:885–887.

21 Gibbs CH, Mahan PE, Lundeen HC, Brehnan K, Walsh EK, Holbrook WB: Occlusal forces during chewing and swallowing as measured by sound transmission. J Prosthet Dent 1981;46:443–449.

22 Waltimo A, Nyström M, Könönen M: Bite force and dentofacial morphology in men with severe dental attrition. Scand J Dent Res 1994;102:92–96.

23 Imfeld T: Dental erosion. Definition, classification and links. Eur J Oral Sci 1996;104:151–155.

24 Kaifu Y, Kasai K, Townsend GC, Richards LC: Tooth wear and the 'design' of the human dentition. A perspective from evolutionary medicine. Yearbook Phys Anthropol 2003;46:47–61.

25 Wright KHR: The abrasive wear resistance of human dental tissues. Wear 1969;14:263–284.

26 Addy M, Hunter ML: Can tooth brushing damage your health? Effects on oral and dental tissues. Int Dent J 2003;53: 177–186.

27 Absi EG, Addy M, Adams D: Dentine hypersensitivity – the effects of toothbrushing and dietary compounds on dentine in vitro: an SEM study. J Oral Rehabil 1992;19:101–110.

28 Dyer D, Addy M, Newcombe RG: Studies in vitro of abrasion by different manual toothbrush heads and a standard toothpaste. J Clin Periodontol 2000;27: 99–103.

29 Wiegand A, Kuhn M, Sener B, Roos M, Attin T: Abrasion of eroded dentine caused by toothpaste slurries of different abrasivities and toothbrushes of different filament diameter. J Dent 2009; 37:480–484.

30 Philpotts CJ, Weader E, Joiner A: The measurement in vitro of enamel and dentine wear by toothpastes of different abrasivity. Int Dent J 2005;55:183–187.

31 Addy M, Hughes J, Pickles M, Joiner A, Huntington E: Development of a method in situ to study toothpaste abrasion of dentine: comparison of 2 products. J Clin Periodontol 2002;29:896–900.

32 Hooper S, West NX, Pickles M, Joiner A, Newcombe RG, Addy M: Investigation of erosion and abrasion of enamel and dentine: a model in situ using toothpastes of different abrasivity. J Clin Periodontol 2003;30:802–808.

33 Pickles MJ, Joiner A, Weader E, Cooper YL, Cox TF: Abrasion of human enamel and dentine caused by toothpastes of differing abrasivity determined using an in situ wear model. Int Dent J 2005;55: 188–193.

34 Joiner A, Pickles MJ, Tanner C, Weader E, Doyle P: An in situ model to study the toothpaste abrasion of enamel. J Clin Periodontol 2004;31:434–438.

35 Lussi A, Jaeggi T, Gerber C, Megert B: Effect of amine/sodium fluoride rinsing on toothbrush abrasion of softened enamel in situ. Caries Res 2004;38:567–571.

36 Wiegand A, Köwing L, Attin T: Impact of brushing force on abrasion of acid-softened and sound enamel. Arch Oral Biol 2007;52:1043–1047.

37 Attin T, Wegehaupt F, Gries D, Wiegand A: The potential of deciduous and permanent bovine enamel as substitute for deciduous and permanent human enamel: erosion-abrasion experiments. J Dent 2007;35:773–777.

38 Wegehaupt F, Gries D, Wiegand A, Attin T: Is bovine dentine an appropriate substitute for human dentine in erosion/abrasion tests? J Oral Rehabil 2008;35: 390–394.

39 Dababneh RH, Khouri AT, Addy M: Dentine hypersensitivity – an enigma? A review of terminology, epidemiology, mechanisms, aetiology and management. Br Dent J 1999;187:606–611.

40 Koulourides T: Experimental changes of mineral density; in Harris RS (ed): Art and Science of Dental Caries Research. New York, Academic Press, 1968, pp 355–378.

41 Schweizer-Hirt CM, Schait A, Schmidt R, Imfeld T, Lutz F, Mühlemann HR: Erosion und Abrasion des Schmelzes. Eine experimentelle Studie. SSO Schweiz Monatsschr Zahnheilkd 1978;88:497–529.

42 Eisenburger M, Hughes J, West NX, Jandt K, Addy M: Ultrasonication as a method to study enamel demineralization during acid erosion. Caries Res 2000;34:289–294.

43 Millward A, Shaw L, Harrington E, Smith AJ: Continuous monitoring of salivary flow rate and pH at the surface of the dentition following consumption of acidic beverages. Caries Res 1997;31: 44–49.

44 Lussi A, Kohler N, Zero D, Schaffner M, Megert B: A comparison of the erosive potential of different beverages in primary and permanent teeth using an in vitro model. Eur J Oral Sci 2000;108: 110–114.

45 Hunter ML, West NX, Hughes JA, Newcombe RG, Addy M: Relative susceptibility of deciduous and permanent dental hard tissues to erosion by a low pH fruit drink in vitro. J Dent 2000;28:265–270.

46 Lippert F, Parker DM, Jandt KD: Susceptibility of deciduous and permanent enamel to dietary acid-induced erosion studied with atomic force microscopy nanoindentation. Eur J Oral Sci 2004; 112:61–66.

47 Johansson A-K, Sorvari R, Birkhed D, Meurman JH: Dental erosion in deciduous teeth – an in vivo and in vitro study. J Dent 2001;29:333–340.

48 Hunter ML, West NX, Hughes JA, Newcombe RG, Addy M: Erosion of deciduous and permanent dental hard tissue in the oral environment. J Dent 2000;28: 257–263.

49 Meurman JH, Drysdale T, Frank RM: Experimental erosion of dentine. Scand J Dent Res 1991;99:457–462.

50 Kleter GA, Damen JJ, Everts V, Niehof J, ten Cate JM: The influence of the organic matrix on demineralization of bovine root dentin in vitro. J Dent Res 1994;73: 1523–1529.

51 Shellis RP, Barbour ME, Jones SB, Addy M: Effects of pH and acid concentration on erosive dissolution of enamel, dentine and compressed hydroxyapatite. Eur J Oral Sci 2010;118:475–482.

52 Ganss C, Schlueter N, Hardt M, von Hinckeldey J, Klimek J: Effects of toothbrushing on eroded dentine. Eur J Oral Sci 2007;115:390–396.

53 Ganss C, Lussi A, Scharmann I, Weigelt T, Hardt M, Klimek J, Schlueter N: Comparison of calcium analysis, longitudinal microradiography and profilometry for the quantitative assessment of erosion in dentine. Caries Res 2009;43:422–429.

54 Ganss C, Hardt M, Blazek D, Klimek J, Schlueter N: Effects of toothbrushing force on the mineral content and demineralized organic matrix of eroded dentine. Eur J Oral Sci 2009;117:255–260.

55 Vieira A, Overweg E, Ruben JL, Huysmans MC: Toothbrush abrasion, simulated tongue friction and attrition of eroded bovine enamel in vitro. J Dent 2006;34:336–342.

56 Järvinen VK, Rytömaa II, Heinonen OP: Risk factors in dental erosion. J Dent Res 1991;70:942–947.

57 Li H, Liu MC, Deng M, Moazzez R, Bartlett DW: An experiment on the attrition of acid demineralized dentine in vitro. Aust Dent J 2011;56:63–67.

58 Sorvari R, Kiviranta I: A semiquantitative method of recording experimental tooth erosion and estimating occlusal wear in the rat. Arch Oral Biol 1988;33: 217–220.

59 Davis WB, Winter PJ: The effect of abrasion on enamel and dentine after exposure to dietary acid. Br Dent J 1980;148: 253–256.

60 Attin T, Koidl U, Buchalla W, Schaller HG, Kielbassa AM, Hellwig E: Correlation of microhardness and wear in differently eroded bovine dental enamel. Arch Oral Biol 1997;42:243–250.

61 Jaeggi T, Lussi A: Toothbrush abrasion of erosively altered enamel after intraoral exposure to saliva: an in situ study. Caries Res 1999;33:455–461.

62 Eisenburger M, Shellis RP, Addy M: Comparative study of wear of enamel induced by alternating and simultaneous combinations of abrasion and erosion in vitro. Caries Res 2003;37:450–456.

63 Gregg T, Mace S, West NX, Addy M: A study in vitro of the abrasive effect of the tongue on enamel and dentine softened by acid erosion. Caries Res 2004; 38:557–560.

64 Eisenburger M, Shellis RP, Addy M: Scanning electron microscopy of softened enamel. Caries Res 2004;38:67–74.

65 Voronets J, Lussi A: Thickness of softened human enamel removed by toothbrush abrasion: an in vitro study. Clin Oral Invest 2010;14:251–256.

66 Wiegand A, Wegehaupt F, Werner C, Attin T: Susceptibility of acid-softened enamel to mechanical wear – ultrasonication versus toothbrushing action. Caries Res 2007;41:56–60.

67 Wiegand A, Begic M, Attin T: In vitro evaluation of abrasion of eroded enamel by different manual, power and sonic toothbrushes. Caries Res 2006;40:60–65.

68 Shellis RP, Finke M, Eisenburger M, Parker DM, Addy M: Relationship between enamel erosion and flow rate. Eur J Oral Sci 2005;113:232–238.

69 Ganss C, Klimek J, Borkovski N: Characteristics of tooth wear in relation to different nutritional patterns including contemporary and medieval subjects. Eur J Oral Sci 2002;110:54–60.

70 Attin T, Buchalla W, Putz B: In vitro evaluation of different remineralization periods in improving the abrasion resistance of previously abraded bovine dentine against tooth-brushing abrasion. Arch Oral Biol 2001;46:871–874.

71 Attin T, Siegel S, Buchalla W, Lennon AM, Hannig C, Becker K: Brushing abrasion of softened and remineralised dentin: an in situ study. Caries Res 2004; 38:62–66.

72 Hara AT, Turssi CP, Teixeira ECN, Serra MC, Cury JA: Abrasive wear on eroded root dentine after different periods of exposure to saliva in situ. Eur J Oral Sci 2003;111:423–427.

73 Schlueter N, Ganss C, Pötschke S, Klimek J, Hannig C: Enzyme activities in the oral fluids of patients suffering from bulimia: a controlled clinical trial. Caries Res 2012;46:130–139.

74 Schlueter N, Hardt M, Klimek J, Ganss C: Influence of the digestive enzymes trypsin and pepsin in vitro on the progression of erosion in dentine. Arch Oral Biol 2010;55:294–299.

75 Schlueter N, Glatzki J, Klimek J, Ganss C: Erosive-abrasive tissue loss in dentine under simulated bulimic conditions. Arch Oral Biol 2012;57:1176–1182.

76 Buzalaf MAR, Kato MT, Hannas AR: The role of matrix metalloproteinases in dental erosion. Adv Dent Res 2012;24: 72–76.

77 Kato MT, Leite AL, Hannas AR, Buzalaf MAR: Gels containing MMP inhibitors prevent dental erosion in situ. J Dent Res 2010a;89:468–472.

78 Kato MT, Leite AL, Hannas AR, Oliveira RC, Pereira JC, Tjäderhane L, Buzalaf MAR: Effect of iron on metalloproteinase inhibition and on the prevention of dentine erosion. Caries Res 2010b;44: 309–316.

79 Kato MT, Leite AL, Hannas AR, Calabria MP, Magalhães AC, Pereira JC, Buzalaf MAR: Impact of protease inhibitors on dentin matrix degradation by collagenase. J Dent Res 2012;91:1119–1123.

80 Magalhães AC, Wiegand A, Rios D, Hannas A, Attin T, Buzalaf MAR: Chlorhexidine and green tea extract reduce dentin erosion and abrasion in situ. J Dent 2009;37:994–998.

81 Litonjua LA, Andreana S, Bush PJ, Tobias TS, Cohen RE: Noncarious cervical lesions and abfractions. A re-evaluation. J Am Dent Assoc 2003;134:845–850.

82 Litonjua LA, Andreana S, Patra AK, Cohen RE: An assessment of stress analyses in the theory of abfraction. Biomed Mater Eng 2004;14:311–321.

83 Hur B, Kim HC, Park JK, Versluis A: Characteristics of non-carious cervical lesions – an ex vivo study using microcomputed tomography. J Oral Rehabil 2011;38:469–474.

84 Wood ID, Kassir ASA, Brunton PA: Effect of lateral excursive movements on the progression of abfraction lesions. Oper Dent 2009;34:273–279.

85 Daley TJ, Harbrow DJ, Kahler B, Young WG: The cervical wedge-shaped lesion in teeth: a light and electron microscope study. Aust Dent J 2009;54:212–219.

86 Litonjua LA, Bush PJ, Andreana S, Tobias TS, Cohen RE: Effects of occlusal load on cervical lesions. J Oral Rehabil 2004;31:225–232.

87 Palamara D, Palamara JEA, Tyas MJ, Pintado M, Messer HH: Effect of stress on acid dissolution of enamel. Dent Mater 2001;17:109–115.

88 Staninec M, Nalla RK, Hilton JF, Ritchie RO, Watanabe LG, Nonomura G, Marshall GW, Marshall SJ: Dentin erosion simulation by cantilever beam fatigue and pH change. J Dent Res 2005;84:371–375.

89 Nyström M, Könen M, Alaluusua S, Evälahti M, Vartiovaara J: Development of horizontal tooth wear in maxillary anterior teeth from five to 18 years of age. J Dent Res 1990;69:1765–1770.

90 Johansson A, Fareed K, Omar R: Analysis of possible factors influencing the occurrence of occlusal tooth wear in a young Saudi population. Acta Odontol Scand 1991;49:139–145.

91 Johansson A, Kiliaridis S, Haraldson T, Omar R, Carlsson GE: Covariation of some factors associated with occlusal tooth wear in a selected high-wear sample. Scand J Dent Res 1993;101:398–406.

92 Lussi A, Schaffner M: Progression of and risk factors for dental erosion and wedge-shaped defects over a 6-year period. Caries Res 2000;34:182–187.

93 Khan F, Young WG, Daley TJ: Dental erosion and bruxism. A tooth wear analysis. Aust Dent J 1998;43:117–127.

94 Johansson AK, Omar R, Carlsson GE, Johansson A: Dental erosion and its growing importance in clinical practice: from past to present. Int J Dent 2012; 2012:632907.

95 Levitch LC, Bader JD, Shugars DA, Heymann HO: Non-carious cervical lesions. J Dent 1994;22:195–207.

96 Nguyen C, Ranjitkar S, Kaidonis JA, Townsend GC: A qualitative assessment of non-carious cervical lesions in extracted human teeth. Aust Dent J 2008; 53:46–51.

97 Khan F, Young WG, Shahabi S, Daley TJ: Dental cervical lesions associated with occlusal erosion and attrition. Aust Dent J 1999;44:176–186.

98 Bartlett DW, Shah P: A critical review of non-carious cervical (wear) lesions and the role of abfraction, erosion and abrasion. J Dent Res 2006;85:306–312.

99 Bader JD, McClure F, Scurria MS, Shugars DA, Heymann HO: Case-control study of non-carious cervical lesions. Community Dent Oral Epidemiol 1996;24:286–291.

100 Piotrowski BT, Gillette WB, Hancock EB: Examining the prevalence and characteristics of abfraction-like cervical lesions in a population of US veterans. J Am Dent Assoc 2001;132:1694–1701.

101 Oginni AO, Olusile AO, Udoye CI: Non-carious cervical lesions in a Nigerian population: abrasion or abfraction? Int Dent J 2003;53:275–279.

102 Young WG, Khan F: Sites of dental erosion are saliva-dependent. J Oral Rehabil 2002;29:35–43.

103 Hellwig E, Lussi A, Goetz F: Influence of human saliva on the development of artificial erosions. Caries Res 2013;47:553–558.

104 Bashir E, Lagerlöf F: Effect of citric acid clearance on the saturation with respect to hydroxyapatite in saliva. Caries Res 1996;30:213–217.

105 Correr C, Alonso RC, Correa MA, Campos EA, Baratto-Filho F, Puppin-Rontani RM: Influence of diet and salivary characteristics on the prevalence of dental erosion among 12-year-old schoolchildren. J Dent Child 2009;76:181–187.

106 Wang P, Zhou Y, Zhu Y, Lin HC: Unstimulated and stimulated salivary characteristics of 12- to 13-year-old schoolchildren with and without dental erosion. Arch Oral Biol 2011;56:1328–1332.

107 Piangprach T, Hengtrakool C, Kukiattrakoon B, Kediarune-Leggat U: The effect of salivary factors on dental erosion in various age groups and tooth surfaces. J Am Dent Assoc 2009;140:1137–1143.

108 Zwier N, Huysmans MC, Jager DH, Ruben J, Bronkhorst EM, Truin GJ: Saliva parameters and erosive wear in adolescents. Caries Res 2013;47:548–552.

109 Sánchez GA, Fernandez De Preliasco MV: Salivary pH changes during soft drinks consumption in children. Int J Paediatr Dent 2003;13:251–257.

110 Johansson AK, Lingström P, Birkhed D: Comparison of factors potentially related to the occurrence of dental erosion in high- and low-erosion groups. Eur J Oral Sci 2002;110:204–211.

111 Carlsson GE, Johansson A, Lundqvist S: A follow-up study of 18 subjects with extensively worn dentitions. Acta Odontol Scand 1985;43:83–90.

112 Mulic A, Bjørg Tveit A, Songe D, Sivertsen H, Skaare AB: Dental erosive wear and salivary flow rate in physically active young adults. BMC Oral Health 2012;12:8.

113 Yoshikawa H, Furuta K, Ueno M, Egawa M, Yoshino A, Kondo S, Nariai Y, Ishibashi H, Kinoshita Y, Sekine J: Oral symptoms including dental erosion in gastroesophageal reflux disease are associated with decreased salivary flow volume and swallowing function. J Gastroenterol 2012;47:412–420.

114 Moazzez R, Bartlett D, Anggiansah A: Dental erosion, gastro-oesophageal reflux disease and saliva: how are they related? J Dent 2004;32:489–494.

115 Corrêa MC, Lerco MM, Cunha Mde L, Henry MA: Salivary parameters and teeth erosions in patients with gastro-esophageal reflux disease. Arq Gastroenterol 2012;49:214–218.

116 Saksena R, Bartlett DW, Smith BG: The role of saliva in regurgitation erosion. Eur J Prosthodont Restor Dent 1999;7:121–124.

117 Wiegand A, Bliggenstorfer S, Magalhaes AC, Sener B, Attin T: Impact of the in situ formed salivary pellicle on enamel and dentine erosion caused by different acids. Acta Odontol Scand 2008;66:225–230.

118 Amaechi BT, Higham SM: Thickness of acquired salivary pellicle as a determinant of the sites of dental erosion. J Dent Res 1999;78:1821–1828.

119 Hannig M, Balz M: Protective properties of salivary pellicles from two different intraoral sites on enamel erosion. Caries Res 2001;35:142–148.

120 Wetton S, Hughes J, Newcombe RG, Addy M: The effect of saliva derived from different individuals on the erosion of enamel and dentine. A study in vitro. Caries Res 2007;41:423–426.

121 Bruvo M, Moe D, Kirkeby S, Vorum H, Bardow A: Individual variations in protective effects of experimentally formed salivary pellicles. Caries Res 2009;43:163–170.

122 Hannig M, Balz M: Influence of in vivo formed salivary pellicle on enamel erosion. Caries Res 1999;33:372–379.

123 Wetton S, Hughes JA, West NX, Addy M: Exposure time of enamel and dentine to saliva for protection against erosion: a study in vitro. Caries Res 2006;40:213–217.

124 Hannig M: The protective nature of the salivary pellicle. Int Dent J 2002;52:417–423.

125 Attin T, Knöfel S, Buchalla W: In situ evaluation of different remineralization periods to improve the abrasion resistance of previously eroded enamel. Caries Res 2001;35:216–222.

Dr. R.P. Shellis, PhD
Department of Preventive, Restorative and Pediatric Dentistry
School of Dental Medicine, University of Bern
Freiburgstrasse 7
CH–3010 Bern (Switzerland)
E-Mail peter.shellis@btinternet.com

Lussi A, Ganss C (eds): Erosive Tooth Wear. Monogr Oral Sci. Basel, Karger, 2014, vol 25, pp 46–54
DOI: 10.1159/000359937

Challenges in Assessing Erosive Tooth Wear

Vasileios Margaritis[a] · June Nunn[b]

[a]College of Health Sciences, Walden University, Minneapolis, Minn., USA; [b]Department of Special Care Dentistry, Dublin Dental University Hospital, Dublin, Ireland

Abstract

Indices for assessing erosive wear are expected to deliver more than is expected of an ideal index: simple with defined scoring criteria so that it is reproducible, reflective of the aetiology of the condition and accurately categorizing shape, area and depth of affect, both at a point in time (prevalence) and longitudinally (incidence/increment). In addition, the differential diagnosis of erosive wear is complex, as it usually co-exists with other types of tooth wear. Therefore, a valid recording of erosive wear at an individual as well as at a population level without a thorough history with respect to general health, diet and habits is a challenge. The aims of this chapter are to describe the potential methodological challenges in assessing erosive wear, to critique the strengths and limitations of the existing erosion indices and to propose the adoption of a validated erosion index for the purpose for which it is intended.   © 2014 S. Karger AG, Basel

Indices for assessing erosive wear are expected to deliver more than is expected of an ideal index: simple with defined scoring criteria so that it is reproducible, reflective of the aetiology of the condition and accurately categorizing shape, area and depth of affect, both at a point in time (prevalence) and longitudinally (incidence/increment) [1]. In addition, the content validity is often theoretically flawed (partial vs. full-mouth recording) as can be the construct validity – for example, when there is little convergence or discriminant validity between a general index of tooth wear and aspects of erosive tooth wear only [2]. Thus arises the difficulty in selecting an index that is internationally comparable and acceptable – a dilemma that is reflected in the burgeoning number of new indices. Also, the literature on this topic is replete with terminology that is used interchangeably, especially tooth wear and erosion. In addition, the differential diagnosis of erosive wear is difficult, as it usually co-exists with other types of tooth wear. Therefore, a valid recording of erosive wear at individual as well as at population level without a thorough history with respect to general health, diet and habits is challenging.

The aims of this chapter are to describe methodological challenges in assessing erosive wear, to critique the strengths and limitations of the existing erosion indices and to propose the adoption of a validated erosion index for the purpose for which it is intended.

Validity and Reliability Challenges

An ideal erosive wear index, as a valid and reliable instrument, should have the highest level of isomorphism, that is, the degree of fit between a measuring instrument and the disease or phenomenon being measured [3]. Therefore, specific quality criteria should be met in order for the researchers to provide evidence that the developed erosive wear indices are appropriate, valid and reliable.

Validity

Validity of an instrument reflects to what extent it measures what it is supposed to measure [2]. Although there are different types of validity, if an erosion index displays a high level of content and construct validity, significant methodological issues will have been adequately addressed. *Content validity* describes whether all aspects that are relevant to grasp the construct of interest have been considered at the highest possible level. Regarding an erosive wear index, the erosion of surfaces of all teeth has to be considered; therefore partial recording indicates low content validity [2]. Although the inclusion of all teeth appears to increase the content validity of an erosion index, there is still the challenge of the researcher's subjective evaluation of the appropriateness for measuring erosive wear *(face content validity)* [3]. Therefore, lack of consensus between investigators regarding the clinical features of erosion may significantly affect the content validity of an instrument. For example, the morphological criteria for occlusal/incisal surfaces are not exclusively associated with erosive tissue loss [4]; thus experts in the field should reach minimum agreement as to the clinical criteria that should be included in an index. On the other hand, *construct validity* is established by relating the instrument to a general theoretical framework [3] and is subdivided into *discriminant* and *convergent validity*. Regarding erosion assessment, *convergent validity* is very difficult to confirm. The results obtained by the new instrument cannot be correlated with the results of an established instrument that measures similar aspects and specifically erosive wear, as this established instrument simply does not yet exist. A potential solution to this may be that the new instrument could be compared to criteria/results obtained from a randomized controlled trial or other evidence-based procedure or to criteria that are determined by a minimum consensus of a panel of experts. On the other hand, an instrument possesses *discriminant validity* if the results of this instrument are not too highly correlated with the results of an established instrument that measures a different construct – for example, abrasive wear. In other words, this type of validity reflects the degree of differential diagnosis of the index/instrument under study. With regard to erosive wear, a potentially high correlation between tooth erosion and wedge-shaped defects might indicate insufficient discriminant validity [2]. Therefore, an ideal erosion index should include specific instead of general clinical criteria (e.g. percentage of hard tissue loss) in order to achieve the maximum discriminant validity. Both convergent and discriminant validity have to be given for a confirmation of construct validity.

Sensitivity and Specificity

Another significant challenge in assessing erosive wear is the achievement of the highest possible level of sensitivity and specificity of an erosion index. The sensitivity of this index indicates its ability to detect dental erosion lesions [2]. In contrast, an erosion instrument with high specificity is able to indicate the absence of dental erosion if dental erosion is not present [2]. Assessment of both sensitivity and specificity requires the comparison with a gold standard, which as mentioned earlier does not exist. Therefore, an attainable way to accomplish this comparison is the one described to confirm face validity.

Reliability

Reliability reflects the extent to which an instrument contains errors that appear between observations – measured either for one observer at different times (intra-examiner reliability) or between multiple examiners at points in time (inter-examiner reliability) [3]. Reliability can be relatively easily addressed if there is appropriate training and calibration of all potential examiners prior to the assessments, focusing on specific clinical criteria that must be applied in given circumstances. This training should include the detection of erosion lesions in photographs as well as in patients. The period of time between the two assessments should be fairly long – for example, 1 month – otherwise the examiners may remember their former ratings. On the other hand, if the time interval between the two assessments is too long, changes in the erosion status might affect the reliability estimates.

Diagnostic Criteria Challenges

As has been previously explained, specific and internationally accepted diagnostic criteria are necessary for the development of a valid and reliable erosion index. However, the validity of current diagnostic criteria for erosive wear has not been systematically studied, even though there is consensus about their definition [5]. Shallow defects located coronal from the cemento-enamel junction may predominantly occur as an effect of chronic acid exposure and most probably might be pathognomonic for dental erosion [5]. On the contrary, grooving of incisal surfaces and cupping of cusps are the most uncertain criteria because they can be an effect of various chemical and physical factors [5]. Therefore, experts in the field should reach agreement on what clinical criteria would be included in an index to exclusively record erosive wear. In order to successfully differentiate clinical diagnosis of dental erosion, having the patient's reports about acid exposure may be helpful and could support the diagnosis 'erosion' [6]. However, in many cases the acid exposure lies in the past, or the patient is not aware of or does

not report an acid exposure. Therefore, any potential aetiological factors/criteria obtained by a thorough history should be validated and standardized in more epidemiological studies, using modern epidemiological approaches [7].

The use of exposed dentine as a diagnostic criterion is under debate. The main benefit of using this criterion is that it is generally interpreted as a relatively severe finding and therefore it may be useful for the assessment of the progression rate and for therapeutic purposes. However, studies indicate that the visual diagnosis of exposed dentine may be challenging, particularly in the cervical area [8]; thus this criterion should be avoided whenever possible, especially in epidemiological studies.

Another significant challenge regarding erosive diagnostic criteria is the definition of pathological and age-related erosion; thus the use of the same erosion index for all ages could be problematic. Tooth wear of the permanent dentition, including attrition and abrasion, is expected to be more obvious at older ages. Furthermore, erosive wear as a result of chemical dissolution could become more severe at older ages because of the coexistence of other types of tooth wear [6]. This observation emphasizes the need to integrate aetiological/pathognomonic criteria in a clinical erosion index in order to reduce the false positive cases as much as possible.

Erosion Indices: Benefits and Limitations

The first indices to describe this condition set out to assess the prevalence of tooth wear and, specifically, erosion of adult teeth. The earliest of these was devised by Eccles [9] and later modified with more descriptive criteria to enable the classification of the effects of erosion per se by site and severity, as graded according to the depth and area of tooth tissue involved (table 1). Smith and Knight [10] later developed an index that would assess tooth wear (tooth wear index, TWI) – again

Table 1. Indices suggested by Smith and Knight, referring to tooth wear in general, and Eccles, including diagnostic criteria for erosive tooth wear

Score/class	Surface	Criteria
TWI according to Smith and Knight [10], 1984		
0	B/L/O/I	No loss of enamel surface characteristics
	C	No loss of contour
1	B/L/O/I	Loss of enamel surface characteristics
	C	Minimal loss of contour
2	B/L/O	Loss of enamel exposing dentine for less than one third of the surface
	I	Loss of enamel just exposing dentine
	C	Defect <1 mm deep
3	B/L/O	Loss of enamel exposing dentine for more than one third of the surface
	I	Loss of enamel and substantial loss of dentine
	C	Defect <1–2 mm deep
4	B/L/O	Complete loss of enamel, or pulp exposure, or exposure of secondary dentine
	I	Pulp exposure or exposure of secondary dentine
	C	Defect >2 mm deep, or pulp exposure, or exposure of secondary dentine
Index according to Eccles [9], 1979		
Class I		Early stages of erosion; absence of developmental ridges; smooth, glazed surface occurring mainly on labial surfaces of maxillary incisors and canines
Class II	F	Dentine is involved for less than one third of the surface
		Type 1: ovoid or crescentic, concave lesion at the cervical region of the surface, which should be differentiated from wedge-shaped lesions Type 2: irregular lesion entirely in the crown, which has a punched-out appearance where the enamel is absent from the floor
Class IIIa	F	More extensive destruction of dentine particularly of the anterior teeth; most of the lesions affect a large part of the surface, but some are localized and hollowed out
Class IIIb	L	Lesions of the surfaces for more than one third of their area; incisal edges become translucent due to loss of dentine; the dentine appears smooth and in some cases is flat or hollowed out; gingival and proximal margins have a white, etched appearance
Class IIIc	I/O	Incisal edges or occlusal surfaces are involved in dentine flattening or cupping; restorations are seen raised above the surrounding tooth surface; incisal edges appear translucent due to undermined enamel
Class IIId	All	Severely affected teeth, where both labial and lingual surfaces are extensively involved

B = Buccal or labial; C = cervical; F = facial; I = incisal; L = lingual or palatal; O = occlusal.

in adults (table 1). There followed modifications of the latter index for use in epidemiological screening on children [11, 12] expressly for the assessment of erosive wear, as well as a new index to qualitatively assess dental erosion in a full-mouth recording. At the other end of the age scale, Donnachie and Walls [13] advocated for greater sensitivity of the TWI to take account of the extremes of tooth wear. Other indices have focused on the aetiology of erosive wear; the index by Lussi [14] (table 2), applicable across the age ranges, is a modification of the original proposed by Linkosalo and Markkanen [15], who developed their index for use with lactovegetarians, and has been used extensively by other workers in Europe.

As has previously been mentioned, whilst there is an acceptance in the literature that there are characteristic presentations that can be ascribed to erosive wear – for example, cupping perhaps and 'proud' restorations – validation of these criteria does not exist, based as they are on case series and individual observations, combined with possible signs and symptoms such as tooth sensitivity, rather than having been systematically derived [16]. Many clinicians and researchers involved in the development and subsequent application of these indices have indicated that, irrespective of whether the index of choice is to assess prevalence or incidence, the reliance on dentine exposure to indicate the extent and or severity of the erosive or general wear process in dental tissues is not reliable [8]. This is verified when examiners assess dentine exposure on extracted teeth that are subsequently sectioned for validation purpose [17].

From the literature, recent studies conducted by different research groups using frequently cited indices (table 3) quote tooth wear in primary teeth involving dentine to range in prevalence between 0 and 82%, with a direct relationship between increasing prevalence and age. This relationship is not reproduced in the permanent dentition [18]. However, inter-examiner reproducibility of recording with these indices is poor – for example,

a kappa value of 0.02–1.00 using a modification of the Smith and Knight TWI [19] to 0.47 using a modification of the index by Lussi [20]. Very few data are available on intra-examiner reproducibility. Nevertheless, El Aidi et al. [21] achieved a high intra-examiner agreement (0.86 on mouth level) using the Van Rijkom et al. [20] modified version of the Lussi index when conducting a 3-year longitudinal study. This modified version discriminates between erosive lesions and pure attrition, considering smooth bordered wear as erosive wear, while sharp-bordered faceted wear was recorded as pure attrition [20].

Indices: Monitoring and Treatment Indication

Indices that assess erosion in large population studies potentially lack the sensitivity and specificity to be useful to longitudinally record erosion for populations or for individual patient use. Oilo et al. [22] devised a qualitative index based on treatment need not dissimilar to restorative indices developed for the same purpose. Patients with signs and symptoms of wear were assigned a score that determined whether or not they received treatment.

Whatever the unreliability of the detection of the exposure of dentine, early enamel loss is even more unpredictable, so that intervention studies aimed at prevention may not reliably use this criterion. Other indices that are weighted more towards assessment of dentine involvement focus on treatment. The recently described basic erosive wear examination (BEWE) index [23] is orientated towards detection of erosion per se, with a scoring system that advocates for prevention +/– intervention. It has a simple scoring system based on sextants not dissimilar to the approach adopted for periodontal screening indices. It thus offers the potential for researchers to have a screening tool and for clinicians to be able to monitor progression, or not, of erosion. Also, overestimation of the prevalence of dental erosion can be prevented

Table 2. Frequently used erosion indices for the assessment of erosive tooth wear in children, adolescents and adults

Surface/score	Criteria
Erosion index according to Lussi [14]	
Facial	
0	No erosion Surface with a smooth, silky-glazed appearance; absence of developmental ridges possible
1	Loss of surface enamel; intact enamel found cervical to the lesion; concavity in enamel, the width of which clearly exceeding its depth, thus distinguishing it from toothbrush abrasion; undulating borders of the lesions are possible; dentine is not involved
2	Involvement of dentine for less than half of the tooth surface
3	Involvement of dentine for more than half of the tooth surface
Occlusal/oral	
0	No erosion Surface with a smooth, silky-glazed appearance Absence of developmental ridges possible
1	Slight erosion; rounded cusps; edges of restorations rising above the level of adjacent tooth surface; grooves on occlusal aspects Loss of surface enamel; dentine is not involved
2	Severe erosion; more pronounced signs than grade 1 Dentine is involved
Index used in the UK National Survey of Children's Dental Health [12] and in the UK National Diet and Nutrition Surveys [19]	
Depth	
0	Normal Loss of surface characterization – enamel only; on incisor teeth there is loss of developmental ridges resulting in a smooth, glazed or 'ground glass' appearance On occlusal surfaces the cusps appear rounded and there may be depressions producing cupping
2	Enamel and dentine – loss of enamel, exposing dentine; on incisors this may resemble a 'shoulder preparation' parallel to the crest of the gingivae, particularly on palatal surfaces The incisors may appear shorter and there may be chipping of the incisal edges On occlusal surfaces cupping and rounding-off of cusps is evident Restorations may be raised above the level of adjacent tooth surface
3	Enamel, dentine and pulp – loss of enamel and dentine resulting in pulp exposure
9	Assessment cannot be made
Area	
0	Normal
1	Less than one third of surface involved
2	One third to up to two thirds of surface involved
3	More than two thirds of surface involved
9	Assessment cannot be made

Erosion index according to Lussi: facial, lingual and occlusal surfaces of all teeth except third molars. Index used in the UK National Survey of Children's Dental Health: only facial and lingual surfaces of primary and permanent maxillary incisor teeth, and in the UK National Diet and Nutrition Surveys: additionally, occlusal surfaces of the molar teeth.

Table 3. The most recently cited indices used in the assessment of erosive wear

Index/authors	Target group	Tooth wear or erosion only	Based on: area shape depth	Presumes aetiology: yes/no	Purpose	Reproducibility: inter-examiner minimum strength of agreement	Frequency of use
Erosion index Eccles [9], 1979	adults	E	A+D+S	Y – industrial sources of acid	prevalence	good[1]	5
TWI Smith and Knight [10], 1984	adults	TW	A+D	N	prevalence	good	11
Modified TWI Millward [11], 1994	children	TW	A+D	N	prevalence	good	2
Modified TWI O'Brien [12], 1994	children/ adolescents	E	A+D	N	prevalence	good	2
O'Sullivan [29], 2000	children	E	A+D	N	prevalence	good	6
Lussi index Modified from Linkosalo and Markkanen [14], 1996	children and adults	E	A+D+S	Y	prevalence		13
BEWE index [23], 2008	children and adults	E	D	N	prevalence and monitoring	good	6

PubMed search criteria for frequency of use were publication year (2000–2013) and use by different research groups. E = Erosion only; TW = tooth wear; A = area; S = shape; D = depth; Y = yes; N = no.
[1] K value at least 0.61; interpretation by Altman [30].

using this index by presenting the recorded data as frequencies of each participant's cumulative score. However, when applied in a general dental practice setting, whilst its specificity is high, the sensitivity was low for moderate-severe erosion. With more severe wear, both the sensitivity and specificity exceed 90% but both inter- and intra-examiner reliability are only moderate [24]. Despite the assertion that assessment of early erosion and, at the other extreme, dentine exposure are difficult, some authors have indicated that the BEWE is most reliable at recording no erosion or extensive dentine involvement [25]. However, BEWE cut-off values have to be reconsidered, since they appeared not to reflect the severity of erosion lesions compared to other erosion indices [6]. A recent report [26] undertaken as part of the 2009 national survey of adult dental health in the UK used the

opportunity to compare the results using the standard assessment of tooth wear included in these national surveys with the BEWE. From the results it appeared that both indices categorized the severity of tooth wear, but there was only agreement on the severity in half of the cases. This was not unexpected since BEWE scores the most severe erosion by sextant and the national adult dental health epidemiological assessment is based on anterior teeth only. The author concluded that the variation between the UK national survey criteria and BEWE were too great for BEWE to be a suitable alternative in any future UK survey.

The more recently described exact tooth wear index [27], based on the TWI and collapsible to both the latter and the BEWE, aims to separate out the assessment of enamel and dentine tissue loss in relation to tooth wear in young adults. The objective of the authors in doing so is to distinguish their index from the indices that have been developed predominantly to assess the need for operative intervention, categorizing as they do different levels of involvement of dentine but often fewer grades of enamel affects. The authors argue that for the purposes of prevention a more sensitive assessment of enamel loss (often at the population level), with four separate categories of enamel involvement based on area, is required.

By contrast, yet another newly devised erosion index, the evaluating index of dental erosion [6], seeks to discriminate between no or some erosion – the latter dichotomized into with or without dentine involvement. However, the latter assessment also includes aetiological variables, which in the literature are associated with erosion, although other authors consider these factors as potentially associated [19, 28].

With the exception of the BEWE, no index would appear to record very widespread (area) loss of enamel and only minimal dentine exposure; rather, dentine involvement is weighted more heavily in most scoring systems, despite the lack of reproducibility around its recording [8]. The widespread loss of enamel is important as a threshold for the instigation of preventive advice, which, to an extent, the BEWE acknowledges [23]. Ganss et al. [17] ask the more important question – how significant is cupping with minimal dentine exposure relative to more widespread tooth tissue loss? This also may suppose that there must be greater loss of dental tissue when dentine is exposed, ignoring the fact that the thickness of enamel varies across the tooth crown [8].

Rather like periodontal indices, many of these scoring systems take no account of current or ceased historical erosive activity so that it is difficult to determine a strategy to appropriately address the clinical scenario with which the patient presents. Is the condition still active? Are we looking at a past, quiescent condition?

Conclusions and Future Perspectives

- Erosive wear and tooth wear are often used and recorded interchangeably; therefore research should focus on the development of an erosion-specific index
- Indices to assess erosive wear are often based on an assessment of all aspects of tooth wear (abrasion, attrition, abfraction) since it is difficult, in the ageing dentition, to discriminate between these
- Lack of consensus between investigators regarding the clinical features of erosion may significantly affect the construct and content validity of an instrument
- A combined index using both clinical and dietary/behavioural/biological criteria could be significantly accurate in erosive lesion assessment
- Reproducibility in the application of erosion indices is poor and detection of dentine exposure is not as reliable as was previously thought
- A different index for epidemiological assessment of erosive wear is probably required for longitudinal assessment/individual patient monitoring

References

1 Bardsley PF: The evolution of tooth wear indices. Clin Oral Investig 2008; 12(suppl 1):S15–S19.

2 Berg-Beckhoff G, Kutschmann M, Bardehle D: Methodological considerations concerning the development of oral dental erosion indices: literature survey, validity and reliability. Clin Oral Investig 2008;12(suppl 1):S51–S58.

3 Frankfort-Nachmias C, Nachmias D: Research Methods in the Social Sciences, ed 7. New York, Worth, 2008, vol 141, pp 149–154.

4 Ganss C, Klimek J, Borkowski N: Characteristics of tooth wear in relation to different nutritional patterns including contemporary and medieval subjects. Eur J Oral Sci 2002;110:54–60.

5 Ganss C: How valid are current diagnostic criteria for dental erosion? Clin Oral Investig 2008;12(suppl 1):S41–S49.

6 Margaritis V, Mamai-Homata E, Koletsi-Kounari H, Polychronopolou A: Evaluation of three different scoring systems for dental erosion: a comparative study in adolescents. J Dent 2011;39: 88–93.

7 Margaritis V, Mamai-Homata E, Koletsi-Kounari H: Novel methods of balancing covariates for the assessment of dental erosion: a contribution to validation of a synthetic scoring system for erosive wear. J Dent 2011;39:361–367.

8 Holbrook P, Ganss C: Is diagnosing exposed dentine a suitable tool for grading erosive loss? Clin Oral Investig 2008; 12(suppl 1):S33–S39.

9 Eccles JD: Dental erosion of non-industrial origin. A clinical survey and classification. J Prosthet Dent 1979;42:649–653.

10 Smith BG, Knight JK: An index for measuring the wear of teeth. Br Dent J 1984; 156:435–438.

11 Millward A, Shaw L, Smith AJ, Rippin JW, Harrington E: The distribution and severity of tooth wear and the relationship between erosion and dietary constituents in a group of children. Int J Paediatr Dent 1994;4:151–157.

12 O'Brien M: Children's dental health in the United Kingdom 1993. Office of Population Censuses and Surveys. London, Her Majesty's Stationery Office, 1994.

13 Donnachie MA, Walls AWG: The tooth wear index: a flawed epidemiological tool in an ageing population group. Community Dent Oral Epidemiol 1996; 24:152–158.

14 Lussi A: Dental erosion clinical diagnosis and case history taking. Eur J Oral Sci 1996;104(part 2):191–198.

15 Linkosalo E, Markkanen H: Dental erosions in relation to lactovegetarian diet. Scand J Dent Res 1985;93:436–441.

16 Young A, Amaechi B, Dugmore C, Holbrook P, Nunn J, Schiffner U, Lussi A, Ganss C: Current erosion indices – flawed or valid? Summary. Clin Oral Investig 2008;12(suppl 1):S59–S63.

17 Ganss C, Klimek J, Lussi A: Accuracy and consistency of the visual diagnosis of exposed dentine on worn occlusal/incisal surfaces. Caries Res 2006;40: 208–212.

18 Kreulen CM, Van 't Spijker A, Rodriguez JM, Bronkhurst EM, Creugers NHJ, Bartlett DW: Systematic review of the prevalence of tooth wear in children and adolescents. Caries Res 2010;44:151–159.

19 Walker A, Gregory J, Bradnock G, Nunn JH, White D: National Diet and Nutrition Survey: young people 4 to 18 years. Volume 2. Report of the Oral Health Survey. London, TSO, 2000.

20 Van Rijkom HM, Truin GJ, Frencken JE, Konig JG, van 't Hof MA, Bronkhurst EM, Roeters FJ: Prevalence, distribution and background variables of smooth bordered tooth wear in teenagers in The Hague, The Netherlands. Caries Res 2002;36:147–154.

21 El Aidi H, Bronkhorst EM, Huysmans MC, Truin GJ: Dynamics of tooth erosion in adolescents: a 3-year longitudinal study. J Dent 2010;38:131–137.

22 Oilo D, Dahl BL, Hatle G, Gad AL: An index for evaluating wear of teeth. Acta Odontol Scand 1987;45:361–365.

23 Bartlett D, Ganss C, Lussi A: Basic Erosive Wear Examination (BEWE): a new scoring system for scientific and clinical needs. Clin Oral Investig 2008; 12(suppl 1):S65–S68.

24 Dixon B, Sharif MO, Ahmed F, Smith AB, Seymour D, Brunton PA: Evaluation of the basic erosive wear examination (BEWE) for use in a general dental practice. Br Dent J 2012;213:670–673.

25 Mulic A, Tveit AB, Wang NJ, Hove LH, Espelid I, Skaare AB: Reliability of two clinical scoring systems for dental erosive wear. Caries Res 2010;44:294–299.

26 Chadwick BL: British adults tooth wear prevalence depends on the index used. Int Assoc Dent Res Conf, Brazil, 2012.

27 Fares J, Shirodaria S, Chiu K, Ahmad N, Sherriff M, Bartlett D: A new index of tooth wear. Reproducibility and application to a sample of 18- to 30-year-old university students. Caries Res 2009;43: 119–125.

28 Hamasha AA, Zawaideh FI, Al-Hadithy RT: Risk indicators associated with dental erosion among Jordanian school children aged 12–14 years of age. Int J Paediatr Dent 2013, DOI:10.1111/ipd.12026, Epub ahead of print.

29 O'Sullivan EA: A new index for the measurement of erosion in children. Eur J Paediatr Dent 2000;1:69–74.

30 Altman DG: Practical statistics for medical research. London, Chapman and Hall, 1991.

V. Margaritis, PhD
Lead Contributing Faculty, College of Health Sciences
Walden University, 100 Washington Ave. South, Suite 900
Minneapolis, MN 55401 (USA)
E-Mail vasileios.margaritis@waldenu.edu

Lussi A, Ganss C (eds): Erosive Tooth Wear. Monogr Oral Sci. Basel, Karger, 2014, vol 25, pp 55–73
DOI: 10.1159/000360973

Prevalence, Incidence and Distribution of Erosion

Thomas Jaeggi · Adrian Lussi

Department of Preventive, Restorative and Pediatric Dentistry, School of Dental Medicine, University of Bern, Bern, Switzerland

Abstract

There is evidence that the presence of erosion is growing steadily. Due to different scoring systems, samples and examiners, it is difficult to compare the different studies. Preschool children from 2 to 5 years showed erosion on deciduous teeth in 1 to 79% of the subjects. Schoolchildren (aged from 5 to 9 years) already had erosive lesions on permanent teeth in 14% of the cases. In the adolescent group (aged between 9 and 20 years), 7 to 100% of the persons examined showed signs of erosion. Incidence data (the increase in the number of subjects presenting signs of dental erosion) was evaluated in four of these studies and presented average annual values between 3.5 and 18%, depending on the initial age of the examined sample. In adults (aged from 18 to 88 years) prevalence data ranged between 4 and 100%. Incidence data are scarce in this age group, and only one study was found analysing the increase of affected surfaces, showing an incidence of 5% for the younger and 18% for older age groups. In general, males present more erosive tooth wear than females. The distribution showed a predominance of affected occlusal surfaces (mandibular first molars) followed by facial surfaces (anterior maxillary teeth). Oral erosion was frequently found on maxillary incisors and canines. Overall, prevalence data are not homogeneous. Nevertheless, there is a trend towards a more pronounced rate of erosion in younger age groups. Furthermore, a tendency was found for more erosive lesions with increasing age and these erosions progressed with age.

© 2014 S. Karger AG, Basel

Erosive tooth wear is a common condition in developed societies. The lesions are often found independent of the age of the population examined. It is difficult to compare the results of epidemiological studies because of different examination standards used (calibration of examiners, scoring system, number and site of teeth) and different non-homogeneous groups examined (age, gender, number of examined individuals, geographical location). It is easier to recruit schoolchildren for clinical examinations than adults. Therefore, more studies have been undertaken on children and adolescents than on adults. Nevertheless, it is important to record erosive tooth lesions in all age groups to gather data about the prevalence, distribution and incidence of erosion.

If we want to understand the occurrence and distribution of erosive lesions, we have to be aware of the different aetiological factors such as reflux, vomiting and diet [1–7]. These causes are discussed in other chapters. In this chapter relevant literature was identified by searching PubMed using the MeSH terms (dental OR enamel OR dentin) AND (erosion OR tooth wear). Studies dealing with the prevalence and incidence of dental erosion were included.

Susceptibility to Erosive Tooth Wear in Children and Adults

There are some differences in the anatomical structure of deciduous teeth compared with permanent teeth. The enamel of deciduous teeth is less thick than that of the permanent dentition. Therefore, the erosive process reaches the dentine earlier, leading to more advanced lesions developing following an exposure to acids. Currently, there is contradictory evidence concerning the higher susceptibility of deciduous teeth compared with permanent teeth [8–12; see chapter by Carvalho et al., this vol., pp. 262–278]. The mechanical resistance of deciduous enamel is lower than that of permanent teeth due to its reduced hardness [13]. Therefore, substance loss in deciduous teeth can be more pronounced than in permanent teeth following erosive tooth wear. Conversely, functional and parafunctional forces in children are, in general, fewer than those found in adults. In summary, the differences in susceptibility to erosive tooth wear between children and adults seem to be small.

Prevalence, Incidence and Distribution of Erosion in Children and Adolescents

Dental Erosion in Preschool and Young School Children
Clinical Studies with Partial Recording of the Teeth
A study of 987 children aged between 2 and 5 years from 17 kindergarten schools showed that 309 (31%) had evidence of erosion and 123

(13%) of them showed involvement of dentine and/or pulp. The measurement of the erosion was confined to primary maxillary incisors [14]. Murakami et al. [15] (2011) examined a total of 967 children aged 3–4 years. The palatal surfaces of the upper incisors and the occlusal surfaces of the lower molars were screened as index surfaces for the assessment of erosive tooth wear. The percent of preschool children who had at least 1 tooth with erosive tooth wear was 51.6%. Most lesions were confined to enamel (93.9%). Another dental examination was carried out on 1,949 children aged 3–5 years in China, and a total of 112 children (5.7%) showed erosion on their primary maxillary incisors; 95 (4.9%) were judged to have erosion confined to enamel and 17 (0.9%) were scored as having erosion extending into dentine or pulp. A significantly higher prevalence of erosion was observed in children who had frequently consumed fruit drinks as babies and whose parents had a higher education level [16]. Harding et al. [17] (2003) found a link between low socio-economic status, frequent consumption of fruit squash and carbonated drinks and the occurrence of dental erosion. In this sample of 202 children (aged 5 years), 47% showed dental erosion, with 21% of lesions in an advanced state (erosion affecting the dentine or pulp). Only palatal and labial surfaces of primary maxillary teeth were assessed. A random sample of 1,002 schoolchildren (aged 5 years) was examined by Nayak et al. The prevalence of dental erosion was approximately 29%, with a higher prevalence observed in females [18]. Mangueira et al. [19] (2009) investigated 983 children aged 6–12 years for dental erosion. Measurement of erosion was confined to primary and permanent maxillary incisors; 19.9% of the children exhibited dental erosion. From this total, 61.8% of the lesions were found in the primary and 38.2% in the permanent dentition. Significant higher prevalence was observed in males and in children with a higher socio-economic level.

Clinical Studies with Full Mouth Recording

As part of a twin study in Australia, dental erosion was investigated in the primary dentition of 2- to 4-year-old twin and singleton children. The prevalence by subject was 77% in monozygotic, 74% in dizygotic and 75% in controls. Of the teeth scored, 12% had mild, 10% moderate and 1% severe lesions with more pronounced defects in the older age group. Dental erosion was observed most frequently in primary first molars (33%), followed by second molars (18%) and canines (18%), lateral incisors (16%), and central incisors (15%) [20]. Millward et al. [21] (1994) examined a total of 178 children aged 4 years and found that almost half of them showed signs of erosion. Frequently, the palatal surfaces of the maxillary incisors were affected, with lesions reaching the dentine. The authors investigated the socio-economic status and found a greater prevalence of dental erosion in the higher socio-economic groups. Moimaz et al. [22] (2013) investigated the occurrence of deciduous tooth erosion in 1,993 preschool children aged 4–6 years. Dental erosion was observed only in 0.6% of the children and no association was found between erosion and sex, age or toothbrushing frequency. The highest prevalence was observed in children aged 6 years (58.3%) and the most affected sextants were the fourth (22.9%) and sixth (20.0%). The lingual and occlusal tooth surfaces were most frequently affected. In another study, 463 children (aged 2–7 years) from 21 kindergartens were examined. Prevalence data in the different age groups were as follows: 23.8% (2–3 years), 27.4% (4 years), 30.4% (5 years) and 39.5% (6–7 years). Prevalence of erosion amounted to 32% and increased with increasing age of the children. Dentine erosion with at least 1 tooth affected was observed in 13.2% of the children. Erosive lesions were only found on primary teeth: maxillary incisors (15.5–25%), maxillary canines (10.5–12%), mandibular canines (5.5–6%) and molars (3.5–5%), as well as maxillary molars (1–5%). Erosions of the primary first and second molars were mostly seen on occlusal surfaces (75.9%), involving enamel or dentine but not the pulp. In incisors and canines, erosive lesions were often located incisally (51.2%) or affected multiple surfaces (28.9%) [23]. A random and stratified sample of 605 Greek preschool children was clinically examined for dental erosion using the basic erosive wear examination (BEWE). The prevalence of dental erosion was 78.8% and the mean BEWE was 3.64. Dental erosion was related to good oral hygiene and high socio-economic level [24]. A stratified cluster sample of 243 children (aged 5–7 years) was examined using the tooth wear index (TWI) of Smith and Knight [69]. Only 1.6% of the children were free from tooth wear; 51.8% exhibited mild tooth wear in the enamel, 41.6% moderate tooth wear involving dentine, 4.1% severe tooth wear into the dentine, and 0.8% severe tooth wear with pulp involvement. Maxillary canines were the most affected teeth (83.2%) and occlusal/incisal the most affected surfaces (52.7%) [25].

The prevalence, severity and distribution of erosive lesions in children living in rural Switzerland were investigated. A total of 42 children were examined, aged between 5 and 9 years. All children had 1 or more erosive lesions confined to enamel on the occlusal surface and 48% of them showed at least 1 lesion extending into dentine; 14% of the children had 1 or more erosive lesions detected on the occlusal surfaces of permanent teeth. Facial and oral erosions were scarce and involved deciduous teeth only; 10% had lesions on facial surfaces and 7% on palatal surfaces; all were confined to enamel. Erosion extending into dentine occurred on the facial surfaces in 5% of the children and on the palatal surfaces in 2%. The facial erosive lesions were mostly located on the primary central incisors. The most commonly affected tooth surfaces were the occlusal surfaces of the deciduous molars. Oral erosions were seldom found on the permanent maxillary incisors [26].

Dental Erosion in Older Children and Adolescents

Study with Assessment of Models
Ganss et al. [27] (2001) examined a large sample of pre-orthodontic study models of adolescents (1,000 individuals, mean age 11.4 ± 3.3 years); they included all surfaces of primary teeth. Moderate erosive lesions were found in 70.6% (facial/oral surfaces: shallow concavities less than one third of the surface; occlusal surfaces: small pits and slightly rounded cusps, moderate cupping) and advanced erosion in 26.4% of the children (facial/oral surfaces: deeper or more extended concavities – more than one third; occlusal surfaces: severe cupping and grooving). The majority of lesions were found on the occlusal or incisal surfaces (molars and canines). In the permanent dentition, 11.6% of the individuals had at least 1 tooth with moderate erosion and 0.2% with advanced erosion. The most affected teeth were the first molars in the mandibular jaw. After a period of 5 years, 265 of the children were followed up by examination of their final study models. The incidence of erosion for permanent teeth was as follows: individuals presenting at least 1 tooth with moderate erosion had an incidence from 5.3 to 23%, whereas the incidence of advanced erosive lesions was between 0.4 and 1.5% [27]. The longitudinal observation revealed that subjects with erosive lesions in their deciduous dentition had a significantly greater risk (relative risk of 3.9) of presenting erosive lesions in their permanent dentition.

Clinical Studies with Partial Recording of the Teeth
Truin et al. [28] (2005) evaluated the prevalence of erosive wear among 12-year-old children in The Hague, the Netherlands. The examination was limited to the palatal surfaces of incisors and canines and the occlusal surfaces of first molars in the permanent dentition. Overall, 24% of the 12-year-olds exhibited signs of erosion; 11% of the children presented erosive wear on first molars and 9% of them also had a maxillary front tooth affected. No significant differences were found between the prevalence of erosion and the different socio-economic status groups examined. However, more boys (28%) than girls (18%) had erosion in any form [28]. The same group examined a sample of 814 students 3 years later. The percentage (24%) of 12-year-olds with dental erosion in 2005 remained unchanged compared with 2002 [29]. A random sample of the same age group (12-year-olds, 791 subjects) was investigated in Libya. Dental erosion was observed in 40.8% of subjects, where 32.5% were in enamel, 8.0% affected dentine and 0.3% of subjects had lesions affecting the pulp [30]. In a cross-sectional study, Vargas-Ferreira et al. [31] (2010) investigated 944 children aged 11–14 years representative of Santa Maria, Brazil. The prevalence of dental erosion was low (7.2%) and confined to enamel. In the UK, examination of the incisors and molars of 1,753 12-year-old children showed a prevalence of tooth erosion of 59.7%, with 2.7% exhibiting exposed dentine. Significantly more erosion was detected in boys than girls. In addition, those with caries experience were found to have more erosion, as were more Caucasians compared with those of Asian origin. Socio-economically advantaged Caucasian children had significantly less tooth erosion than the other examined groups. The culture of the children examined appeared to influence the prevalence of erosion. The distribution of erosive lesions was as follows: erosion occurred most frequently on the palatal surfaces of maxillary incisors (49%) and maxillary molars (53%), as well as the buccal surfaces of mandibular molars (50%). Dentine was exposed to the greatest extent on the occlusal surfaces of mandibular molars (2.2%). Tooth erosion was symmetrical around the midline [32]. The same authors re-examined 1,308 children of the same sample 2 years later and found an incidence of erosion of 12.3%. A total of 161 children who had no evidence of erosion at 12 years developed ero-

sion over the subsequent 2 years. Erosion was present in 56.3% of 12-year-olds and in 64.1% by the age of 14. The proportion of subjects with exposure of deep enamel increased from 4.9 to 13.1%, and those with involved dentine from 2.4 to 8.7%. Boys showed significantly more erosion than girls at both ages, as did Caucasian compared with Asian children in both age groups [33]. Convenience samples of 129 children (aged 11–13 years) in the USA and of 125 children in the UK were examined. Only the palatal and facial surfaces of the maxillary incisors were assessed, and prevalence data were as follows: 41% of the US and 37% of the UK children showed dental erosion. The lesions were mostly confined to enamel [34]. Chadwick et al. [35] (2005) measured the prevalence of palatal erosion of the central maxillary incisors of 197 schoolchildren (aged 11–13 years) with a replica technique. They found 58.5% low erosions (none to limited, normal wear), 28.7% moderate erosions (obvious change in anatomical form but no need for treatment) and 12.3% severe erosions (marked change in anatomical form and need for treatment). Each subject was recorded at baseline and after 9 and 18 months. They concluded that evidence of previous palatal erosion did not predict future erosion. In a cross-sectional survey 1,499 children aged 12–13 years were examined. Signs of dental erosion on at least 1 tooth surface occurred in 416 children (27.3%). The prevalence of erosion in 12- and 13-year-old children was 25.5 and 29.0%, respectively [36]. Bardolia et al. [37] (2010) investigated the prevalence of erosive tooth wear in 13- to 14-year-old children on the Isle of Man. A modified partial recording index was used in which the labial, incisal and oral surfaces of the 12 anterior teeth and the occlusal surface of the first molars were assessed. The number of children with at least 1 surface with exposed dentine was 320 (51%). In London, a cross-section design study containing 525 schoolchildren aged 14 years showed a prevalence of 16.9% for facial and 12% for palatal surface erosion (only the maxil-

lary incisors were examined) [38]. In the North West of England a total of 2,385 children (aged 14 years, 48% male, 52% female) were examined for tooth wear. Tooth wear was scored on all surfaces of the maxillary and mandibular 6 anterior teeth and on the occlusal surfaces of the first molars. A total of 1,276 children (53%) had at least 1 tooth surface (mean 2 surfaces) with exposed dentine. Significantly more males than females had dentine exposed. Incisal or occlusal wear into dentine was seen most frequently on central incisors and mandibular first molars [39]. A single-centre cluster random sample of 414 adolescents (12 and 16 years old) was assessed on dental erosion on the buccal and palatal surfaces of the permanent maxillary incisors and on the occlusal surfaces of the permanent first molars. The prevalence was 20% and erosion was restricted to enamel. No significant differences between the presence of erosion and gender, type of school and mean family income was found [40]. In another study, 609 individuals were screened with a simplified partial recording system using 4 permanent or 6 primary surfaces as markers. Severe erosion extending into dentine on 1 or more maxillary anterior teeth/molars was found to be 13.3% in the group aged 5–6 years, 11.9% in the group aged 13–14 years and 22.3% in the group aged 18–19 years. The total prevalence was 16.4% [41]. McGuire et al. [42] (2009) examined 1,962 children aged 13–19 years for any evidence of dental erosion. All incisors, canines and the first molars were assessed; 45.9% of the children had erosive tooth wear in at least 1 tooth. Females had significantly lower rates of erosive tooth wear compared with males. The percentage of children with dental erosion increased significantly with age.

Clinical Studies with Full Mouth Recording
A representative, nationwide study in Iceland included approximately 20% of all 6-, 12- and 15-year-old children of the country, adding to a total sample of 2,251 children. Dental erosion was recorded in all erupted permanent teeth. No ero-

sion was found in the permanent teeth of 6-year-olds, but erosion was present in 15.7% of 12-year-olds and in 30.7% of 15-year-olds, significantly more frequently in boys than girls. The teeth most commonly scored as having erosion were the mandibular first molars, and by 15 years of age erosion was being recorded frequently on the palatal surfaces of maxillary incisors [43]. Caglar et al. [44] (2005) investigated the occurrence of erosive defects in a sample of 153 schoolchildren (aged 11 years) in Istanbul, Turkey; 28% of them exhibited dental erosion but no relationship was found between erosion and possible related sources. In another study, a total of 83 children (46 girls, 37 boys) between the ages of 7 and 14 years were examined for dental erosion. A total of 47.4% of the children in the group aged 7–11 years and 52.6% in the group aged 12–14 years exhibited dental erosion. The most often affected teeth were the maxillary incisors [45]. The prevalence of dental erosion was assessed in children and adolescents of a private dental practice in Brazil. Of the 232 participants, aged 2–20 years, 25.4% showed erosion. In both primary and permanent dentitions, the occlusal surface was the most commonly affected by erosive lesions (77.1%) [46]. A cross-sectional study was carried out involving 389 children (mean age 12 years). The prevalence of dental erosion was 26%. No significant difference in prevalence was found between boys and girls. Enamel loss was the most prevalent type of dental erosion (65%) [47]. Zhang et al. [48] (2014) investigated a stratified random sample of 12-year-old children in 7 primary schools in Hong Kong on dental caries and erosion. Of the 600 children (316 boys, 284 girls) 75% had at least some sign of erosion, but no severe erosion. Dental erosion was more severe among the children who had caries experience and consumed fruit juice. Tooth erosion was recorded 3 times with 1.5-year intervals in a sample of 622 children aged 10–12 years at baseline. The prevalence was as follows: 30.4% (11-year-olds), 38.3% (12 years), 40.6% (13 years), 42.6% (14 years) and 44.2% (15 years). A signifi-

cantly higher prevalence was found in boys than girls. The incidence of dental erosions investigated (percentage of the sound population developing erosion) was as follows: 26.5% (11-year-olds), 15.8% (12 years), 10.9% (13 years) and 6.4% (14 years). A decreasing incidence of dental erosion was observed, but the progression of erosion increased with age. In children with erosion, molars (especially mandibular occlusal surfaces) and the upper anterior teeth were predominately affected. On tooth level, the incidence decreased significantly with increasing age for upper incisors and lower first molars [49]. A longitudinal study of dental erosion in 73 girls aged 12 years showed that 68% had dental erosion at the beginning of the investigation. After 1.5 years 65 girls were re-examined and 95% showed the clinical appearance of erosive lesions. Therefore the incidence was 27%. The mean number of teeth affected was 2.2 at the start of the investigation and 5.6 after 18 months [50]. Milosevic et al. [51] (1994) examined a total of 1,035 children (mean age 14 years) in 10 schools in Liverpool, UK. It was found that 305 of them had tooth wear lesions with involvement of dentine, mainly incisally; 8% also exhibited exposed dentine on occlusal and/or palatal surfaces; the occlusal surfaces of the first mandibular molars and the palatal aspects of the maxillary incisors were mainly affected. Statistical evaluation showed significantly more erosion in males than in females. Al-Dlaigan et al. [52] (2001) established the prevalence of erosion in a cluster random sample of 418 teenagers (aged 14 years, 209 girls, 209 boys) in Birmingham, UK. They found that 48% of the children had erosion within enamel, 51% had erosion within enamel with possible slight involvement of dentine and 1% had erosion with advanced involvement of dentine. They postulated a relationship between low socioeconomic status and the occurrence of erosion. The majority of tooth surfaces showed evidence of enamel erosion on both maxillary and mandibular teeth on the facial and oral aspects. Defects with visible dentine involvement were mainly found on the incisal edges of most anterior teeth, whereas dentinal erosions were most common on the maxillary and mandibular facial surfaces of anterior teeth. Significantly more males than females showed these lesions [52]. In Reykjavik, Iceland, 20% of a cohort sample of 15-year-olds was examined (n = 278). The investigators found that a total of 21.6% of the subjects suffered from dental erosion, and two thirds of these were male. Enamel erosion was found in 72% of the cases, 23% showed dentinal erosion and 5% had severe dentinal erosion [53]. Kaczmarek et al. [54] (2012) evaluated the frequency and severity of dental erosion in 15-year-old adolescents. A total of 180 subjects of both sexes were examined with the BEWE scoring system. The frequency of dental erosion was 36.1%. The sixth and fourth followed by the third and first sextant were commonly affected. Van Rijkom et al. [55] (2002) investigated the prevalence and distribution of smooth-bordered tooth wear in teenagers in The Hague, the Netherlands. A sample of 345 teenagers aged 10–13 years and 400 aged 15 and 16 years were examined clinically. The investigation was based on a modification of the index of Lussi et al. [56] (1991). In the younger age group 3% of the subjects showed visible smooth wear on enamel; only 1 subject (0.3%) had deep smooth enamel wear. In the older age group, 30% of the subjects had visible smooth wear of enamel – deep smooth wear of enamel was found in 11% and there was 1 case of smooth wear into dentine. In the majority of subjects, first molars and maxillary anterior teeth were affected. The prevalence of visible smooth wear was significantly higher in boys than in girls and it tended to increase with increasing socio-economic status. To describe the prevalence of eroded tooth surfaces among 15- to 17-year-old schoolchildren in a Danish city, 558 subjects were examined for dental erosions. It was found that 14% of the children had more than 3 surfaces affected; the palatal surfaces were affected more so than the facial surfaces. No evidence of lesions in dentine was observed [57].

Reviewing the data from the national dental surveys of young people in the UK, a trend towards a higher prevalence of erosion in children aged between 3.5 and 4.5 years was found. Overall, the prevalence data from cross-sectional national studies indicated that erosion increased with age of children and adolescents over time. In addition, dietary habits, the presence or absence of gastroesophageal reflux and socio-demographic parameters had some influence on dental erosion [58].

An overview of the localization of erosion in children and adolescents is given in table 1. Prevalence and incidence data are listed in table 2. In conclusion, the results from several epidemiological studies involving erosive tooth wear in children and adolescents show that, with increasing mean age of the population group examined, a trend to more erosive lesions was detected; males seem to develop more erosion than females, and lesions involve mostly the palatal surface of the maxillary incisors and the occlusal surface of the mandibular first molars. The relationship between the presence of erosive lesions and the socio-economic status of the population groups investigated remains controversial.

Prevalence, Incidence and Distribution of Erosion in Adults

Studies with Assessment of Extracted Teeth or Models
As early as 1972, Sognnaes et al. [59], in a sample of 10,827 extracted teeth, found 18% with signs of erosion-like lesions. They noted that mandibular teeth had a higher frequency of such lesions than the corresponding maxillary teeth (21% compared with 13%). The highest percentage of erosion-like lesions was found in mandibular incisors (28%). Khan et al. [60] (2001), in a cross-sectional study, investigated the presence, absence and relative size of cupped lesions on cusps and occlusal fissures of premolar and permanent mo-

Table 1. Localization of erosion in children and adolescents: an overview of different epidemiological studies listed in the order of age of the examined subjects

Author(s)	Year	Age, years	Localization
Taji et al. [20]	2010	2–4	Most frequent in first molars, followed by second molars and canines, lateral and central incisors
Millward et al. [21]	1994	4	Palatal surfaces of the maxillary incisors
Moimaz et al. [22]	2013	4–6	Lingual and occlusal surfaces of the fourth and sixth sextants
Wiegand et al. [23]	2006	2–7	Primary dentition: maxillary incisors and canines followed by mandibular canines and molars and maxillary molars (occlusal and incisal surfaces) Permanent dentition: none of the incisors or first molars showed signs of erosion
Mantonanaki et al. [24]	2013	5	Maxillary anterior teeth followed by mandibular molars
Gatou and Mamai-Homata [25]	2012	5–7	Primary dentition: maxillary (and mandibular) anterior teeth (canines); incisal and occlusal surfaces most affected
Jaeggi and Lussi [26]	2004	5–9	Primary dentition: occlusal surfaces of all teeth (predominantly molars); facial and oral surfaces of the maxillary incisors (scarce) Permanent dentition: occlusal surfaces of the first molars
Arnadottir et al. [43]	2010	6–15	Permanent dentition: mandibular (and maxillary) first molars followed by maxillary anterior teeth; especially cup-like lesions on the cusps of lower first molars
Caglar et al. [45]	2011	7–14	Maxillary anterior teeth
Ganss et al. [27]	2001	8–14	Primary dentition: occlusal (incisal) surfaces of molars and canines Permanent dentition: occlusal surfaces of mandibular first molars
El Aidi et al. [49]	2010	10–12 (13–16)	Molars (especially occlusal surfaces of mandibular molars) and the upper anterior teeth were predominantly affected; the incidence decreased significantly with age for upper incisors and lower first molars
Nahás Pires Corrêa et al. [46]	2011	2–20	Primary and permanent dentition: occlusal surfaces of all teeth
Milosevic et al. [51]	1994	14	Palatal and incisal surfaces of maxillary incisors; occlusal surfaces of the first mandibular molars
Al-Dlaigan et al. [52]	2001	14	Low erosion: majority of tooth surfaces; moderate erosion: incisal edges of anterior teeth; sever erosion: maxillary and mandibular facial surfaces of anterior teeth
Kaczmarek et al. [54]	2012	15	Sixth and fourth, followed by third and first sextant
Van Rijkom et al. [55]	2002	10–13 15–16	First molars and maxillary anterior teeth
Larsen et al. [57]	2005	15–17	Palatal surfaces of maxillary incisors

Table 2. Prevalence and incidence of erosion in children and adolescents (percent of examined subjects): an overview of different epidemiological studies listed in the order of age of the examined subjects

Author(s)	Year	Sample			Erosion prevalence	Erosion incidence	Conclusion
		age, years	n	examination			
Taji et al. [20]	2010	2–4	128	clinical	77%/74%/ 75%	–	Dental erosion in 77% monozygotic, 74% dizygotic twins and 75% in controls; 12% with mild, 10% with moderate and 1% with severe erosion
Al-Malik et al. [14]	2002	2–5	987	clinical	31%	–	1/3 with erosion, and 1/3 to 1/2 of them showed involvement of dentine or pulp
Murakami et al. [15]	2011	3–4	967	clinical	51.6%	–	Most lesions were confined to enamel (93.9%)
Luo et al. [16]	2005	3–5	1,949	clinical	5.7%	–	4.9% with erosion confined to enamel, 0.9% with involvement of dentine or pulp
Millward et al. [21]	1994	4	178	clinical	50%	–	Almost half of the examined children showed erosion
Moimaz et al. [22]	2013	4–6	1,993	clinical	0.6%	–	Prevalence of deciduous tooth erosion was low; no association with sex, age or toothbrushing
Wiegand et al. [23]	2006	2–3 4 5 6–7	463	clinical	23.8% 27.4% 30.4% 39.5%	–	Prevalence of erosion amounted to 32% and increased with increasing age; dentine erosion could be observed in 13.2%
Harding et al. [17]	2003	5	202	clinical	47%	–	21% of the erosive lesions with involvement of dentine or pulp
Nayak et al. [18]	2010	5	1,002	clinical	29%	–	Higher prevalence in females
Mantonanaki et al. [24]	2013	5	605	clinical	78.8%	–	Dental erosion was related to good oral hygiene and high socio-economic level
Gatou and Mamai-Homata [25]	2012	5–7	243	clinical	51.8%/ 41.6%/ 4.1%/0.8%	–	51.8% exhibited mild (within enamel), 41.6% moderate (involving dentine), 4.1% deep dentinal and 0.8% pronounced tooth wear (pulp involvement)
Jaeggi and Lussi [26]	2004	5–9	42	clinical	100%/ 14.3%	–	100% of the children with enamel erosion, 47.6% with dentinal erosion, 14.3% already with erosion on permanent teeth
Mangueira et al. [19]	2009	6–12	983	clinical	19.9%	–	61.8% of the lesions in primary and 38.2% in permanent dentition

Table 2. Continued

Author(s)	Year	Sample			Erosion prevalence	Erosion incidence	Conclusion
		age, years	n	examination			
Arnadottir et al. [43]	2010	6–15	2,251	clinical	0%/15.7%/ 30.7%	–	6-year-olds: no erosion, 12-year-olds: 15.7%, 15-year-olds: 30.7%
Caglar et al. [44]	2005	11	153	clinical	28%	–	No significant differences in prevalence data between girls and boys
Caglar et al. [45]	2011	7–14	83	clinical	47.4%/ 52.6%	–	47.4% of the age group 7–11 years and 52.6% of the age group 12–14 years exhibited dental erosion
Ganss et al. [27]	2001	8–14	1,000	models	70.6%/ 11.6%	–	Primary teeth: 70.6% with moderate erosion, 26.4% with advanced erosion; permanent teeth: 11.6% (moderate erosion) and 0.2% (advanced erosion);
		16	265	models	–/23%	–/18% within 5 years	permanent teeth (longitudinally): increase of erosion from 5.3 to 23% (moderate erosion) and from 0.4 to 1.5% (advanced erosion)
Nahás Pires Corrêa et al. [46]	2011	2–20	232	clinical	25.4%	–	Erosion showed association with frequent consumption of soft drinks, candies and fruits
Dugmore and Rock [32]	2004	12	1,753	clinical	59.7%	–	2.7% of the erosive lesions with involvement of dentine
Truin et al. [28]	2005	12	324	clinical	24%	–	24% of the children showed signs of erosion
Truin et al. [29]	2007	12	814	clinical	24%	–	No increase in dental erosion in 12-year-olds within 3 years
Correr et al. [47]	2009	12	389	clinical	26%	–	No significant differences in prevalence data between girls and boys
Huew et al. [30]	2012	12	791	clinical	40.8%	–	Enamel erosion in 32.5%, dentinal erosion in 8.0% and erosion into pulp in 0.3% of examined subjects
Zhang et al. [48]	2014	12	600	clinical	75%	–	75% of the children had some sign of erosion, but no severe erosion
Deery et al. [34]	2000	11–13	129 (USA) 125 (UK)	clinical	41% (USA) 37% (UK)	–	Erosion was mostly confined to enamel
Chadwick et al. [35]	2005	11–13	197	clinical (replica technique)	100%	–	58.5% with low erosion, 28.7% with moderate erosion, 12.3% with severe erosion

Table 2. Continued

Author(s)	Year	Sample age, years	n	examination	Erosion prevalence	Erosion incidence	Conclusion
Vargas-Ferreira et al. [31]	2010	11–14	944	clinical	7.2%	–	Erosion was confined to enamel
El Aidi et al. [49]	2010	11 12 13 14 15	622	clinical	30.4% 38.3% 40.6% 42.6% 44.2%	26.5% 15.8% 10.9% 6.4%	Incidence over a period of 1.5 years (% of the sound population); incidence of children with new erosion decreased with age; progression of erosion with age in children with erosion
Wang et al. [36]	2010	12/13	1,499	clinical	25.5%/ 29.0%	–	At least 1 tooth surface with signs of erosion
Nunn et al. [50]	2001	12/13.5	73/65	clinical	68%/95%	27% after 1.5 years	Mean number of affected teeth rose from 2.2 to 5.6
Dugmore and Rock [33]	2003	12/14	1,308	clinical	56.3%/ 64.1%	12.3% within two years	Deep enamel erosions increased from 4.9 to 13.1% and with dentine involvement from 2.4 to 8.7%
Bardolia et al. [37]	2010	13–14	629	clinical	51%	–	Percent of children with exposed dentine
Milosevic et al. [51]	1994	14	1,035	clinical	30%	–	30% with involvement of dentine; more males than females showed tooth wear lesions
Williams et al. [38]	1999	14	525	clinical	17%[1]/12%[1]	–	17% of facial and 12% of palatal surfaces of maxillary incisors with erosion
Al-Dlaigan et al. [52]	2001	14	418	clinical	100%	–	48% with low erosion, 51% with moderate erosion, 1% with severe erosion
Bardsley et al. [39]	2004	14	2,385	clinical	53%	–	53% had at least 1 tooth with exposed dentine
Gurgel et al. [40]	2011	12/16	414	clinical	20%	–	Only erosion confined to enamel
Arnadottir et al. [53]	2003	15	278	clinical	21.6%	–	72% of the erosions confined to enamel, 23% reaching the dentine, 5% reaching deep into dentine
Kaczmarek et al. [54]	2012	15	180	clinical	36.1%	–	The dental erosion risk was low in the examined group
Van Rijkom et al. [56]	2002	10–13 15–16	345 400	clinical	3% 30%/11%	–	3% of the younger and 30% of the older age group showed visible smooth wear; 11% of the older age group had deep enamel lesions
Larsen et al. [57]	2005	15–17	558	clinical	14%	–	14% more than 3 surfaces of erosion

Table 2. Continued

Author(s)	Year	Sample			Erosion prevalence	Erosion incidence	Conclusion
		age, years	n	examination			
Hasselkvist et al. [41]	2010	5–6 13–14 18–19	135 227 247	clinical	13.3% 11.9% 22.3%	– 	Total prevalence for all age groups was 16.4%; 34.4% of boys aged 18–19 years had 1 or more teeth with severe erosion
McGuire et al. [42]	2009	13–19	1,962	clinical	45.9%	–	At least 1 tooth with dental erosion; erosive tooth wear increased with age

[1] Percent of examined tooth surfaces.

lar teeth using image analysis of study models. The frequencies of the following five types of lesions on the tooth sites were scored as follows: unaffected (46%), small (17%), medium (8%), large cuspal-cupped (4%) and fissure involvement by cupping (3%); 22% of the possible tooth sites were absent. The influence of age was evaluated by comparison of the models of 59 younger (aged 13–27) and 57 older subjects (aged 28–70). They found a linear increase in lesion number and size with age. However, cupped lesions often occurred on mandibular first molar cusp tips, and attained greater extension in adults under 27 years compared with older subjects. They concluded that the mandibular first permanent molar is an indicator for the age of onset and severity of dental erosion [60].

Studies with Partial Recording of the Teeth
Isaksson et al. [61] (2013) examined the molars and maxillary incisors of 494 Swedish individuals aged 20 years. Erosion was present in 75% of subjects, and 18% had extensive lesions. Swedish young adults had a high prevalence of dental erosion, but the level of severe erosion was low. A large-scale multicentre study with the aim of assessing the prevalence of tooth wear on buccal/facial and lingual/palatal tooth surfaces in a sample of young adults, aged 18–35 years, was carried out

in Europe. Calibrated examiners measured tooth wear, using the BEWE in 3,187 patients from 7 European countries. Each individual was characterized by the highest BEWE score recorded for any scoreable surface. The prevalence of more severe tooth wear categorized as BEWE scores 2 and 3 was 26.1 and 3.3%, respectively, with at least 1 tooth affected; 26.5% of the individuals in the younger age group (18–25 years) and 31.4% in the older age group (26–35 years) showed significant erosion. Large differences in prevalence data between different countries were observed [62]. Xhonga et al. [63] (1972) investigated the progression of erosive tooth wear in 14 patients with erosion-like patterns (aged between 26 and 65 years). They found an average daily rate of progression of approximately 1 μm. In another study, a random selection of 95 males with a mean age of 20.9 years was scored. Only the maxillary anterior teeth were included. They concluded that 28% of the teeth in this sample showed pronounced dental erosion [64]. In another study, 30 randomly selected individuals (age range 24–55 years) with a mean age of 39 years were used as a comparison group; 12 index surfaces per person were examined. Erosive wear was recorded in 20% of the individuals of this group, mostly confined to enamel [65]. From the community of Jönköping (Sweden) 585 randomly selected dentate individuals were screened for occlusal and incisal tooth wear. The age of the people examined was 20–80 years. The results showed an increase of severity and prevalence of wear with age. Men presented with more teeth and with more occlusal wear than women. The factors significantly related to tooth wear were as follows: number of teeth present, age, sex, occurrence of bruxism, use of snuff, and saliva buffer capacity [66].

Clinical Studies with Full Mouth Recording

Mulic et al. [67] (2012) assessed 1,456 subjects (aged 18 years) for erosive tooth wear in Oslo, Norway and found that 38% of the examined young adults had at least 1 tooth with erosive lesions. In addition to gender (males), dietary habits such as frequent consumption of fruit juice and sugary soft drinks, and the occurrence of reflux and vomiting, appeared to be risk indicators for erosive wear. In a two-centre study, Xhonga and Valdmanis [68] (1983) examined a total of 527 randomly selected patients for erosive tooth wear (aged 14–88 years). Erosion-like lesions were divided into three groups: minor, moderate and severe. This study suggested that the prevalence in the USA was about 25% for erosive tooth wear. Minor lesions (prevalence about 20%) were found most often in premolar and anterior teeth. Moderate lesions were scarce (prevalence about 4%) and equally distributed. Severe lesions (prevalence about 25%) were found predominantly in molar regions, followed by premolars. In a case-control study in the Metropolitan Helsinki area 100 controls (mean age 36.3 years, range 17–83 years) were randomly selected by dentists; 5 of these control subjects had erosion. Therefore, the prevalence of dental erosion in patients of this area was 5%. Although only 5 of the examined individuals showed erosive defects, most of them admitted to having regular exposure to acid. Dietary exposure was present in 21 cases, gastric exposure in 19 and both types of exposure in 5 cases; 55 of the controls did not exceed any of the exposure limits [2]. A study in England using the TWI by Smith and Knight [69, 70] investigated the prevalence of

tooth wear in 1,007 dental patients. More than 93,500 tooth surfaces were examined and overall 5.1% had wear which exceeded the threshold values. Only 9 patients had completely unworn dentitions. The 15- to 26-year age group showed 5.73% of tooth surfaces which were worn to an unacceptable degree; the three intermediate groups (age groups 26–35, 36–45 and 46–55 years) had values between 3.37 and 4.62%, the 56- to 65-year age group had 8.19%, and the over 65-year age group had 8.84% of the surfaces with pathological tooth wear. In particular, the older age groups had higher levels of unacceptable tooth wear, and men tended to have slightly more wear than women [71]. Bartlett et al. [72] (2011) investigated the association of tooth wear, diet and dietary habits in adults aged 18–30 years. A modified index based on the TWI of Smith and Knight was used. All tooth surfaces were examined and graduated for wear on enamel and then on dentine. The 1,010 participants had a mean age of 21.9 years, of whom 70% were female and 30% male. Results showed all subjects had evidence of wear on enamel, with 20.1% showing enamel loss of more than one third of the surface on at least 1 tooth. Tooth wear with involvement of dentine on at least 1 tooth surface was found in 7.9% of the participants. Enamel wear was generalized, occurring mostly on the anterior teeth and the first molars. Dentine wear was most frequently observed on the incisal surfaces of the upper and lower incisors. Tooth wear was associated with a number of acidic dietary products and drinking habits. The TWI index of a random sample of adults aged 45 years and over from Newcastle upon Tyne (UK) was assessed by Donachie and Walls [73] (1995). A total of 586 subjects were dentate and able to undergo the examinations. Results showed significantly increasing wear levels with increasing age for all cervical and occlusal/incisal tooth surfaces. Especially in the older age cohort, occlusal/incisal surfaces showed some of the highest mean wear scores. With the exception of palatal surfaces of maxillary anterior teeth, no significant variation in tooth wear with age was found for buccal or palatal surfaces. The mean wear scores were greater in males than females. Only small variation was found between subjects of different social classes. Manaf et al. [74] (2012) investigated a total of 150 undergraduate students for dental erosion at University Kebangsaan, Malaysia (33 males and 117 females, aged 19–24 years). The BEWE was used to assess the occurrence of dental erosion; 68% of subjects had tooth erosion. Preventive measures such as dietary advice may reduce the occurrence of tooth erosion among this age group. Jaeggi et al. [75] (1999) assessed a sample of 417 Swiss army recruits (aged between 19 and 25 years). Clinical examination showed dental erosions on all tooth surfaces with the most pronounced defects found on occlusal surfaces; 82% of the screened recruits had erosive lesions within enamel on these tooth surfaces. Occlusal lesions with involvement of dentine were found in 128 recruits (30.7%). Facial defects occurred in 60 cases (14.4%, enamel erosion) and 2 cases (0.5%, dentinal erosion). Palatal erosions were scarce, with only 3 individuals affected (0.7%). The localization of the erosive lesions were as follows: facial erosions were frequent on canines and premolars of both jaws, occlusal erosions on first molars and premolars of both jaws and palatal erosions on maxillary anterior teeth. Lussi et al. [56] (1991) examined the frequency and severity of erosion on all tooth surfaces of 391 randomly selected persons from two age groups: 26–30 and 46–50 years. Erosions confined to enamel were found on facial surfaces in 11.9% of the younger and 9.6% of the older subjects, whereas more pronounced erosive defects (erosion with involvement of dentine) were found in 7.7% of the younger and 13.2% of the older age group. On average, 3.5 teeth per person in the younger and 2.8 teeth per person in the older age group were affected. Occlusally, erosions confined to enamel were found in 35.6% of the younger and 40.1% of the older persons. At least 1 severe erosive lesion was observed in 29.9% of the younger and 42.6% of the older sample. Therefore, 3.2 teeth per per-

son in the younger and 3.9 teeth per person in the older group showed these advanced lesions. Statistical analyses revealed a significant impact of the consumption of erosive drinks and foodstuffs on facial and occlusal erosions. Slight erosive defects (erosion confined to enamel) were found on the palatal surfaces in 3.6% of the younger and 6.1% of the older examined individuals. Severe palatal erosions were scarce and highly associated with chronic vomiting [56]. To determine the progression of erosive defects the same authors re-examined 55 persons 6 years later. They found a distinct progression of erosion on facial and occlusal surfaces. The increase in the defects was more pronounced in the older age group. The prevalence of occlusal erosions involving dentine rose from 3 to 8% (younger age group) and from 8 to 26% (older age group). An increase in facial erosions was observed over the entire dentition but especially in premolar and molar areas. The increase in erosion with denudation of dentine ranged from 4.2% (tooth 16) to 17.6% (tooth 15), with no differences between maxillary and mandibular jaws. The increase in occlusal lesions in the premolar and molar areas was even more marked: for dentinal erosion from 0.1% (tooth 35) to 33.4% (tooth 14), again with no differences between maxillary and mandibular jaws. Oral erosions were detected only in the maxillary jaw. The most marked increase in oral erosion was found in the central incisors (from 6 to 10%). Although all patients initially were personally informed about the risk factors for the development and progression of erosive lesions, they did not change their nutritional habits. Statistical analyses showed that 28% of the variability of the progression of erosion could be explained with the consumption of nutritional acids and age. Further, it was shown that one third of the patients accounted for about two thirds of the total progression. Four or more nutritional acidic intakes per day were associated with higher progression when it was combined with low buffer capacity of stimulated saliva and hard toothbrushes (p < 0.01) [76]. A cross-sectional, descriptive and ana-

Table 3. Localization of erosion in adults: an overview of different epidemiological studies listed in the order of age of the examined subjects

Author(s)	Year	Age, years	Localization
Sognnaes et al. [59]	1972	–	Mandibular teeth (21%) with a higher frequency than the corresponding maxillary teeth (13%); with 28% mandibular incisors showed the most lesions
Xhonga and Valdmanis [68]	1983	14–88	Minor erosions: premolars and anterior teeth Severe erosions : molars and premolars
Jaeggi et al. [75]	1999	19–25	Facial erosions: maxillary and mandibular canines and premolars Occlusal erosions: maxillary and mandibular first molars and premolars Palatal erosions: maxillary incisors and canines
Bartlett et al. [72]	2011	18–30	Enamel wear: anterior teeth and first molars Dentine wear: incisal surfaces of the upper and lower incisors
Lussi et al. [56]	1991	26–30 46–50	Facial erosions: maxillary and mandibular canines and premolars Occlusal erosions: maxillary and mandibular premolars and molars Palatal erosions: maxillary incisors and canines
Lussi et al. [11]	2000	32–36 52–56	Facial erosions: increase, especially on premolar and molar surfaces Occlusal erosions: increase, especially on canine, premolar and molar surfaces Palatal erosions: increase, especially on maxillary central incisor surfaces
Vered et al. [77]	2014	15–60	Upper anterior sextant: 19.8% showed hard tissue loss (13.4% with BEWE 2; 6.4% with BEWE 3) Other sextants: 5% or less showed hard tissue loss

lytic survey was conducted among 500 subjects of five age groups (15–60 years) in Israel. Dental erosion was measured with the BEWE scoring system. Overall, 50% of the examined subjects showed erosive tooth wear. Among them, 10% had distinct erosion of over 50% of the dental surface. Total BEWE score differences were statistically significant by age group; as the age increased, the mean total BEWE scores increased significantly (p < 0.001). The association between acidic foods and erosion was evident among the younger population (p = 0.038). Multiple regression analyses revealed significant association of erosive tooth wear with age (p < 0.001) and diet (p = 0.044). The distribution of dental erosion among the survey participants according to the worst BEWE scores of different sextants revealed that the upper anterior sextant was most affected, with 19.8% of the par-

ticipants showing hard tissue loss on this sextant compared with a maximum of 5% for the other sextants [77]. In a nationwide representative study in Germany, Schiffner et al. [78] (2002) investigated the prevalence of non-carious cervical lesions involving two age groups: 35–44 and 65–74 years. They found that 42.1% of the younger and 46.3% of the older individuals showed at least 1 of these lesions (mean number of lesions per subject for the two groups: 2.2 and 2.5 teeth, respectively). Erosion confined to enamel was found in 6.4% of the younger and 4.1% of the older age group. Advanced erosion with involvement of dentine was present in 4.3% of the younger and 3.8% of the older individuals. Cervical wedge-shaped defects were found in 31.5% of the younger and 35% of the older population group. There was a significantly higher prevalence of non-carious cervical lesions

Table 4. Prevalence and incidence of erosion in adults (percent of examined tooth surfaces): an overview of different epidemiological studies listed in the order of age of the examined subjects

Author(s)	Year	Sample			Erosion prevalence	Erosion incidence	Conclusion
		age, years	n	examination			
Sognnaes et al. [59]	1972	–	10,827	extracted teeth	18%[1]	–	Mandibular teeth (21%) with higher frequency of erosion than the corresponding maxillary teeth (13%)
Mulic et al. [67]	2012	18	1,456	clinical	38%[2]	–	Associations to gender (males), dietary habits, reflux and vomiting
Xhonga and Valdmanis [68]	1983	14–88	527	clinical	25%[2]	–	Minor and severe erosions predominant
Isaksson et al. [61]	2013	20	494	clinical	75%[2]/18%[2]	–	High prevalence of erosion in young adults, but low severe erosion
Johansson et al. [64]	1996	21	95	clinical	28%[1]	–	Pronounced erosion (only maxillary anterior teeth were scored)
Manaf et al. [74]	2012	19–24	150	clinical	68%[2]	–	A high prevalence was observed in the sample under study
Jaeggi et al. [75]	1999	19–25	417	clinical	F: 14.4%/0.5% O: 82.0%/30.7% P: 0.7%/0.0%	–	Prevalence data: enamel/ dentinal erosions are listed; occlusal erosions most frequent
Bartlett et al. [72]	2011	18 – 30	1,010	clinical	100%[2]/7.9%[2]	–	All participants with at least 1 tooth with enamel tooth wear; 7.9% with dentinal tooth wear
Bartlett et al. [62]	2013	18–25 26–35	1,341 1,846	clinical	26.5%[2] 31.4%[2]	–	Large differences in prevalence of erosive tooth wear between different countries
Lussi et al. [56]	1991	26–30 46–50	194 197	clinical	F: 11.9%/7.7% O: 35.6%/29.9% P: 3.6%/0.0% F: 9.6%/13.2% O: 40.1%/42.6% P: 6.1%/2.0%	–	Prevalence data: enamel/dentinal erosions are listed; increase of number and severity of erosive lesions with increasing age
Mulic et al. [65]	2011	24–55	30	clinical	20%[2]	–	Dental erosion most frequently confined to enamel
Lussi et al. [76]	2000	32–36 52–56	55	clinical	O: 8% O: 26%	O: 5% O: 18%	Occlusal erosions involving dentine Progression of erosion on facial and occlusal surfaces especially in the older age group
Smith and Robb [71]	1996	15–26 26–55 56–65 >65	1,007	clinical	5.7% 3.3%–4.6% 8.2% 8.8%	–	Percent of tooth surfaces with pathological level of tooth wear in relation to age
Vered et al. [77]	2014	15–18 25–28 35–38 45–48 55–60	500	clinical	36.6%[2] 42.0%[2] 55.8%[2] 53.1%[2] 61.9%[2]	–	Percent of subjects with BEWE scores of 1 and more increased with age (p = 0.002) Association of erosive tooth wear with age and diet
Schiffner et al. [78]	2002	35–44 65–74	655 1,027	clinical	6.4%[2]/4.3%[2] (42.1%[2]) 4.1%[2]/3.8%[2] (46.3%[2])	–	Prevalence data: facial enamel/dentinal erosions are listed, as well as total of non-carious cervical lesions

Erosion prevalence: F = Facial; O = occlusal; P = palatal.
[1] Percent of examined teeth. [2] Percent of examined subjects.

in men than in women. Considering the reduced number of teeth, a significant increase in the presence of these alterations was found in older subjects.

An overview of the localization of erosion in adults is given in table 3. Prevalence and incidence data are summarized in table 4.

Conclusion

As mentioned previously, it is difficult to make comparisons between studies because of the different indices used and also because of the different teeth assessed in the samples [see chapter by Margaritis and Nunn, this vol., pp. 46–54]. This is compounded by the multifactor nature of tooth wear. Tooth surface substance loss has different causes: erosion, attrition, abrasion and abfraction all contribute to the functional loss and aging of the teeth [79]. Prevalence data show that erosive tooth wear is a common condition. It can start as soon as the first dental surface reaches the oral cavity by exposure to extrinsic or intrinsic acid. Primary and permanent teeth are equally involved. In addition, if mechanical stress loads the tooth surface, the progression of the defects increases further. Erosive tooth wear can be found on all tooth surfaces but is most common on occlusal and facial surfaces of all maxillary and mandibular teeth and on palatal surfaces of the maxillary anterior teeth.

Systematic (cross-sectional) prevalence data and incidence studies are scarce and therefore a conclusion about the occurrence, progression and distribution of erosive tooth wear cannot be made easily. There are some indications that the prevalence of erosive tooth wear shows an increase, especially in younger age groups. The main explanation for this could be the change in nutritional habits and lifestyle. For the future, it is important to collect more data and obtain additional information about this condition, preferably using an internationally accepted, standardized and validated index. It appears that differences of the distribution within the dentition in the different studies are difficult to explain. Factors such as the influence of the tongue movement (lip pressure, etc.) in different languages should be included in future studies. It would be of benefit if systematic investigations were undertaken on all age groups, all social classes and the population of different geographic regions and cultures. Erosive tooth wear is a growing condition of the oral cavity and it is essential that adequate preventive measures are implemented on a risk group level.

References

1 Osatakul S, Sriplung H, Puetpaiboon A, Junjana CO, Chamnongpakdi S: Prevalence and natural course of gastroesophageal reflux symptoms: a 1-year cohort study in Thai infants. J Pediatr Gastroenterol Nutr 2002;34:63–67.

2 Järvinen VK, Rytömaa II, Heinonen OP: Risk factors in dental erosion. J Dent Res 1991;70:942–947.

3 Linnet V, Seow WK: Dental erosion in children: a literature review. Pediatr Dent 2001;23:37–43.

4 Dahshan A, Patel H, Delaney J, Wuerth A, Thomas R, Tolia V: Gastroesophageal reflux disease and dental erosion in children. J Pediatr 2002;140:474–478.

5 O'Sullivan EA, Curzon ME, Roberts GJ, Milla PJ, Stringer MD: Gastroesophageal reflux in children and its relationship to erosion of primary and permanent teeth. Eur J Oral Sci 1998;106:765–769.

6 Lussi A, Jaeggi T, Zero D: The role of diet in the aetiology of dental erosion. Caries Res 2004;38:34–44.

7 Dugmore CR, Rock WP: A multifactorial analysis of factors associated with dental erosion. Br Dent J 2004;196:283–286.

8 Hunter ML, West NX, Hughes JA, Newcombe RG, Addy M: Erosion of deciduous and permanent dental hard tissue in the oral environment. J Dent 2000;28:257–263.

9 Amaechi BT, Higham SM, Edgar WM: Factors influencing the development of dental erosion in vitro: enamel type, temperature and exposure time. J Oral Rehabil 1999;26:624–630.

10 Hunter ML, West NX, Hughes JA, Newcombe RG, Addy M: Relative susceptibility of deciduous and permanent dental hard tissues to erosion by a low pH fruit drink in vitro. J Dent 2000;28:265–270.

11 Lussi A, Kohler N, Zero D, Schaffner M, Megert B: A comparison of the erosive potential of different beverages in primary and permanent teeth using an in vitro model. Eur J Oral Sci 2000;108:110–114.

12 Lussi A, Schaffner M, Jaeggi T, Grüninger A: Erosion. Clinical aspects – diagnosis – risk factors – prevention – therapy. Schweiz Monatsschr Zahnmed 2005;115: 917–935.

13 Attin T, Koidl U, Buchalla W, Schaller HG, Kielbassa AM, Hellwig E: Correlation of microhardness and wear in differently eroded bovine dental enamel. Arch Oral Biol 1997;42:243–250.

14 Al-Malik MI, Holt RD, Bedi R: Erosion, caries and rampant caries in preschool children in Jeddah, Saudi Arabia. Community Dent Oral Epidemiol 2002;30: 16–23.

15 Murakami C, Oliveira LB, Sheiham A, Nahás Pires Corrêa MS, Haddad AE, Bönecker M: Risk indicators for erosive tooth wear in Brazilian preschool children. Caries Res 2011;45:121–129.

16 Luo Y, Zeng XJ, Du MQ, Bedi R: The prevalence of dental erosion in preschool children in China. J Dent 2005; 33:115–121.

17 Harding MA, Whelton H, O'Mullane DM, Cronin M: Dental erosion in 5-year-old Irish school children and associated factors: a pilot study. Community Dent Health 2003;20:165–170.

18 Nayak SS, Ashokkumar BR, Ankola AV, Hebbal MI: Distribution and severity of erosion among 5-year-old children in a city in India. J Dent Child 2010;77:152–157.

19 Mangueira DF, Sampaio FC, Oliveira AF: Association between socioeconomic factors and dental erosion in Brazilian schoolchildren. J Public Health Dent 2009;69:254–259.

20 Taji SS, Seow WK, Townsend GC, Holcombe T: A controlled study of dental erosion in 2- to 4-year-old twins. Int J Paediatr Dent 2010;20:400–409.

21 Millward A, Shaw L, Smith A: Dental erosion in four-year-old children from differing socioeconomic backgrounds. ASDC J Dent Child 1994;61:263–266.

22 Moimaz SA, Araújo PC, Chiba FY, Garbín CA, Saliba NA: Prevalence of deciduous tooth erosion in childhood. Int J Dent Hyg 2013;11:226–230.

23 Wiegand A, Müller J, Werner C, Attin T: Prevalence of erosive tooth wear and associated risk factors in 2–7-year-old German kindergarten children. Oral Dis 2006;12:117–124.

24 Mantonanaki M, Koletsi-Kounari H, Mamai-Homata E, Papaioannou W: Dental erosion prevalence and associated risk indicators among preschool children in Athens, Greece. Clin Oral Investig 2013;17:585–593.

25 Gatou T, Mamai-Homata E: Tooth wear in the deciduous dentition of 5–7-year-old children: risk factors. Clin Oral Investig 2012;16:923–933.

26 Jaeggi T, Lussi A: Erosionen bei Kindern im frühen Schulalter. Schweiz Monatsschr Zahnmed 2004;114:876–881.

27 Ganss C, Klimek J, Giese K: Dental erosion in children and adolescents – a cross-sectional and longitudinal investigation using study models. Community Dent Oral Epidemiol 2001;29:264–271.

28 Truin GJ, Van Rijkom HM, Mulder J, Van't Hof MA: Caries trends 1996–2002 among 6- and 12-year-old children and erosive wear prevalence among 12-year-old children in The Hague. Caries Res 2005;39:2–8.

29 Truin GJ, Frencken JE, Mulder J, Kootwijk AJ, Jong ED: Prevalence of caries and dental erosion among school children in The Hague from 1996–2005. Ned Tijdschr Tandheelkd 2007;114:335–342.

30 Huew R, Waterhouse PJ, Moynihan PJ, Maguire A: Dental erosion among 12-year-old Libyan schoolchildren. Community Dent Health 2012;29:279–283.

31 Vargas-Ferreira F, Piovesan C, Praetzel JR, Mendes FM, Allison PJ, Ardenghi TM: Tooth erosion with low severity does not impact child oral health-related quality of life. Caries Res 2010;44:531–539.

32 Dugmore CR, Rock WP: The prevalence of tooth erosion in 12-year-old children. Br Dent J 2004;196:279–282.

33 Dugmore CR, Rock WP: The progression of tooth erosion in a cohort of adolescents of mixed ethnicity. Int J Paediatr Dent 2003;13:295–303.

34 Deery C, Wagner ML, Longbottom C, Simon R, Nugent ZJ: The prevalence of dental erosion in a United States and a United Kingdom sample of adolescents. Pediatr Dent 2000;22:505–510.

35 Chadwick RG, Mitchell HL, Manton SL, Ward S, Ogston S, Brown R: Maxillary incisor palatal erosion: no correlation with dietary variables? J Clin Pediatr Dent 2005;29:157–164.

36 Wang P, Lin HC, Chen JH, Liang HY. The prevalence of dental erosion and associated risk factors in 12–13-year-old school children in Southern China. BMC Public Health 2010;10:478.

37 Bardolia P, Burnside G, Ashcroft A, Milosevic A, Goodfellow SA, Rolfe EA, Pine CM: Prevalence and risk indicators of erosion in thirteen- to fourteen-year-olds on the Isle of Man. Caries Res 2010; 44:165–168.

38 Williams D, Croucher R, Marcenes W, O'Farrell M: The prevalence of dental erosion in the maxillary incisors of 14-year-old schoolchildren living in Tower Hamlets and Hackney, London, UK. Int Dent J 1999;49:211–216.

39 Bardsley PF, Taylor S, Milosevic A: Epidemiological studies of tooth wear and dental erosion in 14-year-old children in North West England. Part 1. The relationship with water fluoridation and social deprivation. Br Dent J 2004;197: 413–416.

40 Gurgel CV, Rios D, Buzalaf MA, da Silva SM, Araújo JJ, Pauletto AR, de Andrade Moreira Machado MA: Dental erosion in a group of 12- and 16-year-old Brazilian schoolchildren. Pediatr Dent 2011; 33:23–28.

41 Hasselkvist A, Johansson A, Johansson AK: Dental erosion and soft drink consumption in Swedish children and adolescents and the development of a simplified erosion partial recording system. Swed Dent J 2010;34:187–195.

42 McGuire J, Szabo A, Jackson S, Bradley TG, Okunseri C: Erosive tooth wear among children in the United States: relationship to race/ethnicity and obesity. Int J Paediatr Dent 2009;19:91–98.

43 Arnadottir IB, Holbrook WP, Eggertsson H, Gudmundsdottir H, Jonsson SH, Gudlaugsson JO, Saemundsson SR, Eliasson ST, Agustsdottir H: Prevalence of dental erosion in children: a national survey. Community Dent Oral Epidemiol 2010;38:521–526.

44 Caglar E, Kargul B, Tanboga I, Lussi A: Dental erosion among children in an Istanbul public school. J Dent Child 2005;72:5–9.

45 Caglar E, Sandalli N, Panagiotou N, Tonguc K, Kuscu OO: Prevalence of dental erosion in Greek minority school children in Istanbul. Eur Arch Paediatr Dent 2011;12:267–271.

46 Nahás Pires Corrêa MS, Nahás Pires Corrêa F, Nahás Pires Corrêa JP, Murakami C, Mendes FM: Prevalence and associated factors of dental erosion in children and adolescents of a private dental practice. Int J Paediatr Dent 2011; 21:451–458.

47 Correr GM, Alonso RC, Correa MA, Campos EA, Baratto-Filho F, Puppin-Rontani RM: Influence of diet and salivary characteristics on the prevalence of dental erosion among 12-year-old schoolchildren. J Dent Child 2009;76: 181–187.

48 Zhang S, Chau AM, Lo EC, Chu CH: Dental caries and erosion status of 12-year-old Hong Kong children. BMC Public Health 2014;14:7.

49 El Aidi H, Bronkhorst EM, Huysmans MC, Truin GJ: Dynamics of tooth erosion in adolescents: a 3-year longitudinal study. J Dent 2010;38:131–137.

50 Nunn JH, Rugg-Gunn A, Gordon PH, Stephenson G: A longitudinal study of dental erosion in adolescent girls (ORCA abstract 97). Caries Res 2001;35:296.

51 Milosevic A, Young PJ, Lennon MA: The prevalence of tooth wear in 14-year-old school children in Liverpool. Community Dent Health 1994;11:83–86.

52 Al-Dlaigan YH, Shaw L, Smith A: Dental erosion in a group of British 14-year-old school children. Part I. Prevalence and influence of differing socioeconomic backgrounds. Br Dent J 2001;190:145–149.

53 Arnadottir IB, Saemundsson SR, Holbrook WP: Dental erosion in Icelandic teenagers in relation to dietary and lifestyle factors. Acta Odontol Scand 2003; 61:25–28.

54 Kaczmarek U, Czajczynska-Waszkiewicz A, Skladnik-Jankowska J: Prevalance of dental erosion in 15-year-old subjects from Lower Silesia province. J Stoma 2012;65:359–369.

55 Van Rijkom HM, Truin GJ, Frencken JE, König KG, Van't Hof MA, Bronkhorst EM, Roeters FJ: Prevalence, distribution and background variables of smooth-bordered tooth wear in teenagers in The Hague, The Netherlands. Caries Res 2002;36:147–154.

56 Lussi A, Schaffner M, Hotz P, Suter P: Dental erosion in a population of Swiss adults. Community Dent Oral Epidemiol 1991;19:286–290.

57 Larsen MJ, Poulsen S, Hansen I: Erosion of the teeth: prevalence and distribution in a group of Danish school children. Eur J Paediatr Dent 2005;6:44–47.

58 Nunn JH, Gordon PH, Morris AJ, Pine CM, Walker A: Dental erosion – changing prevalence? A review of British national children's surveys. Int J Paediatr Dent 2003;13:98–105.

59 Sognnaes RF, Wolcott RB, Xhonga FA: Dental erosion. I. Erosion-like patterns occurring in association with other dental conditions. J Am Dent Assoc 1972; 84:571–576.

60 Khan F, Young WG, Law V, Priest J, Daley TJ: Cupped lesions of early onset dental erosion in young southeast Queensland adults. Aust Dent J 2001;46: 100–107.

61 Isaksson H, Birkhed D, Wendt LK, Alm A, Nilsson M, Koch G: Prevalence of dental erosion and association with lifestyle factors in Swedish 20-year olds. Acta Odontol Scand, Epub ahead of print.

62 Bartlett DW, Lussi A, West NX, Bouchard P, Sanz M, Bourgeois D: Prevalence of tooth wear on buccal and lingual surfaces and possible risk factors in young European adults. J Dent 2013;41:1007–1013.

63 Xhonga FA, Wolcott RB, Sognnaes RF: Dental erosion. II. Clinical measurements of dental erosion progress. J Am Dent Assoc 1972;84:577–582.

64 Johansson AK, Johansson A, Birkhed D, Omar R, Baghdadi S, Carlsson GE: Dental erosion, soft-drink intake, and oral health in young Saudi men, and the development of a system for assessing erosive anterior tooth wear. Acta Odontol Scand 1996;54:369–378.

65 Mulic A, Tveit AB, Hove LH, Skaare AB: Dental erosive wear among Norwegian wine tasters. Acta Odontol Scand 2011; 69:21–26.

66 Ekfeld A: Incisal and occlusal tooth wear and wear of some prosthodontic materials. An epidemiological and clinical study. Swed Dent J Suppl 1989;65:1–62.

67 Mulic A, Skudutyte-Rysstad R, Tveit AB, Skaare AB: Risk indicators for dental erosive wear among 18-year-old subjects in Oslo, Norway. Eur J Oral Sci 2012;120:531–538.

68 Xhonga FA, Valdmanis S: Geographic comparisons of the incidence of dental erosion: a two centre study. J Oral Rehabil 1983;10:269–277.

69 Smith BG, Knight JK: An index for measuring the wear of teeth. Br Dent J 1984; 156:435–438.

70 Donachie MA, Walls AW: The tooth wear index: a flawed epidemiological tool in an ageing population group. Community Dent Oral Epidemiol 1996; 24:152–158.

71 Smith BG, Robb ND: The prevalence of toothwear in 1,007 dental patients. J Oral Rehabil 1996;23:232–239.

72 Bartlett DW, Fares J, Shirodaria S, Chiu K, Ahmad N, Sherriff M: The association of tooth wear, diet and dietary habits in adults aged 18–30 years old. J Dent 2011;39:811–816.

73 Donachie MA, Walls AW: Assessment of tooth wear in an ageing population. J Dent 1995;23:157–164.

74 Manaf ZA, Lee MT, Ali NH, Samynathan S, Jie YP, Ismail NH, Bibiana Hui Ying Y, Wei Seng Y, Yahya NA: Relationship between food habits and tooth erosion occurrence in Malaysian University students. Malays J Med Sci 2012; 19:56–66.

75 Jaeggi T, Schaffner M, Bürgin W, Lussi A: Erosionen und keilförmige Defekte bei Rekruten der Schweizer Armee. Schweiz Monatsschr Zahnmed 1999;109: 1171–1182.

76 Lussi A, Schaffner M: Progression of and risk factors for dental erosion and wedge-shaped defects over a 6-year period. Caries Res 2000;34:182–187.

77 Vered Y, Lussi A, Zini A, Gleitman J, Sganz-Cohen HD: Dental erosive wear assessment among adolescents and adults utilizing the basic erosive wear examination (BEWE) scoring system. Clin Oral Investig, Epub ahead of print.

78 Schiffner U, Micheelis W, Reich E: Erosionen und keilförmige Zahnhalsdefekte bei deutschen Erwachsenen und Senioren. Dtsch Zahnarztl Z 2002;57:102–106.

79 Nunn JH: Prevalence of dental erosion and the implications for oral health. Eur J Oral Sci 1996;104:156–161.

Dr. T. Jaeggi
Department of Preventive, Restorative and Pediatric Dentistry
School of Dental Medicine, University of Bern, Freiburgstrasse 7
CH–3010 Bern (Switzerland)
E-Mail thomasjaeggi@bluewin.ch

Lussi A, Ganss C (eds): Erosive Tooth Wear. Monogr Oral Sci. Basel, Karger, 2014, vol 25, pp 74–98
DOI: 10.1159/000359938

Prevalence of Erosive Tooth Wear in Risk Groups

Nadine Schlueter[a] · Anne Bjørg Tveit[b]

[a]Department of Conservative and Preventive Dentistry, Dental Clinic, Justus Liebig University Giessen,
Giessen, Germany; [b]Department of Cariology and Gerodontology, Institute of Clinical Dentistry,
Faculty of Dentistry, University of Oslo, Oslo, Norway

Abstract

Individuals have different risks for developing erosive lesions depending on background, behavioural, dietary and medical variables. It is anticipated that people with regular impact of gastric juice, i.e. patients with eating disorders and gastroesophageal reflux disease (GERD) have a specially high risk of developing dental erosions; the same could be true for those with special diets, regular consumption of acidic beverages, medicine and drug intake and occupational exposure to acids. Eating disorders are associated with an increased occurrence, severity and risk for dental erosion, even though not all bulimic patients show a pathological level of tooth wear. There seems also to be a tendency that in the case of GERD, erosion is more common and more severe than in healthy controls. Regarding exogenous causes, many studies, though not all, document a positive association between the consumption of acidic beverages and dental erosions and there seems to be a dose-response relationship; however, further studies are necessary for a final statement. The same applies for the association between drug or medication intake or special diet and erosion prevalence. Though only few studies exist, there seems to be a tendency for an increase of erosion prevalence amongst persons abusively consuming alcohol. Some studies show an increased risk for dental erosion for employees testing wine or working in acid processing factories. Even though some associations between acid impact and erosion prevalence appear clear, the number of studies is small. There is a lack of controlled prevalence studies, making it difficult to give final statements for all risk groups.
© 2014 S. Karger AG, Basel

The dental hard tissue undergoes multiple chemical and mechanical impacts during the whole life, which can lead to wear and tear. Though dental erosive wear is a multifactorial condition, it is still not conclusively clarified as to which factors contribute to the manifestation of erosion. However, there are indications that in particular the frequency of acidic challenges plays an important role [see chapter by Lussi and Hellwig, this vol., pp. 220–229], potentially increasing the risk for developing erosion.

Risk is defined as the probability that an event will occur within a given period of time [1] and is used to express the probability of a particular outcome (i.e. disease) to occur following an exposure [2]. A risk factor may be defined as 'an environmental, behavioural, or biological factor confirmed by temporal sequence, usually in longitudinal studies, which, if present, directly increases the probability of a disease occurring, and if absent or removed reduces the probability' [3].

Aetiology of erosion is manifold and individuals have different risks for developing erosive lesions depending on background, behavioural, dietary and medical variables. Examples of risk groups could be persons suffering from underlying diseases, such as gastroesophageal reflux disease (GERD), eating disorders (anorexia nervosa, AN, bulimia nervosa, BN, and rumination) and chronic alcohol abuse or alcohol dependence. Special nutrition habits (high consumption of soft or sports drinks), special diets (vegetarian, vegan or raw food diet) or the regular intake of drugs, medications and food supplements can also increase the risk for dental erosion. The same applies for persons with an occupational exposure to acids.

The following chapter aims to report the prevalence of dental erosion in the defined risk groups. Since epidemiological studies do not exist for all risk groups, and there are great variations between studies regarding the selection of study population, age groups, number of examiners, indices used and diagnostic thresholds, the challenge is to draw final conclusions from these papers.

Gastroesophageal Reflux Disease

GERD is defined as a condition in which the gastroduodenal content regularly reaches the oesophagus and then probably the oral cavity. It possibly interferes with the oral tissues, causing symptoms which can impair the quality of life [4, 5]. A chronic symptomatic reflux can be diagnosed at 4–7% in the general population [6]; however, the prevalence for the so-called silent reflux (asymptomatic reflux) is about 25% [7], meaning that these persons potentially have a high risk for dental erosion. For a detailed description of intrinsic causes of erosion, see chapter by Moazzez and Bartlett [this vol., pp. 180–196]. A PubMed search with the terms (dental OR enamel OR dentin) AND (erosion OR tooth wear) AND (reflux OR gastro) revealed 250 hits, from which 34 deal with the prevalence of dental erosion in persons with GERD; 6 studies deal with GERD in patients with other underlying diseases (Sjögren's syndrome, patients with cerebral palsy and disabled persons), which were excluded since no clear distinction between GERD-related wear and other wear factors was made, and 1 study was excluded since data about erosion occurrence were collected by questionnaires; all other assessments were performed clinically. Various age groups were investigated, which can be categorized into children (age range between 1 and <18 years; 11 studies) and adults (age range between 18 and 79 years; 16 studies). Out of the 27 studies considered (table 1), 3 studies from the children's and 2 from the adults' groups did not include a control group. In the children's group, between 11 and 98% of the included persons in the GERD and 14 and 75% in the control group showed any sign of erosion at least at one tooth. If erosion is assessed on a tooth-based level, the range was between 11 and 19% for deciduous teeth and between 4 and 10% for permanent teeth in the GERD group. Values for control were between 5 and 10% for deciduous and between 0.8 and 2% for permanent teeth. Studies without controls showed values within the same range. For adults the range of erosion prevalence in the GERD group was comparable to the children's group; between 9 and 75% showed any sign of erosion at least at one tooth; in the control group the prevalence was distinctly lower at between 0 and 40%. The tooth-based results also showed a higher occurrence of erosion in persons with GERD than in the control group. The uncontrolled studies showed a lower prevalence, ranging between 6 and 24%. In particular, if one considers the severity of erosion, persons with GERD often show higher severity grades than controls. Some studies found that the most affected surface of teeth in persons with GERD is the palatal surface of the upper front teeth, which is in clear contrast to the occurrence of

Table 1. Cross-sectional and non-randomized case-control studies investigating the prevalence of erosion in persons suffering from gastroesophageal reflux disease

Author	Mean age, years	Test group, n	Control, n	Diagnosis of reflux	Index	Results based on
Children						
Bartlett et al. [68], 1998	12	132	78	quest.	TWI	indiv.
Ersin et al. [109], 2006	6.5	38	42	2	E&J	indiv.
						teeth
Farahmand et al. [110], 2013	5.9	54	58	quest.	Aine	indiv.
Linnett et al. [111], 2002	6.5	52	52	medical records	Aine	indiv.
						teeth
Murakami et al. [112], 2011	3.5	75	890	quest.	O'Brian	indiv.
Nunn et al. [113], 2003				quest.	mod. TWI	indiv.
Vargas-Ferreira et al. [114], 2011		105	839	quest.	O'Sullivan	teeth
Wild et al. [115], 2011	14.0	59	20	2	yes/no (simpl. TWI)	erosion per tooth
						indiv.
Aine et al. [116], 1993	*8.1*	*17*	*–*	*self-report of symptoms, 2*	*Aine*	*indiv.*
Dahshan et al. [117], 2002	*10.4*	*37 (24 GERD)*	*–*	*4*	*Aine*	*indiv.*
O'Sullivan et al. [118], 1998	*4.9*	*53*	*–*	*pH-monitoring*	*own*	*indiv.*
Adults						
Benages et al. [119], 2006		181	72	not named	E&J	indiv.
Correa et al. [120], 2012	33.4	30	30	clinically, 1, 3	E&J	teeth
Di Fede et al. [121], 2008	46.9	200	100	2, 4	TWI	indiv.
Gregory-Head et al. [122], 2000		10	10	2	TWI	teeth
Jensdottir et al. [53], 2004	35	23	57	2, 3, 4	yes-no mod. Lussi	indiv.
Moazzez et al. [123], 2005	43.3	31	7	2, 3	mod. TWI	indiv.
						teeth

Prev. test	Prev. control	Sign.	Comment
11%	14%	no	results calculated on the basis of study data, not only persons with GERD included
76%	24%	yes	
19% (prim.)	5% (prim.)	yes	
10% (perm.)	2% (perm.)	yes	
98%	19%	yes	
46% (perm.)	40% (perm.)	no	
14%	10%	yes	
20% (prim.)	20% (prim.)	no	
4% (perm.)	0.8% (perm.)	yes	
67%	51%	yes	prevalence calculated on basis of study data; only palatal surfaces of incisor and occlusal surfaces of molars were scored
79%	62%	yes	reanalysis of surveys: national survey of children's dental health (n = 17,061), NDNS (n = 1,451 + n = 1,726)
11%	6%	–	prevalence calculated on the basis of study data (study population minus persons with GERD)
0.19	0.11	yes	
85%	75%	no	
87%	–	–	*similar occurrence of erosion in persons with primary and permanent dentition*
83.3%	–	–	
17%	–	–	*erosion severity and number of teeth affected by erosion increased with age*
48%	13%	yes	severity and number of erosion in GERD group higher than in control; different location
4.7 teeth	0.06 teeth	yes	
9%	13%	no	no association of GERD and erosion, but association of GERD and xerostomia
mean TWI score 0.95±0.55	mean TWI score 0.30±0.28	yes	
35%	40%	no	
29%	0%	–	only palatal surfaces were investigated
71%	0%	–	

Table 1. Continued

Author	Mean age, years	Test group, n	Control, n	Diagnosis of reflux	Index	Results based on
Moazzez et al. [124], 2004	44.0	104	31	2, 3	mod. TWI	teeth
Mulic et al. [26], 2012	18	198	1,199	quest.	VEDE	indiv.
Muñoz et al. [125], 2003	47.8	181	72	2, 4	Hattab mod. E&J	indiv.
Oginni et al. [126], 2005	38	125	100	quest.	TWI	indiv.
Schroeder et al. [127], 1995	52	20	10	2	E&J	indiv.
Tantbirojn et al. [128], 2012	31	12	6	diagnosis of a physician	not named	indiv.
						teeth
Wang et al. [129], 2010	45.3	88	36	1, 2, 3	TWI	indiv.
Yoshikawa et al. [130], 2012	68.8	40	30	self-report, 1	mod. TWI	indiv.
						teeth
Järvinen et al. [131], 1988		*109*	*–*	*1*	*E&J*	*indiv.*
	51.9	*20*			*E&J*	*indiv.*
	52.4	*24*			*E&J*	*indiv.*
Meurman et al. [132], 1994	*50.2*	*117*	*–*	*4*	*E&J*	*indiv.*

Studies displayed in italics included no control group. 1 = Endoscopy; 2 = 24-hour oesophageal pH-metry; 3 = oesophageal manometry; 4 = oesophago-gastro-duodenoscopy; E&J = Eccles and Jenkins; TWI = Smith and Knight tooth wear index; NDNS = National Diet and Nutrition Surveys; OR = odds ratio; prev. test = prevalence in the test group suffering from GERD; prev. control = prevalence in the control group; indiv. = individuals; sign. = significance (indicates whether differences between test group and control group reached significance); quest. = questionnaire; simpl. = simplified; mod. = modified; prim. = primary; perm. = permanent.

erosion in the general population, whereas others found no difference between both groups (for details see table 1). Subsuming the results, it appears difficult to give a final conclusion. The results are sometimes contradictory, probably due to the use of different diagnostic methods to select the GERD group or even due to the use of different indices; however, there seems to be a tendency that in the case of GERD erosion is more common and in particular more severe than in healthy controls.

Prev. test	Prev. control	Sign.	Comment
24% (30% pal. surfaces)	8% (0% pal. surfaces)	yes	
49%	35%	yes	prevalence calculated on the basis of data of study (study population (n = 1,456) minus persons with GERD minus persons with vomiting) OR for erosion in case of GERD: 2.0
48%	13%	yes	higher severity and more teeth affected in patients with GERD than in controls
16%	5%	yes	higher TWI score in persons with GERD
55%	10%	yes	severity and number of erosion in GERD group higher than in control
75%	17%	–	study on surface loss progression, loss per tooth (mm^3) in persons with erosion 3- to 10-fold higher than in controls
38	1	–	
49%	14%	yes	occurrence of erosion associated with occurrence of respiratory symptoms (no resp. symp: 37% erosion, occasionally: 44%, frequent: 65%)
24%	0%	–	
2.4%	0%	–	
6%	–	–	*prevalence of erosion in patients with reflux esophagitis, duodenal ulcer, gastric ulcer, cholecystectomy*
20%	–	–	*prevalence of erosion only in patients with reflux esophagitis*
13%	–	–	*prevalence of erosion only patients with duodenal ulcer*
24%	–	–	*Duration of disease in patients with erosion longer (17.4 vs. 8.0 years)*

Eating Disorders

Eating disorders are divided into AN, BN and eating disorders not otherwise specified (EDNOS, according to the Diagnostic and Statistical Manual of Mental Disorders, DSM-V, ed. 5). EDNOS includes individuals with symptoms of AN or BN who do not fulfil all the diagnostic criteria, as well as individuals with binge eating disorder (BED). These eating disorders affect the regulation of food intake such as restricted dietary choice and induced vomiting and thereby could have an impact on oral health.

Prevalence of eating disorders has been reported from different countries. A study based on the National Comorbidity Survey Replication (NCS-R), a nationally representative survey of the US population, estimated that the lifetime prevalence of eating disorders ranged from 0.6 to 4.5% in 2007 (AN 0.6%, BN 1.0%) [8]. In the age group 13–18 years the lifetime prevalence was 0.3% (AN) and 0.9% (BN), respectively [9].

Comparable results were found for Europe; in Norway, the lifetime prevalence of BED was between 1.5 and 3.2%, of BN between 0.4 and 1.6% and of AN between 0.2 and 0.7%. EDNOS had a lifetime prevalence between 3.0 and 15% [10, 11]. Recent studies from Finland and Germany reported comparable values (Finland: AN 1.3%, BN 1.1% and EDNOS 1.0% [12]; German children and adolescents: AN 0.14%, BN 0.11% [13]). In general, the majority (>90%) of individuals that get AN or BN are females [13, 14].

Persons suffering from an eating disorder are at higher risk for dental erosion, especially those with an eating disorder in combination with vomiting (BN) since gastric juice is highly erosive [15]. Those suffering from AN are at higher risk for both exogenous-caused erosion due to dietary habits (restrictive diet) and endogenous-caused erosion due to vomiting episodes, which occur in some anorectic patients (bulimic AN or anorectic BN). Many patients who experience self-induced vomiting have reported a large consumption of soft drinks, whereas many anorectics have reported a diet characterized by a high consumption of citrus fruits, apples and juices [16], both potentially increasing the erosion risk.

In general, there are only few studies dealing with the prevalence of erosion in persons showing eating disorders. Many of the publications present case reports; most of the prevalence studies include only a small number of cases, reducing their validity.

Several studies showed significantly higher values of erosive tooth wear in patients suffering from eating disorders compared to a control group [17–23]. In the study by Öhrn et al. [20], 81 outpatients from a psychiatric clinic for eating disorders had dental examination [20]. The oral status of the patients with diagnosed eating disorders was generally worse than that of an age-matched reference group, and was characterized by significantly higher frequencies of erosive tooth wear in addition to caries and low unstimulated salivary flow rate, low buffer capacity in stimulated saliva and high counts of lactobacilli and mutans streptococci. Erosive tooth wear was found in all but 2 individuals with eating disorders (98%), while in the reference group the wear was minor and less frequent. Of the 81 patients with eating disorders, loss of tooth structure suggestive of erosion involving the dentine was found in 45 patients (56%) [20].

A controlled cross-sectional study involved 1,203 randomly selected female students aged 15–18 years [24] and identified 72 (6%) with a score indicating a high chance to meet the criteria for BN; 20 (1.7%) were identified not only with a high chance to meet the bulimia criteria but also with a high risk. Dental erosions were found in 45% of those with eating disorders compared to 8.8% among controls. Such relations were also found in 2 further studies investigating groups of young females with BN compared to control groups [22, 23]. Nearly the same values for erosion were found in a group of 79 women hospitalized because of chronic eating disorder (42% showing erosion) and 48 age-matched healthy women (4% showing erosion). Additionally, a higher severity of dental erosions was found among those with eating disorder. No erosions that affected the dentine were found in the control group, but were in 26% of the examined maxillary anterior teeth and 21% of the posterior teeth in the eating disorder group. In this study not only persons with BN but also those with other eating disorders have been investigated. The group showing vomiting of those with eating disorders had a higher level of dental erosions compared to the non-vomiting group, even though the difference did not reach statistical significance [21].

Hellström [16] (1977) examined 39 patients who had been suffering from AN for periods ranging from 1 to 20 years, including both patients with and without vomiting episodes. Likewise, in the above-mentioned study [21] a marked difference in erosion was found between the group that vomited (27 patients) and the group that did not (12 patients). Dental erosions occurred in nearly all vomiting patients, mostly in a severe form. Also, the localization differed between both groups. The buccal type of erosion was rare in the non-vomiting patients but common in those who had vomiting. Perimolysis (loss of enamel and dentine on the lingual surfaces of the teeth as a result of chemical and mechanical effects caused mainly by regurgitation of gastric contents and aggravated by the movement of the tongue [25]) was found only in the vomiting group; 23 out of 27 (85%) had erosions on lingual and occlusal surfaces and 15 (56%) had severe lesions involving deeper layers of enamel and dentine [16]. These findings clearly indicate that vomiting increases the probability of developing erosion [23, 26] and may be the most serious risk factor for those with eating disorders.

Though vomiting has clearly been related to the occurrence of erosive wear, the study by Robb et al. [18] showed that those who suffered from AN but did not vomit also had more erosions than a control population. However, there are also studies showing contradictory results. None of 23 women with AN in the study by Shaughnessy et al. had dental erosions even though 26% of them reported a history of binge eating/purging activity [18]. Several further studies show that not all persons suffering from eating disorders show dental erosion [17, 19, 27], even if the risk is quite high. A Finnish study found that 13 of 35 bulimics (37%) did not have any dental erosion [19]. In another study from the UK it has been found that among bulimics who induced vomiting, 14 out of 33 (42%) had such lesions; the corresponding finding for those who did not induce vomiting was 2 out of 7 (29%). For the anorectics (both the purging and non-purging type), 6 out of 18 (33%) had a pathological level of tooth wear [17]. In several studies no linear association was found between frequency or duration of vomiting and dental erosion [17, 18, 28].

Generally, it is difficult to evaluate the risk of various dietary factors, vomiting and/or unfavourable saliva factors for patients with eating disorders. Information about self-induced vomiting, frequency and duration are associated with uncertainties, because many patients feel ashamed of their eating disorders. It is often a general finding that persons with eating disorders are well educated and well informed about the condition. However, patients with vomiting/binge eating behaviour have a 5.5-times higher risk of dental erosions than those without such behaviour; persons with eating disorders in general, independent of the type, had an up to 8.5-times increased risk of having dental erosion and show dental erosive lesions more often with a longer history of eating disorders [23].

In conclusion, eating disorders are associated with an increased occurrence, severity and risk for dental erosion related to both exogenous and endogenous acids. In particular, the regular impact of gastric juice in the case of vomiting seems to be the major risk factor for developing erosion in persons suffering from eating disorders.

Special Diet

Approximately 1–9% of the western society live on a vegetarian diet [29] and approximately 0.1% on a vegan diet [30]. These diets normally include a higher consumption of vegetables and fruits, i.e. approximately 30% higher consumption of fruits amongst vegetarians compared to omnivores [31] or up to a 96% proportion of fruit consumption in persons living on a raw food diet [32]. As it has been assumed that a high frequency of fruit intake is a risk factor for the development of dental erosion [see chapters by Barbour and Lussi, this vol., pp. 143–154, and Lussi and Hellwig, this vol., pp. 220–229], such diets may lead to a higher occurrence of erosive defects [33, 34].

Epidemiological studies dealing with special diet and erosion are rare and sometimes show contradictory results. The PubMed search with the terms (dental OR enamel OR dentin) AND (erosion OR tooth wear) AND (vegetarian OR vegan OR raw food OR nutrition) revealed 86 hits of which only 6 were relevant; 1 of these studies deals with the occurrence and severity of erosion in a group of persons living on a raw food diet. In this study the prevalence of erosion was generally high (98% of individuals in the raw food group, 87% in the control group); however, the severity of erosion was clearly higher in the raw food group (61% severe erosion compared to 32% in the control group) and the percentage of surfaces affected of all investigated surfaces was higher amongst the raw food consumers (24 vs. 7% in the control group) [32].

The other 5 studies deal with the impact of vegetarian nutrition on erosion prevalence. The number of cases in all studies is small, reducing the validity of these studies. Except for 1 study showing a higher prevalence in vegetarian persons (77 vs. 0% in a control group) and an association between consumption of acidic food and the occurrence of erosion [35], no significant increase was found in the other studies (48% of vegetarian children showed distinct erosive defects vs. 51% of controls [36]; 39 vs. 24% in adults [37]). No association between the type of consumed foodstuff [36, 37] or the duration [37, 38] of the vegetarian diet and the prevalence of erosion was found, albeit some studies have shown an increased risk for the development of erosion in the case of a vegetarian diet (OR up to 6.7) [39, 40].

High Consumption of Acidic Beverages

Acidic drinks are thought to be one of the most important factors leading to dental erosive wear, especially considering that the consumption of such drinks has increased greatly over the past decades [41–43]. In particular, adolescents and young adults consume large volumes of soft drinks and fruit juices up to nearly 1 litre per capita and day [41, 44], which are commonly believed to be causal factors for dental erosive lesions [34, 45, 46]. Furthermore, the frequency and duration of acid attacks, as well as the manner of consumption of erosive foods and beverages, is said to influence the severity of the erosive lesions [34, 47–49].

The PubMed Search using the terms (dental OR enamel OR dentin) AND (erosion OR tooth wear) AND (acidic beverages OR soft drinks) revealed a tremendous number of studies, all dealing with the impact of foodstuffs and drinks on erosion. However, from the 431 papers found, 401 were excluded since they show in vitro or in situ results or case reports. Only clinical studies were included. Most of these studies included children and adolescents. Studies on adults are rather seldom. Prevalence studies on the occurrence of erosion in persons highly consuming soft drinks or acidic beverages do not exist; there are only studies investigating the association between the consumption of specific food stuffs or drinks and the occurrence of erosion and studies investigating the risk for dental erosion in the case of consuming these comestibles. Among these studies a huge variety in indices used for assessing erosion and in types of questionnaires used for collecting data about nutritional behaviour and habits was found, making it difficult to compare the results. Data exist from all continents, resulting in an additional problem since the consumption customs highly vary between and even within one continent. A further problem is that in some studies the prevalence of erosion in the investigated groups is very low, making it difficult to find any association between the occurrence of erosion and eating habits. In other studies nearly everybody showed erosion; in this case an association of the occurrence of erosion with numerous types of the ingested food stuffs and drinks can easily be found, even with actual non-erosive food. All the above-mentioned issues might be the reason for some contradictory results of the studies found.

In a study from the UK, structured dietary histories were taken from 309 age- and gender-matched children either with or without erosion to determine the type and frequency of intake of acidic foods and drinks, together with any drinking habits that prolonged exposure of the teeth to dietary acids [50]. They showed that the children with erosion drank acidic beverages significantly more frequently. A comparable significant positive association between erosive wear and consumption of carbonated soft drinks has also been found in several other studies from around the world, independent of the consumption customs in the respective country [26, 34, 51–62]. Some of the studies even found an association with non-erosive food [33, 63–65], perhaps as a result of a high level of occurrence of erosion in the group investigated [63, 65].

The total contact time between acidic drink and teeth also seems to play a role. The consumption of acidic fruit juices and sugary soft drinks several times daily increased the risk of dental erosive wear [see chapter by Barbour and Lussi, this vol., pp. 143–154], indicating a dose-response relationship (greater consumption places the dentition at a greater risk) [26]. A similar association has also been detected by several other authors [34, 53, 63]. Swishing of drinks has also been found as a factor increasing the risk for dental erosion [66], supporting the theory on a dose-response relationship.

In contrast to the above-mentioned studies, El Aidi et al. [67] did not identify a significant positive association between erosive wear and carbonated soft drinks. This is in accordance with several other studies [56, 64, 66, 68–71]. Correr et al. [56] also revealed no relationship between dental erosion and consumption of acidic fruit juices and beverages. However, they say that it should be noted that the sample size in the study was small, which is, in general, a problem of several other studies.

While the consumption of soft drinks has increased during the past decades [41] but has stayed on this high level over the last 5–10 years [43], the consumption of sports and energy drinks has distinctly increased within the last decade by approximately 60% [72]. This might be an additional risk factor for erosion. However, only 1 study actually found a 4-fold increase in the risk [34], whereas some studies have demonstrated that sports drinks consumed during exercise are not associated with erosive lesions [26, 70, 73–75]. The lack of association could be explained by the small number of responders consuming sports drinks in the mentioned studies. Less than once per week consumption was registered by 87% of the 18-year-olds, while only 3 of the physically active young adults had a high consumption of sports drinks. It may be that the physically active participants, although regularly exercising but not necessarily competitively, did not use nutrient replacements and were possibly aware of the fact that the sports drinks do not offer more benefit than water [73].

Longitudinal studies investigating the progression or the incidence of erosion are rather seldom; 1 such study was performed in The Netherlands by El Aidi et al. [67]. As mentioned, no positive association between erosive wear and carbonated soft drinks was detected and also only a vague association between the incidence of erosive wear and a special type of foodstuff or drink was found; solely the intake of alcoholic mixed drinks was significantly associated. In a Swiss study the progression of non-carious dental hard tissue defects has been investigated over a period of 6 years. It has clearly been shown that the progression was correlated with the consumption of dietary acids [76].

There seems to be a gender-specific risk for developing erosion. In an Icelandic study, male teenagers had a nearly 3-fold increased risk for getting erosion compared to females [77]. Different risk indicators for dental erosive wear among males and females were revealed in a Norwegian study [26]. For males, only engagement in vocational studies and frequent consumption of sugary soft drinks were significantly associated with erosive wear; for females, reported vomiting or reflux and the consumption of fruit juice were found to be significantly linked to the presence of lesions [26].

In conclusion, the majority of studies have documented a positive association between the consumption of acidic beverages and dental erosions. There seems to be a dose-response relationship.

However, there are also studies showing an association not only with the typical acidic food stuffs and drinks but also with actually non-erosive food such as yoghurt or other milk products, whereas other studies showed that the consumption of milk [67, 71, 78] and yoghurt [67] was associated with a lower prevalence of dental erosion, which adds to the controversy of the results. In some of the studies that could not reveal any associations between the consumption of soft drinks or other acidic beverages, the consumption was lower than in other studies or the sample sizes were small, reducing the validity of these studies. In general, there is a need for research in this field using standardised questionnaires for the collection of nutritional habits and behaviours and standardised indices for the assessment of erosion in groups with adequate sample sizes.

Drugs and Medications

Acidic drugs, medications and food supplements, such as acetylicsalicylic acid (ASA), iron tablets or vitamin supplements, are common and potentially erosive. However, the erosive potential can only occur if the contact time between teeth and the preparation is long enough. This could be the case if taken as effervescent or chewing tablets [see chapter by Hellwig and Lussi, this vol., pp. 155–162]. Other medications could potentially contribute to the development of gastric reflux or can reduce the flow of saliva, which possibly can also increase the risk for the development of erosive defects [see chapter by Hara and Zero, this vol., pp. 197–205]. However, the number of controlled epidemiological studies on this issue is small – mostly case reports have been published. A PubMed search with the terms (dental OR enamel OR dentine) AND (erosion OR tooth wear) AND (medication OR drugs) revealed 249 hits, of which only 9 were relevant; most articles were excluded since they dealt with in vitro studies, or presented review articles or case reports. Therefore, it is difficult to make final statements on the association of erosion and the intake of medications.

The intake of asthma medication in the form of inhalation aerosols has often been associated with the occurrence of dental erosion, since the content of the inhalers might have an acidic pH. Other authors attribute an oesophagus sphincter relaxation effect to the β_2-sympathomimetic agent, which might lead to a higher risk for gastroesophageal reflux. However, only 1 controlled study including 20 test and 20 control persons (mean age 13) has shown an association with the severity of erosion. In the test group, nobody showed mild erosion, one third showed moderate and two thirds showed severe erosion. On the other side no severe erosion was found in the control group but 50% had mild and 50% had moderate erosion [79]. An increased risk for developing erosion in children (age 4–16) suffering from asthma was found by McDerra et al. [80]. A further 2 studies, however, on 268 asthmatic and 1,331 healthy children (aged 12 years) [81] and on 33 asthmatic and 20 healthy adults [82], respectively, showed no differences in erosion prevalence (59% for children and 45% for adults in the asthma group, and 60 and 40%, respectively, in the control group).

The occurrence of erosion after the regular intake of ASA and vitamin C preparations has only been reported in case reports. In this context 1 study from the 1980s has indeed shown that chewing ASA tablets is highly associated with the occurrence of erosion (n = 25; erosion prevalence 100%), but not the swallowing of ASA tablets (n = 17; erosion prevalence 0%) [83].

It is also often speculated that the intake of illicit drugs leads to dental erosion due to the reduction of the saliva flow rate and the acidity of the substance itself. However, only 1 case report showed erosion in patients with illicit drug abuse [84], whereas others show an association with bruxism [85, 86] rather than with erosion.

In conclusion, no final statement about the association between drug or medication intake and the occurrence of erosion can be made, since there is not enough data from valid controlled studies available and the assumption that there is a clear association is only based on case reports.

Alcohol Use Disorders

The prevalence for alcohol use disorders in the general population worldwide is estimated at 1.7% (WHO, 2003); however, the prevalence can be much higher in developed countries, as shown for the USA in the DSM-IV survey on alcohol abuse and dependence. In this study up to 9% of younger male adults (aged 18–29) showed alcohol abuse and even 13% of this group showed alcohol dependence [87]. It is often reported that chronic alcoholism is associated with a higher prevalence of erosion, either due to the direct effect of consumed alcoholic drinks or due to the effect of regular vomiting or an alcohol-induced gastroesophageal reflux. However, the number of studies dealing with this issue is quite low and the PubMed search with the terms (dental OR enamel OR den-

tine) AND (erosion OR tooth wear) AND (alcoholism OR alcohol abuse OR alcohol misuse) revealed 21 hits, from which only 7 were relevant. The studies are very heterogeneous in index (tooth wear index, TWI, Eccles and Jenkins index, yes-no decision maker, not further specified), number of individuals (34–195) and type of recording (individual, tooth or surface based). The age of the persons investigated ranged between 20 and 68 years with a similar distribution in all studies. Only 2 of 7 studies included a control group. In these studies an increase of erosion prevalence was found in alcoholic persons compared to controls. The study of Robb and Smith [88] used the TWI, recording not only erosion but all types of wear; 92% of the persons examined showed tooth wear, whereas only 65% of the controls did so (p ≤ 0.01). If calculated on the basis of the surface-based data, 9.9% of tooth surfaces of the alcoholic patients and only 1.8% of the controls showed signs of wear (p ≤ 0.001). A similar result was found in the study of Dukic et al. [89], showing 17.3 teeth with erosive lesion per person in the alcoholic group and 6.5 in the controls (p ≤ 0.01) in a yes-no decision model. Prevalence in the other studies was 47% [90] and 33% [91] (individual based) – the latter study investigated not only the misuse of alcohol but also of illicit drugs – and 23% [92] and 49% [93] (surface based). An association with low saliva pH [89] and with symptoms of GERD or vomiting was found in 1 study [92]; 2 studies showed that the upper palatal surfaces of the front teeth were the most affected [88, 93].

Even if only few studies exist, there seems to be a tendency for an increase of wear prevalence amongst persons showing an abusive consumption of alcohol.

Occupation

It is often assumed that in the western society occupational-caused erosion is a marginal phenomenon due to occupational health and safety mea-

Table 2. Cross-sectional and non-randomized case-control studies investigating the prevalence of erosion in factory workers

Author	Country	Occupation	Test group, n	Control, n	Type of acid	Acid conc., mg/m³	Employment period
Amin et al. [133], 2001	Jordan	phosphate industry	37	31	phosphoric, sulphuric, hydrofluoric, fluosilicic,	–	9.5 years
		battery industry	24	15	sulphuric	–	11.3 years
Arowojolu [134], 2001	Nigeria	battery industry	38	67	sulphuric	–	–
Chikte and Josie-Perez [135], 1999	South Africa	electro-winning facility	103	–	sulphuric	0.3–1	4.2 (1 month–24 years)
			102	–	sulphuric	0.1–0.3	4.2 (1 month–24 years)
Chikte et al. [136], 1998	South Africa	electro-plating factory	58	–	sulphuric	–	0.25–22 years
Gamble et al. [137], 1984	USA	battery industry	245 (5 plants A–E)	–	sulphuric	–	–
			35 (A)	–	sulphuric	0.07	20.2 years
			57 (B)	–	sulphuric	0.14	4.0 years
			38 (C)	–	sulphuric	0.07	10.2 years
			59 (D)	–	sulphuric	0.27	7.5 years
			59 (E)	–	sulphuric	0.14	12.2 years
Kim and Douglass [138], 2003	Korea	34 factories (plating, galvanizing, chemical, dye, petroleum)	943	–	hydrochloric, nitric, sulphuric	–	–
Kim et al. [139], 2006	Korea	42 factories using acids	519	431	hydrochloric, nitric, sulphuric, fluoric, chloric	–	8.6 years (0–35)

Index	Results based on	Prev. test	Prev. control	Sign.	Comment
TWI	teeth (upper front)	80% (25% enamel/ 55% dentine)	47% (20% enamel/ 27% dentine)	yes	only upper front teeth were examined
TWI	teeth (upper front)	100% (54% enamel/ 46% dentine)	81% (61% enamel/ 19% dentine)	yes	most affected surfaces upper central incisors labial
	teeth	41%	3%	yes	
	indiv.	97% (21% enamel/ 76% dentine)	–	–	higher exposure leads to a higher risk for dental erosion (OR 5.5); no relation between acid exposure time and erosion
	indiv.	75% (39% enamel/ 35% dentine)	–	–	
REA	indiv.	76% (47% enamel/ 29% dentine)	–	–	22% tooth loss due to erosion => prevalence 98%; higher exposure leads to a higher risk for dental erosion (OR 5.5); no relation between acid exposure time and erosion
ten Cate	indiv.	14%	–	–	increasing risk with increasing cumulative exposure
		15%	–	–	
		27%	–	–	
		0%	–	–	
		21%	–	–	
		33%	–	–	
ten Cate	teeth	26% (17% enamel/ 8% dentine)	–	–	risk for erosion increases with exposure time; wearing masks reduces risk for erosion
ten Cate	teeth	–	–	–	OR for erosion 1.81, for severe erosion 6.42, for erosion after sulphuric acid exposure 1.94, after multiple acid exposure 3.40

Table 2. Continued

Author	Country	Occupation	Test group, n	Control, n	Type of acid	Acid conc., mg/m^3	Employment period
Lapping [140], 1964	South Africa	manufacturing, packing of sodium acid sulphate	20	–	sulphuric	–	0.25–10 years
Lynch and Bell [141], 1947	not named	manufacturing of guncotton and nitrocellulose	97	–	sulphuric, nitric	–	1 month–3.5 years
			26	–		–	1–3 months
			29	–		–	3 month–1 year
			42	–		–	1–3.5 years
Malcolm and Paul [142], 1961	UK	battery industry	78	44	sulphuric	0.8–16.6	4.9–21.3 years
		battery forming	63			3.0–16.6	
		battery charging	15			0.8–2.5	
Petersen and Gormsen [143], 1991	Germany	battery industry	61	–	sulphuric	0.4–4.1	
			15	–			≤10 years
			46	–			>10 years
Remijn et al. [144], 1982	The Netherlands	galvanizing factory	38	–	hydrochloric	>7 (27% of work-time)	–
Skogedal et al. [145], 1977	Norway	electrolytic zinc factory	12	–	sulphuric	–	2–11 years

Index	Results based on	Prev. test	Prev. control	Sign.	Comment
not named	indiv.	35%	–	–	case series of workers from the factory
not named	indiv.	44%	–	–	increasing prevalence with increasing employment period
not named	indiv.	23%	–	–	
not named	indiv.	38%	–	–	
not named	indiv.	62%	–	–	
own	indiv.	79% (46% enamel/ 33% dentine)	0%	yes	dentures due to erosion occurred often
		87% (46% enamel/ 41% dentine)			
		47% (47% enamel/ 0% dentine)			
ten Cate	indiv.	31%	–	–	severity of erosion increased with exposure time
	teeth	mean no. affected teeth (1.3 enamel/ 0.2 dentine)			
	teeth	mean no. affected teeth (0.9 enamel/ 0.4 dentine)			
ten Cate	indiv.	90% (34% enamel/ 55% dentine)	–	–	incisors only; assessment of erosion on photographs
	teeth	83% (48% enamel/ 34% dentine)			
ten Cate	indiv.	58% (8% enamel/ 50% dentine)	–	–	severity and number of eroded teeth increased with exposure time

Table 2. Continued

Author	Country	Occupation	Test group, n	Control, n	Type of acid	Acid conc., mg/m³	Employment period
Suyama et al. [146], 2010	Japan	battery industry	40	–	sulphuric	0.5–8.0	8.8 years
			28			0.5–1.0	
			8			1.0–4.0	
			4			4.0–8.0	
			15				0–4 years
			8				5–9 years
			7				10–14 years
			7				15–19 years
			3				>20 years
ten Bruggen Cate [96], 1968	Great Britain	battery, galvanizing, planting factories	555	293	various types	–	up to 40 years
		battery industry	70 (form)		sulphuric	–	
			16 (charge)		sulphuric	–	
		galvanizing factory	72 (picklers)		hydrochloric, sulphuric	–	
			35 (non-picklers)		hydrochloric, sulphuric	–	
			132 (other acids)		other acids	–	
		planting factory	76		chromic, nitric, hydrofluoric, phosphoric	–	
Tuominen et al. [147], 1991; Tuominen and Tuominen [148], 1992	Tanzania	fertilizer company	68	61	sulphuric	–	1–19 years
		industry company	20	20	sulphonic	–	1–19 years

Index	Results based on	Prev. test	Prev. control	Sign.	Comment
Japan Dental Assoc.	indiv.	23%	–	–	prevalence increased with acid concentration in the air and with employment period
		18%			
		25%			
		50%			
		0%			
		0%			
		43%			
		57%			
		67%			
ten Cate	indiv.	32% (26% enamel/ 6% dentine)	0%	–	severity of erosion increased with exposure time
		60% (41% enamel/ 19% dentine)			severity of erosion increased with exposure time
		42% (42% enamel/ 0% dentine)			severity of erosion increased with exposure time
		57% (47% enamel/ 10% dentine)			severity of erosion increased with exposure time
		20% (17% enamel/ 3% dentine)			severity of erosion increased with exposure time
		29% (27% enamel/ 2% dentine)			severity of erosion increased with exposure time
		15% (15% enamel/ 0% dentine)			severity of erosion increased with exposure time
E&J	indiv.	63%	38%	yes	prevalence of erosion increased with exposure time
E&J	indiv.	50%	15%	yes	prevalence of erosion increased with exposure time

Table 2. Continued

Author	Country	Occupation	Test group, n	Control, n	Type of acid	Acid conc., mg/m^3	Employment period
Tuominen et al. [149], 1989; Tuominen and Tuominen [150], 1991; [148], 1992	Finland	battery, galvanizing factory	76	81	sulphuric	1–5	1–39 years

E&J = Eccles and Jenkins; TWI = Smith and Knight tooth wear index; REA = rapid epidemiological assessment; OR = odds ratio; acid conc. = concentration of acid measured in the air; prev. test = prevalence in the test group suffering from GERD; prev. control = prevalence in the control group; indiv. = individuals; sign. = significance (indicates whether differences between test group and control group reached significance).

sures. However, this type of destruction of dental hard tissue still occurs in persons working in battery, galvanizing or plating factories; also, persons working as sommeliers or in chemical, pharmaceutical or biotechnological labs or enterprises might be regularly exposed to acids and are therefore at higher risk for dental erosion.

Most of the studies dealing with occupational erosion were performed on workers in battery and galvanizing factories. Those workers are regularly exposed to sulphuric acid and therefore at high risk for dental erosion. The effect of the exposure to other acids, such as hydrochloric, hydrofluoric, nitric or phosphoric acid, was more seldomly analysed. The PubMed search with the terms (dental OR enamel OR dentine) AND (erosion OR tooth wear) AND (occupational OR workers) revealed 90 hits, of which 21 were relevant dealing with the topic of factory workers (table 2) and 3 dealing with the topic of winemakers.

Most of the publications found dealing with factory workers present uncontrolled studies; however, some of them show very high prevalence of erosion in persons working daily with acids. In the older studies, loss of teeth due to erosive lesions was a commonly mentioned condition, possibly leading to an underestimation of the prevalence in these studies. Often, an association between the duration of employ-

ment as well as the concentration of acid in the air or a short distance between worker and acid source and the severity of erosion was found. However, one has to bear in mind that most of the studies are relatively old or have been performed in developing countries. In the past and in particular in developing countries occupational safety measures are often rare and the limit for the maximum allowable concentration of acids in the air in these countries is often higher, probably leading to higher prevalence values in these countries or in older studies. Indeed, most studies have revealed that persons using no or only limited occupational safety measures show severe defects more often. In addition to the data summarised in table 2, there are some isolated studies showing an increased risk for dental erosion for employees working with silicone [94] or proteolytic enzymes [95], at soft drink or munitions factories or as cleaners of dyestuff containers [96].

The potential of wine to cause dental erosion is a result of its fruit-acid content, with tartaric and malic acids being the most abundant [97, 98]. The low pH of wine, which is reported to range from 3 to 4 [99–101] and the low concentrations of P and Ca ions [102] are also of importance for the erosive effect of wine. In addition to the acidity of the wine, tasting habits among the wine tast-

Index	Results based on	Prev. test	Prev. control	Sign.	Comment
E&J	indiv.	26% (12% enamel/ 14% dentine)	11% (6% enamel/ 5% dentine)	yes	prevalence of erosion increased with exposure time

ers are an additional risk factor for dental erosion. Each mouthful of wine is kept and swilled around in the mouth for many seconds which is a more pronounced challenge for the enamel compared with normal drinking habits. In addition, each tasting session last for hours and 20–40 different wines could be tested during a session [97, 101, 103, 104].

Although professional wine tasting is very common all over the world, there are only few case reports [97, 101, 103] and studies, most with a small number of cases, investigating the association between wine intake and dental erosive wear [99, 100, 104].

In a prevalence survey involving 19 Swedish wine tasters, erosive tooth wear was found in 74% of the participants [99]. Of those persons showing erosion, 37% (n = 7) showed erosion in enamel, less than one third of dentine was involved in 26% of cases (n = 5) and 11% (n = 2) had severe tooth erosion (more than one third into dentine). The lesions were mainly found on the labiocervical surfaces of maxillary incisors and canines. The length of time the subjects had been employed as wine tasters varied from 2 to 37 years with a median value of 7 years. The frequency of wine tasting sessions each week varied with the individual, from only 2 to 5 a week. They stated that the occurrence of erosion among full-time wine tasters

was very high and that erosion is an occupational risk for wine tasters [99].

In another study [100], tooth surface loss among 21 winemakers in South Africa was investigated. Only 3 subjects (14%) exhibited erosive tooth wear, but this was 2.5 times greater compared to a non-exposed group. The severity of the exposed dentine was twice that of the non-exposed group. The wine tastings ranged from several tastings per week to 50–150 tastings per day [100].

At a state-owned Norwegian alcoholic beverage retailer, 18 wine tasters were examined for recording possible dental erosions [104]. These wine tasters test all wines for quality, taste and flavour before approval for sale and perform tasting sessions on average on 60 days per year plus a full 10-day course a year involving several wine tasting sessions per day. Erosive wear was recorded in 50% (n = 9) of the wine tasters and in 20% (n = 6) of a comparison group (p = 0.03). The majority of the lesions of the wine tasters involved dentine, while in the comparison group most erosive wear was confined to enamel. There was no statistically significant difference between severity, number of dental erosions and years in the occupation [104].

There are some anecdotic case reports on the harmful effect of regular swimming in chlorinated swimming pool water, showing a rapid loss of dental hard tissue in a very short time [105, 106]. It is assumed that non-buffered swimming pool water can lead to dental erosion, in particular in competitive swimmers, since it might have a low pH and might be under-saturated with respect to hydroxyapatite. However, epidemiological studies on this issue are rare and only 4 studies were found. In a study from India investigating 100 18-year-old swimmers, a high prevalence of erosion (90%) was found; however, no control group was included and no information on the index used, the diagnostic criteria used and the control of the pH of the swimming pool water was given. In 2 other studies from Poland and from the USA, an increase of erosion occurrence was found compared to a control group. However, the prevalence in both studies was generally low (Poland: 26 vs. 10% [107]; USA: 13 vs. 0% [108]). In the last study found, prevalence of tooth wear of 100% (64% of lesions in enamel, 36% of lesions in dentine) was reported [75], but the study did not clearly describe which kind of non-carious-caused substance loss was assessed (TWI, no clear definition of diagnosis criteria). Additionally, a high consumption of acidic sports drinks by the swimmers was recorded, making it difficult to attribute the high prevalence of tooth wear to regular swimming in chlorinated pool water. Therefore, no final conclusion can be made on this issue. It is unlikely that teeth are damaged by well-buffered and pH-controlled chlorinated water; if the pH and the buffering capacity, however, are not controlled and therefore low, the water might pose a risk.

Conclusion

The literature covering the prevalence in risk groups was in some cases scarce, and the results were often contradictory and sometimes uncertain due to the use of different indices and small study groups. However, some links were found. In the case of GERD, erosion seems to be more common and in particular more severe than in healthy controls. Eating disorders are associated with an increased occurrence, severity and risk for dental erosion related to both exogenous and endogenous acids. In particular, the regular impact of gastric juice in the case of vomiting seems to be the major risk factor for developing erosion in those persons.

From epidemiological studies dealing with special diet (e.g. vegetarians), no clear correlation between erosive wear and diet could be found. In most of the studies dealing with the consumption of acidic beverages and dental erosions, a positive association was documented. No association between drug or medication intake and the occurrence of erosion could be found due to lack of data from valid controlled studies. Though only few studies exist, there seems to be a tendency for an increase of erosive wear prevalence amongst persons showing an abusive consumption of alcohol. Most of the publications dealing with factory workers present uncontrolled studies; however, some show a very high prevalence of erosion in persons working daily with acids. The occurrence of erosion among full-time wine tasters is higher than in a comparison group.

The reason why not all persons at high risk have erosive lesion indicates that people have different susceptibility for erosions. It is possible that saliva factors and tooth surface composition may be at least as important as the frequency of acid attack.

In general, there is a need for more research in this field, using standardised questionnaires for the collection of nutrition habits and behaviours and standardised indices for the assessment of erosions in groups with adequate sample sizes.

References

1 Rothman KJ: Epidemiology: An Introduction. New York, Oxford University Press, 2002.
2 Burt BA: Concepts of risk in dental public health. Community Dent Oral Epidemiol 2005;33:240–247.
3 Beck JD: Risk revisited. Community Dent Oral Epidemiol 1998;26:220–225.
4 Moayyedi P, Delaney B: GORD in adults. Clin Evid (online) 2008;2008:pii0403.
5 Jones R, Galmiche JP: Review: what do we mean by GERD? – definition and diagnosis. Aliment Pharmacol Ther 2005;22(suppl 1):2–10.
6 Sonnenberg A, El-Serag HB: Clinical epidemiology and natural history of gastroesophageal reflux disease. Yale J Biol Med 1999;72:81–92.
7 Fass R, Dickman R: Clinical consequences of silent gastroesophageal reflux disease. Curr Gastroenterol Rep 2006;8:195–201.
8 Hudson JI, Hiripi E, Pope HG Jr, Kessler RC: The prevalence and correlates of eating disorders in the National Comorbidity Survey Replication. Biol Psychiatry 2007;61:348–358.
9 Swanson SA, Crow SJ, Le GD, Swendsen J, Merikangas KR: Prevalence and correlates of eating disorders in adolescents. Results from the national comorbidity survey replication adolescent supplement. Arch Gen Psychiatry 2011;68:714–723.
10 Gotestam KG, Agras WS: General population-based epidemiological study of eating disorders in Norway. Int J Eat Disord 1995;18:119–126.
11 Kjelsas E, Bjornstrom C, Gotestam KG: Prevalence of eating disorders in female and male adolescents (14–15 years). Eat Behav 2004;5:13–25.
12 Lahteenmaki S, Saarni S, Suokas J, Saarni S, Perala J, Lonnqvist J, et al: Prevalence and correlates of eating disorders among young adults in Finland. Nord J Psychiatry, Epub ahead of print.
13 Jaite C, Hoffmann F, Glaeske G, Bachmann CJ: Prevalence, comorbidities and outpatient treatment of anorexia and bulimia nervosa in German children and adolescents. Eat Weight Disord 2013;18:157–165.
14 Micali N, Hagberg KW, Petersen I, Treasure JL: The incidence of eating disorders in the UK in 2000–2009: findings from the General Practice Research Database. BMJ Open 2013;3:e002646.

15 Bartlett DW, Coward PY: Comparison of the erosive potential of gastric juice and a carbonated drink in vitro. J Oral Rehab 2001;28:1045–1047.
16 Hellström I: Oral complications in anorexia nervosa. Scand J Dent Res 1977;85:71–86.
17 Milosevic A, Slade PD: The orodental status of anorexics and bulimics. Br Dent J 1989;197:66–70.
18 Robb ND, Smith BG, Geidrys LE: The distribution of erosion in the dentitions of patients with eating disorders. Br Dent J 1995;178:171–175.
19 Rytömaa I, Järvinen V, Kanerva R, Heinonen OP: Bulimia and tooth erosion. Acta Odontol Scand 1998;56:36–40.
20 Öhrn R, Enzell K, Angmar-Månsson B: Oral status of 81 subjects with eating disorders. Eur J Oral Sci 1999;107:157–163.
21 Emodi-Perlman A, Yoffe T, Rosenberg N, Eli I, Alter Z, Winocur E: Prevalence of psychologic, dental, and temporomandibular signs and symptoms among chronic eating disorders patients: a comparative control study. J Orofac Pain 2008;22:201–208.
22 Dynesen AW, Bardow A, Petersson B, Nielsen LR, Nauntofte B: Salivary changes and dental erosion in bulimia nervosa. Oral Surg Oral Med Oral Pathol Oral Radiol Endod 2008;106:696–707.
23 Johansson AK, Norring C, Unell L, Johansson A: Eating disorders and oral health: a matched case-control study. Eur J Oral Sci 2012;120:61–68.
24 Hermont AP, Pordeus IA, Paiva SM, Abreu MH, Auad SM: Eating disorder risk behavior and dental implications among adolescents. Int J Eat Disord 2013;46:677–683.
25 Holst JJ, Lange F: Perimylolysis. A contribution towards the genesis of tooth wasting from nonmechanical causes. Acta Odontol Scand 1939;1:36.
26 Mulic A, Skudutyte-Rysstad R, Tveit AB, Skaare AB: Risk indicators for dental erosive wear among 18-year-old subjects in Oslo, Norway. Eur J Oral Sci 2012;120:531–538.
27 Touyz SW, Liew VP, Tseng P, Frisken K, Williams H, Beumont PJ: Oral and dental complications in dieting disorders. Int J Eat Disord 1993;14:341–347.

28 Milosevic A, Brodie DA, Slade PD: Dental erosion, oral hygiene, and nutrition in eating disorders. Int J Eat Disord 1997;21:195–199.
29 Ruby MB: Vegetarianism. A blossoming field of study. Appetite 2012;58:141–150.
30 Max Rubner-Institut: Nationale Verzehrsstudie II; Ergebnisbericht Teil 1. Bundesforschungsinstitut für Ernährung und Lebensmittel, 2008.
31 Farmer B, Larson BT, Fulgoni VL III, Rainville AJ, Liepa GU: A vegetarian dietary pattern as a nutrient-dense approach to weight management: an analysis of the national health and nutrition examination survey 1999–2004. J Am Diet Assoc 2011;111:819–827.
32 Ganss C, Schlechtriemen M, Klimek J: Dental erosions in subjects living on a raw food diet. Caries Res 1999;33:74–80.
33 Lussi A, Schaffner M, Hotz P, Suter P: Dental erosion in a population of Swiss adults. Community Dent Oral Epidemiol 1991;19:286–290.
34 Järvinen VK, Rytömaa I, Heinonen OP: Risk factors in dental erosion. J Dent Res 1991;70:942–947.
35 Linkosalo E, Markkanen H: Dental erosions in relation to lactovegetarian diet. Scand J Dent Res 1985;93:436–441.
36 Al-Dlaigan YH, Shaw L, Smith AJ: Vegetarian children and dental erosion. Int J Paediatr Dent 2001;11:184–192.
37 Herman K, Czajczynska-Waszkiewicz A, Kowalczyk-Zajac M, Dobrzynski M: Assessment of the influence of vegetarian diet on the occurrence of erosive and abrasive cavities in hard tooth tissues. Postepy Hig Med Dosw (online) 2011;65:764–769.
38 Linkosalo E, Syrjanen S, Alakuijala P: Salivary composition and dental erosions in lacto-ovo-vegetarians. Proc Finn Dent Soc 1988;84:253–260.
39 Rafeek RN, Marchan S, Eder A, Smith WA: Tooth surface loss in adult subjects attending a university dental clinic in Trinidad. Int Dent J 2006;56:181–186.
40 Smith WA, Marchan S, Rafeek RN: The prevalence and severity of non-carious cervical lesions in a group of patients attending a university hospital in Trinidad. J Oral Rehabil 2008;35:128–134.
41 Jacobson MF: Liquid Candy – How Soft Drinks Are Harming Americans' Health. Washington, Center for Science in the Public Interest, 2005.

42 Lussi A, Jaeggi T, Zero D: The role of diet in the aetiology of dental erosion. Caries Res 2004;38(suppl 1):34–44.

43 UNESDA: Statistics on the consumption of non-alcoholic beverages in Europe. 2013. http://www.unesda.org/industry.

44 Max Rubner-Institut: Nationale Verzehrsstudie II; Ergebnisbericht Teil 2. Bundesforschungsinstitut für Ernährung und Lebensmittel, 2008.

45 Margaritis V, Mamai-Homata E, Koletsi-Kounari H, Polychronopoulou A: Evaluation of three different scoring systems for dental erosion: a comparative study in adolescents. J Dent 2011; 39:88–93.

46 Okunseri C, Okunseri E, Gonzalez C, Visotcky A, Szabo A: Erosive tooth wear and consumption of beverages among children in the United States. Caries Res 2011;45:130–135.

47 Johansson AK, Lingström P, Imfeld T, Birkhed D: Influence of drinking method on tooth-surface pH in relation to dental erosion. Eur J Oral Sci 2004;112: 484–489.

48 Johansson AK, Lingstrom P, Birkhed D: Comparison of factors potentially related to the occurrence of dental erosion in high- and low-erosion groups. Eur J Oral Sci 2002;110:204–211.

49 Moazzez R, Smith BGN, Bartlett DW: Oral pH and drinking habit during ingestion of a carbonated drink in a group of adolescents with dental erosion. J Dent 2000;28:395–397.

50 O'Sullivan EA, Curzon ME: A comparison of acidic dietary factors in children with and without dental erosion. ASDC J Dent Child 2000;67:186–192.

51 Millward A, Shaw L, Smith AJ, Rippin JW, Harrington E: The distribution and severity of tooth wear and the relationship between erosion and dietary constituents in a group of children. Int J Paediatr Dent 1994;4:151–157.

52 Dugmore CR, Rock WP: A multifactorial analysis of factors associated with dental erosion. Br Dent J 2004;196:283–286.

53 Jensdottir T, Arnadottir IB, Thorsdottir I, Bardow A, Gudmundsson K, Theodors A, et al: Relationship between dental erosion, soft drink consumption, and gastroesophageal reflux among Icelanders. Clin Oral Invest 2004;8:91–96.

54 El Karim IA, Sanhouri NM, Hashim NT, Ziada HM: Dental erosion among 12–14 year-old school children in Khartoum: a pilot study. Community Dent Health 2007;24:176–180.

55 Waterhouse PJ, Auad SM, Nunn JH, Steen IN, Moynihan PJ: Diet and dental erosion in young people in south-east Brazil. Int J Paediatr Dent 2008;18:353–360.

56 Correr GM, Alonso RC, Correa MA, Campos EA, Baratto-Filho F, Puppin-Rontani RM: Influence of diet and salivary characteristics on the prevalence of dental erosion among 12-year-old schoolchildren. J Dent Child (Chic) 2009;76:181–187.

57 Bardolia P, Burnside G, Ashcroft A, Milosevic A, Goodfellow SA, Rolfe EA, et al: Prevalence and risk indicators of erosion in thirteen- to fourteen-year-olds on the Isle of Man. Caries Res 2010;44: 165–168.

58 Ratnayake N, Ekanayake L: Prevalence and distribution of tooth wear among Sri Lankan adolescents. Oral Health Prev Dent 2010;8:331–337.

59 Wang P, Lin HC, Chen JH, Liang HY: The prevalence of dental erosion and associated risk factors in 12–13-year-old school children in Southern China. BMC Public Health 2010;10:478.

60 Huew R, Waterhouse PJ, Moynihan PJ, Kometa S, Maguire A: Dental erosion and its association with diet in Libyan schoolchildren. Eur Arch Paediatr Dent 2011;12:234–240.

61 Fung A, Brearley ML: Tooth wear and associated risk factors in a sample of Australian primary school children. Aust Dent J 2013;58:235–245.

62 Isaksson H, Birkhed D, Wendt LK, Alm A, Nilsson M, Koch G: Prevalence of dental erosion and association with lifestyle factors in Swedish 20-year-olds. Acta Odontol Scand, Epub ahead of print.

63 Al-Dlaigan YH, Shaw L, Smith A: Dental erosion in a group of British 14-year-old school children. Part II. Influence of dietary intake. Br Dent J 2001;190:258–261.

64 Milosevic A, Bardsley PF, Taylor S: Epidemiological studies of tooth wear and dental erosion in 14-year-old children in North West England. Part 2. The association of diet and habits. Br Dent J 2004;197:479–483.

65 Abu-Ghazaleh SB, Burnside G, Milosevic A: The prevalence and associated risk factors for tooth wear and dental erosion in 15- to 16-year-old schoolchildren in Amman, Jordan. Eur Arch Paediatr Dent 2013;14:21–27.

66 van Rijkom HM, Truin GJ, Frencken JE, König KG, van't Hof MA, Bronkhorst EM, et al: Prevalence, distribution and background variables of smooth-bordered tooth wear in teenagers in the Hague, the Netherlands. Caries Res 2001;36:147–154.

67 El Aidi H, Bronkhorst EM, Huysmans MC, Truin GJ: Multifactorial analysis of factors associated with the incidence and progression of erosive tooth wear. Caries Res 2011;45:303–312.

68 Bartlett DW, Coward PY, Nikkah C, Wilson RF: The prevalence of tooth wear in a cluster sample of adolescent schoolchildren and its relationship with potential explanatory factors. Br Dent J 1998;184:125–129.

69 Williams D, Croucher R, Marcenes W, O'Farrell M: The prevalence of dental erosion in the maxillary incisors of 14-year-old schoolchildren living in Tower Hamlets and Hackney, London, UK. Int Dent J 1999;49:211–216.

70 Sirimaharaj V, Brearley ML, Morgan MV: Acidic diet and dental erosion among athletes. Aust Dent J 2002;47: 228–236.

71 Manaf ZA, Lee MT, Ali NH, Samynathan S, Jie YP, Ismail NH, et al: Relationship between food habits and tooth erosion occurrence in Malaysian University students. Malays J Med Sci 2012;19:56–66.

72 British Soft Drinks Association: The 2012 UK soft drinks report. London, 2012.

73 Coombes JS: Sports drinks and dental erosion. Am J Dent 2005;18:101–104.

74 Mathew T, Casamassimo PS, Hayes JR: Relationship between sports drinks and dental erosion in 304 university athletes in Columbus, Ohio, USA. Caries Res 2002;36:281–287.

75 Milosevic A, Kelly MJ, McLean AN: Sports supplement drinks and dental health in competitive swimmers and cyclists. Br Dent J 1997;182:303–308.

76 Lussi A, Schaffner M: Progression of and risk factors for dental erosion and wedge-shaped defects over a 6-year period. Caries Res 2000;34:182–187.

77 Arnadottir IB, Saemundsson SR, Holbrook WP: Dental erosion in Icelandic teenagers in relation to dietary and lifestyle factors. Acta Odontol Scand 2003; 61:25–28.

78 Nahas Pires Correa MS, Nahas Pires CF, Nahas Pires Correa JP, Murakami C, Mendes FM: Prevalence and associated factors of dental erosion in children and adolescents of a private dental practice. Int J Paediatr Dent 2011;21:451–458.

79   Al-Dlaigan YH, Shaw L, Smith AJ: Is there a relationship between asthma and dental erosion? A case control study. Int J Paediatr Dent 2002;12:189–200.

80   McDerra EJ, Pollard MA, Curzon ME: The dental status of asthmatic British school children. Pediatr Dent 1998;20: 281–287.

81   Dugmore CR, Rock WP: Asthma and tooth erosion. Is there an association? Int J Paediatr Dent 2003;13:417–424.

82   Stensson M, Wendt LK, Koch G, Oldaeus G, Ramberg P, Birkhed D: Oral health in young adults with long-term, controlled asthma. Acta Odontol Scand 2011;69:158–164.

83   Sullivan RE, Kramer WS: Iatrogenic erosion of teeth. ASDC J Dent Child 1983; 50:192–196.

84   Bassiouny MA: Dental erosion due to abuse of illicit drugs and acidic carbonated beverages. Gen Dent 2013;61:38–44.

85   Milosevic A, Agrawal N, Redfearn P, Mair L: The occurrence of toothwear in users of Ecstasy (3,4-methylenedioxymethamphetamine). Community Dent Oral Epidemiol 1999;27:283–287.

86   Nixon PJ, Youngson CC, Beese A: Tooth surface loss: does recreational drug use contribute? Clin Oral Investig 2002;6: 128–130.

87   Grant BF, Dawson DA, Stinson FS, Chou SP, Dufour MC, Pickering RP: The 12-month prevalence and trends in DSM-IV alcohol abuse and dependence: United States, 1991–1992 and 2001–2002. Drug Alcohol Depend 2004;74: 223–234.

88   Robb ND, Smith BG: Prevalence of pathological tooth wear in patients with chronic alcoholism. Br Dent J 1990;169: 367–369.

89   Dukic W, Dobrijevic TT, Katunaric M, Milardovic S, Segovic S: Erosive lesions in patients with alcoholism. J Am Dent Assoc 2010;141:1452–1458.

90   Araujo MW, Dermen K, Connors G, Ciancio S: Oral and dental health among inpatients in treatment for alcohol use disorders: a pilot study. J Int Acad Periodontol 2004;6:125–130.

91   Almas K, Al Wazzan K, Al Hussain I, Al-Ahdal KY, Khan NB: Temporomandibular joint status, occlusal attrition, cervical erosion and facial pain among substance abusers. Odontostomatol Trop 2007;30:27–33.

92   Hede B: Determinants of oral health in a group of Danish alcoholics. Eur J Oral Sci 1996;104:403–408.

93   Manarte P, Manso MC, Souza D, Frias-Bulhosa J, Gago S: Dental erosion in alcoholic patients under addiction rehabilitation therapy. Med Oral Patol Oral Cir Bucal 2009;14:e376–e383.

94   Johansson AK, Johansson A, Stan V, Ohlson CG: Silicone sealers, acetic acid vapours and dental erosion: a work-related risk? Swed Dent J 2005;29:61–69.

95   Westergaard J, Larsen IB, Holmen L, Larsen AI, Jorgensen B, Holmstrup P, et al: Occupational exposure to airborne proteolytic enzymes and lifestyle risk factors for dental erosion – a cross-sectional study. Occup Med (Lond) 2001;51:189–197.

96   ten Bruggen Cate HJ: Dental erosion in industry. Br J Ind Med 1968;25:249–266.

97   Ferguson MM, Dunbar RJ, Smith JA, Wall JG: Enamel erosion related to winemaking. Occup Med (Lond) 1996; 46:159–162.

98   Mok TB, McIntyre J, Hunt D: Dental erosion: in vitro model of wine assessor's erosion. Aust Dent J 2001;46: 263–268.

99   Wiktorsson AM, Zimmerman M, Angmar-Månsson B: Erosive tooth wear: prevalence and severity in Swedish winetasters. Eur J Oral Sci 1997;105: 544–550.

100 Chikte UM, Naidoo S, Kolze TJ, Grobler SR: Patterns of tooth surface loss among winemakers. SADJ 2005; 60:370–374.

101 Gray A, Ferguson MM, Wall JG: Wine tasting and dental erosion. Case report. Aust Dent J 1998;43:32–34.

102 Lussi A, Megert B, Shellis RP, Wang X: Analysis of the erosive effect of different dietary substances and medications. Br J Nutr 2012;107:252–262.

103 Chaudhry SI, Harris JL, Challacombe SJ: Dental erosion in a wine merchant: an occupational hazard? Br Dent J 1997;182:226–228.

104 Mulic A, Tveit AB, Hove LH, Skaare AB: Dental erosive wear among Norwegian wine tasters. Acta Odontol Scand 2011;69:21–26.

105 Dawes C, Boroditsky CL: Rapid and severe tooth erosion from swimming in an improperly chlorinated pool: case report. J Can Dent Assoc 2008;74:359–361.

106 Jahangiri L, Pigliacelli S, Kerr AR: Severe and rapid erosion of dental enamel from swimming: a clinical report. J Prosthet Dent 2011;106:219–223.

107 Buczkowska-Radlinska J, Lagocka R, Kaczmarek W, Gorski M, Nowicka A: Prevalence of dental erosion in adolescent competitive swimmers exposed to gas-chlorinated swimming pool water. Clin Oral Investig 2013;17:579–583.

108 Centerwall BS, Armstrong CW, Funkhouser LS, Elzay RP: Erosion of dental enamel among competitive swimmers at a gas-chlorinated swimming pool. Am J Epidemiol 1986;123:641–647.

109 Ersin NK, Oncag O, Tumgor G, Aydogdu S, Hilmioglu S: Oral and dental manifestations of gastroesophageal reflux disease in children: a preliminary study. Pediatr Dent 2006;28:279–284.

110 Farahmand F, Sabbaghian M, Ghodousi S, Seddighoraee N, Abbasi M: Gastroesophageal reflux disease and tooth erosion: a cross-sectional observational study. Gut Liver 2013;7:278–281.

111 Linnett V, Seow WK, Connor F, Shepherd R: Oral health of children with gastro-esophageal reflux disease: a controlled study. Aust Dent J 2002;47: 156–162.

112 Murakami C, Oliveira LB, Sheiham A, Nahas Pires Correa MS, Haddad AE, Bonecker M: Risk indicators for erosive tooth wear in Brazilian preschool children. Caries Res 2011;45:121–129.

113 Nunn JH, Gordon PH, Morris AJ, Pine CM, Walker A: Dental erosion – changing prevalence? A review of British National children's surveys. Int J Paediatr Dent 2003;13:98–105.

114 Vargas-Ferreira F, Praetzel JR, Ardenghi TM: Prevalence of tooth erosion and associated factors in 11–14-year-old Brazilian schoolchildren. J Public Health Dent 2011;71:6–12.

115 Wild YK, Heyman MB, Vittinghoff E, Dalal DH, Wojcicki JM, Clark AL, et al: Gastroesophageal reflux is not associated with dental erosion in children. Gastroenterology 2011;141:1605–1611.

116 Aine L, Baer M, Mäki M: Dental erosions caused by gastroesophageal reflux disease in children. J Dent Child 1993;60:210–214.

117 Dahshan A, Patel H, Delaney J, Wuerth A, Thomas R, Tolia V: Gastroesophageal reflux disease and dental erosion in children. J Pediatr 2002;140:474–478.

118 O'Sullivan EA, Curzon ME, Roberts GJ, Milla PJ, Stringer MD: Gastroesophageal reflux in children and its relationship to erosion of primary and permanent teeth. Eur J Oral Sci 1998;106: 765–769.

119 Benages A, Muñoz JV, Sanchiz V, Mora F, Minguez M: Dental erosion as extraoesophageal manifestation of gastro-oesophageal reflux. Gut 2006;55: 1050–1551.

120 Correa MC, Lerco MM, Cunha ML, Henry MA: Salivary parameters and teeth erosions in patients with gastroesophageal reflux disease. Arq Gastroenterol 2012;49:214–218.

121 Di Fede O, Di LC, Occhipinti G, Vigneri S, Lo RL, Fedele S, et al: Oral manifestations in patients with gastro-oesophageal reflux disease: a single-center case-control study. J Oral Pathol Med 2008;37:336–340.

122 Gregory-Head BL, Curtis DA, Kim L, Cello J: Evaluation of dental erosion in patients with gastroesophageal reflux disease. J Prosthet Dent 2000;83:675–680.

123 Moazzez R, Anggiansah A, Bartlett DW: The association of acidic reflux above the upper oesophageal sphincter with palatal tooth wear. Caries Res 2005;39:475–478.

124 Moazzez R, Bartlett D, Anggiansah A: Dental erosion, gastro-oesophageal reflux disease and saliva: how are they related? J Dent 2004;32:489–494.

125 Muñoz JV, Herreros B, Sanchiz V, Amoros C, Hernandez V, Pascual I, et al: Dental and periodontal lesions in patients with gastro-oesophageal reflux disease. Dig Liver Dis 2003;35:461–467.

126 Oginni AO, Agbakwuru EA, Ndububa DA: The prevalence of dental erosion in Nigerian patients with gastro-oesophageal reflux disease. BMC Oral Health 2005;5:1–6.

127 Schroeder PL, Filler SJ, Ramirez B, Lazarchik DA, Vaezi MF, Richter JE: Dental erosion and acid reflux disease. Ann Intern Med 1995;122:809–815.

128 Tantbirojn D, Pintado MR, Versluis A, Dunn C, DeLong R: Quantitative analysis of tooth surface loss associated with gastroesophageal reflux disease: a longitudinal clinical study. J Am Dent Assoc 2012;143:278–285.

129 Wang GR, Zhang H, Wang ZG, Jiang GS, Guo CH: Relationship between dental erosion and respiratory symptoms in patients with gastro-oesophageal reflux disease. J Dent 2010;38:892–898.

130 Yoshikawa H, Furuta K, Ueno M, Egawa M, Yoshino A, Kondo S, et al: Oral symptoms including dental erosion in gastroesophageal reflux disease are associated with decreased salivary flow volume and swallowing function. J Gastroenterol 2012;47:412–420.

131 Järvinen V, Meurman JH, Hyvarinen H, Rytömaa I, Murtomaa H: Dental erosion and upper gastrointestinal disorders. Oral Surg Oral Med Oral Pathol 1988;65:298–303.

132 Meurman JH, Toskala J, Nuutinen P, Klemetti E: Oral and dental manifestations in gastroesophageal reflux disease. Oral Surg Oral Med Oral Pathol 1994;78:583–589.

133 Amin WM, Al-Omoush SA, Hattab FN: Oral health status of workers exposed to acid fumes in phosphate and battery industries in Jordan. Int Dent J 2001; 51:169–174.

134 Arowojolu MO: Erosion of tooth enamel surfaces among battery chargers and automobile mechanics in Ibadan: a comparative study. Afr J Med Med Sci 2001;30:5–8.

135 Chikte UM, Josie-Perez AM: Industrial dental erosion: a cross-sectional, comparative study. SADJ 1999;54:531–536.

136 Chikte UM, Josie-Perez AM, Cohen TL: A rapid epidemiological assessment of dental erosion to assist in settling an industrial dispute. J Dent Assoc S Afr 1998;53:7–12.

137 Gamble J, Jones W, Hancock J, Meckstroth RL: Epidemiological-environmental study of lead acid battery workers. III. Chronic effects of sulfuric acid on the respiratory system and teeth. Environ Res 1984;35:30–52.

138 Kim H-D, Douglass CW: Associations between occupational health behaviors and occupational dental erosion. J Public Health Dent 2003;63:244–249.

139 Kim H-D, Hong YC, Koh D, Paik DI: Occupational exposure to acidic chemicals and occupational dental erosion. J Public Health Dent 2006;66:205–208.

140 Lapping D: Dental erosion in a South African chemical industry. S Afr Med J 1964;38:15–16.

141 Lynch JB, Bell J: Dental erosion in workers exposed to inorganic acid fumes. Br J Ind Med 1947;4:84–86.

142 Malcolm D, Paul E: Erosion of the teeth due to sulphuric acid in the battery industry. Brit J Ind Med 1961;18: 63–69.

143 Petersen PE, Gormsen C: Oral conditions among German battery factory workers. Community Dent Oral Epidemiol 1991;19:104–106.

144 Remijn B, Koster P, Houthuijs D, Boleij J, Willems H, Brunekreef B, et al: Zinc chloride, zinc oxide, hydrochloric acid exposure and dental erosion in a zinc galvanizing plant in the Netherlands. Ann Occup Hyg 1982;25:299–307.

145 Skogedal O, Silness J, Tangerud T, Laegreid O, Gilhuus-Moe O: Pilot study on dental erosion in a Norwegian electrolytic zinc factory. Community Dent Oral Epidemiol 1977;5:248–251.

146 Suyama Y, Takaku S, Okawa Y, Matsukubo T: Erosion in workers exposed to sulfuric acid in lead storage battery manufacturing facility. Bull Tokyo Dent Coll 2010;51:77–83.

147 Tuominen ML, Tuominen RJ, Fubusa F, Mgalula N: Tooth surface loss and exposure to organic and inorganic acid fumes in workplace air. Community Dent Oral Epidemiol 1991;19:217–220.

148 Tuominen M, Tuominen R: Tooth surface loss and associated factors among factory workers in Finland and Tanzania. Community Dent Health 1992;9: 143–150.

149 Tuominen M, Tuominen R, Ranta K, Ranta H: Association between acid fumes in the work environment and dental erosion. Scand J Work Environ Health 1989;15:335–338.

150 Tuominen M, Tuominen R: Dental erosion and associated factors among factory workers exposed to inorganic acid fumes. Proc Finn Dent Soc 1991; 87:359–364.

PD Dr. N. Schlueter
Department of Conservative and Preventive Dentistry
Dental Clinic, Justus Liebig University Giessen, Schlangenzahl 14
DE–35392 Giessen (Germany)
E-Mail nadine.schlueter@dentist.med.uni-giessen.de

Lussi A, Ganss C (eds): Erosive Tooth Wear. Monogr Oral Sci. Basel, Karger, 2014, vol 25, pp 99–107
DOI: 10.1159/000359939

The Histological Features and Physical Properties of Eroded Dental Hard Tissues

Carolina Ganss[a] · Adrian Lussi[b] · Nadine Schlueter[a]

[a]Department of Conservative and Preventive Dentistry, Dental Clinic, Justus Liebig University Giessen, Giessen, Germany; [b]Department of Preventive, Restorative and Pediatric Dentistry, School of Dental Medicine, University of Bern, Bern, Switzerland

Abstract

Erosive demineralisation causes characteristic histological features. In enamel, mineral is dissolved from the surface, resulting in a roughened structure similar to an etching pattern. If the acid impact continues, the initial surface mineral loss turns into bulk tissue loss and with time a visible defect can develop. The microhardness of the remaining surface is reduced, increasing the susceptibility to physical wear. The histology of eroded dentine is much more complex because the mineral component of the tissue is dissolved by acids whereas the organic part is remaining. At least in experimental erosion, a distinct zone of demineralised organic material develops, the thickness of which depends on the acid impact. This structure is of importance for many aspects, e.g. the progression rate or the interaction with active agents and physical impacts, and needs to be considered when quantifying mineral loss. The histology of experimental erosion is increasingly well understood, but there is lack of knowledge about the histology of in vivo lesions. For enamel erosion, it is reasonable to assume that the principal features may be similar, but the fate of the demineralised dentine matrix in the oral cavity is unclear. As dentine lesions normally appear hard clinically, it can be assumed that it is degraded by the variety of enzymes present in the oral cavity. Erosive tooth wear may lead to the formation of reactionary or reparative dentine.

© 2014 S. Karger AG, Basel

Erosive wear occurs from the interaction of dental hard tissue surfaces with the surrounding liquid phase and, in the oral environment, with various physical impacts. These interactions are complex and erosive loss is not simply increased by physical forces; rather, the histological changes occurring from acid impacts are the prerequisite that physiological forces (e.g. from chewing or normal physical impacts like adequate toothbrushing) can cause lesions of a clinically typical shape. The histological features of such lesions require specific strategies for prevention or non-invasive therapy that differ fundamentally from those of a carious lesion. Thus, understanding the character of eroded dental hard tissues is essential for applying and developing suitable causal and symptomatic measures.

The histology of sound enamel has been extensively investigated [1]. It is a non-vital, densely packed mineralised structure which is mainly composed of calcium and phosphate in the form of a non-stoichiometric hydroxyapatite. The mineral is organised in rods of hexagonal structure. The dimension of these crystals is difficult to measure, but values for width and thickness in the order of 50–70 and 20–25 nm, respectively, have been published [2]. Other components of

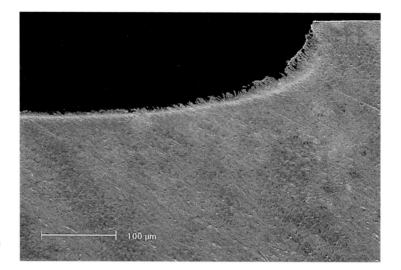

Fig. 1. Cross section (embedded, cut and polished) of an enamel sample from an in vitro experiment [6]. Erosion was performed with 1% citric acid (6 × 5 min/day, 10 days). Substantial bulk mineral loss occurred; on the remaining surface, partial surface demineralisation in the order of approx. 20 μm in depth is clearly visible.

enamel are organic material (2 vol%) and water (11 vol%) [2], making up only a small portion of the tissue. The high mineral content makes the enamel resistant against physical impacts. The value for the hardness of enamel varies depending on the measuring system and the load applied [3] and is also different with respect to the region of the tooth crown as well as with respect to the distance from the surface [4] so that no fixed value exists. Overall, however, the hardness of enamel is sufficient to withstand the majority of physical forces occurring during physiological processes (e.g. chewing) or oral hygiene measures. Thus, it is assumed that even over-vigorous oral hygiene habits would not be relevant for the wear of sound enamel [5].

When erosive demineralisation occurs (see chapter by Shellis et al., this vol., pp. 163–179), mineral is dissolved from the surface, causing a rough irregular structure similar to the etching pattern known from adhesive dentistry. Little is known about how deep the partly demineralised zone reaches; values ranging between a few microns [6] up to around 100 μm [7] have been reported. When the acid exposure continues, bulk enamel loss occurs (fig. 1). On such demineralised enamel surfaces, the microhardness is re-duced. As a consequence, eroded enamel is less resistant against physical forces than the sound tissue and, at least under experimental conditions, enamel loss is distinctly increased under erosive/abrasive conditions compared to erosion or abrasion alone and the amount of abrasive wear is related to the loss of microhardness [8].

Though it has been speculated that the partly demineralised surface zone is easily removed by physical forces, scanning electron microscopy (SEM) studies revealed that signs of demineralisation or etched prism structures are still visible even after toothbrushing [9, 10] (fig. 2).

The histology of experimental enamel erosion produced in in situ or in vitro models is quite well understood, but the erosive demineralisation is much more severe under such conditions compared to the in vivo situation. Respective experimental designs comprise single erosive challenges or cycles of erosion and intervention over one or few weeks [11], resulting in loss values distinctly higher than in vivo. It is therefore reasonable to assume that structural changes occurring under real life conditions are much less pronounced – all the more as in vivo erosive wear is not a straightforward process but consists of bursts and silent periods depending on habits, lifestyle and

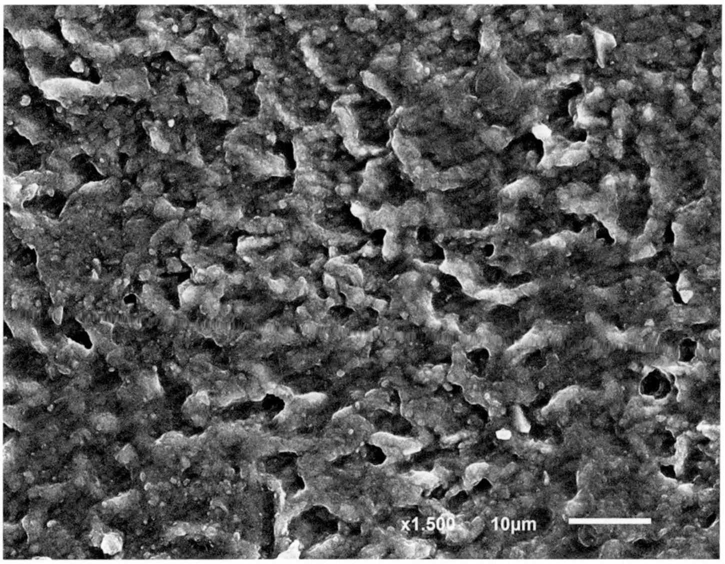

Fig. 2. Surface of an enamel sample from an in situ study [26]. Erosion was performed extra-orally with 0.5% citric acid (6 × 2 min/day, 7 days). Twice daily, the sample was exposed intra-orally to a saliva/NaF toothpaste mixture for 2 min and within this time brushed with a powered toothbrush for 5 s (load 250 g). The last intervention was brushing. The rough surface structure and prism-like pattern as distinct signs of erosive demineralisation are still clearly visible even after the brushing procedure.

general health aspects. Correspondingly, an early replica study revealed different morphologies of erosive wear ranging from irregular and pitted structures to more or less smooth lesion surfaces. It was speculated that the former are related to active lesions whereas the latter characterise inactive stages [12]. So far, there is no information about the physical properties of in vivo lesions, particularly with respect to microhardness. The assumption that in vivo erosive demineralisation is much less severe, however, might also hold true for the loss of microhardness.

Whether these differences between experimental and in vivo lesions are relevant for transposing experimental results to instructions for patients remains elusive.

Dentine is structurally and biologically distinctly different from enamel (for normal histology, see e.g. [1]) as it is a vital and permeable tissue of complex structure. The mineral compound of dentine is also non-stoichiometric hydroxyapatite but, unlike enamel where large crystallites build densely packed prisms, the crystals are much smaller and are associated with the organic component of the tissue [13]. Bulk mineral solely

occurs around the tubules defined as peritubular dentine. Overall, the inorganic portion makes up only around 47 vol%, whereas organic material (mainly collagen) contributes to around 33 vol%. In addition, the amount of water in dentine is high (21 vol%) [2]. From this feature it is clear that the physical properties of sound dentine differ from those of enamel. The elastic modulus is much lower, as is the microhardness [4], the latter making dentine more prone to physical wear. As a consequence, abrasive lesions (e.g. from toothbrushing) occur in dentine rather than in enamel [5].

Experimental erosive demineralisation in dentine leads to a structure distinctly different from that in enamel. Acid impacts cause a rapid dissolution of peri- and intertubular mineral but the organic portion is not degraded [14–16]. The result is that there is no bulk loss; instead, there is a spongy, completely demineralised structure remaining, the surface of which keeps the same level as the original sound tissue as long as it stays hydrated. The border between the demineralised and the mineralised tissue can be sharp (fig. 3) or can consist of a zone of partial demineralisation

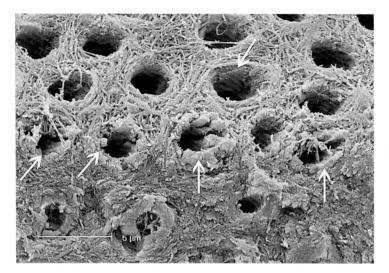

Fig. 3. Cross section (fractured, critical point dried) of a dentine sample from an in vitro experiment [19]. Erosion was performed with HCl (6 × 2 min/day; 9 days) and brushed with a powered tooth brush (2 × 15 s/day, load 300 g). Though the sample was brushed, the fully demineralised organic matrix is still present. Though there are minor signs of partial demineralisation (arrows indicate partly demineralised peritubular dentine), there is a sharp demarcation against the underlying sound tissue.

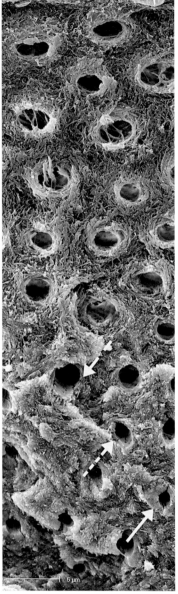

Fig. 4. Cross section (fractured and critical point dried) of a dentine sample from an in vitro experiment [27]. Erosive demineralisation was performed with 1% citric acid for 90 min. In the upper third, dentine is fully demineralised with enlarged tubules and a fluffy intertubular structure. In the middle third, the intertubular dentine appears more dense with signs of mineral, but the peritubular dentine is fully dissolved (broken arrow). Towards the lower third of the picture, the degree of mineralisation increases with some peritubular dentine preserved (dotted arrow); the lower part shows sound dentine with fully mineralised intertubular and completely preserved peritubular dentine (full arrow). The diameter of the tubules is much smaller than in the demineralised parts [in part from Lussi et al.; Caries Res 2011;45(suppl 1):2–12].

covering the underlying sound tissue (fig. 4). This zone of demineralised organic matrix is of importance for several aspects. Firstly, as soon as it reaches a certain thickness, all chemical processes become diffusion controlled. In the case of continuing erosive demineralisation, this means that the mineral loss is not linear but decreases with increasing thickness of the organic surface material [17, 18]. Secondly, active ingredients also have to diffuse through this structure and so far it is not clear how relevant interactions between such substances and collagen are. Thirdly, it has

102

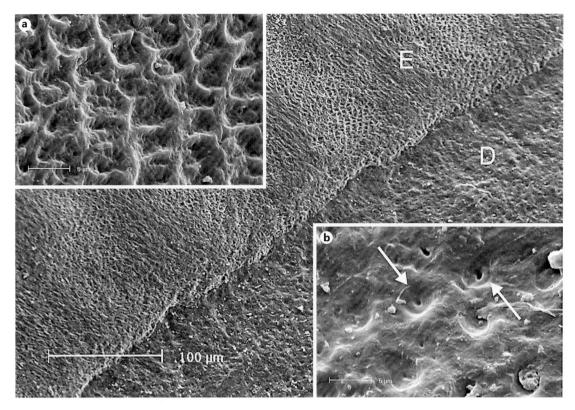

Fig. 5. SEM image from a replica of the palatal surface of an upper canine with exposed dentine. The patient suffered from a severe eating disorder with chronic vomiting for several hours per day. E = Proximal enamel rim, D = exposed dentine. **a** At higher magnification, signs of erosive demineralisation are clearly visible, indicating an active stage of the condition. **b** At higher magnification, patent tubules are visible (arrows). Peritubular dentine is preserved. The level of the surrounding intertubular dentine is only slightly above the peritubular dentine. This feature is distinctly different from experimental erosion and indicates that there is only a very thin, if any, layer of demineralised organic material on the lesion surface even in active stages [in part from Lussi et al.; Caries Res 2011;45(suppl 1):2–12].

been shown that the demineralised organic portion is strikingly resistant against abrasive forces [19] (fig. 3), which is relevant for designing erosion/abrasion experiments with dentine. Finally, this structure may impact the quantification of erosive mineral loss, at least when surface mapping methods are used [3].

Similar to in vivo enamel erosion, there is almost nothing known about the histology of dentine erosion developing in the oral cavity. From clinical experience, such lesions appear hard when scratched with a probe and are shiny, which is in contrast to experimental lesions which are resilient and dull. As demineralised human collagen can be digested by collagenases and other proteolytic enzymes [18, 20, 21], it could be assumed that it does not survive in vivo. The rate of demineralisation is surely much slower than in experiments, so that intraoral proteolysis may be sufficient to remove such structures as soon as the mineral is dissolved. The SEM replica image of a subject with active erosion supports this assumption (fig. 5). If this is the case, solid/liquid interactions in vivo are, similar to enamel, surface controlled rather than diffusion controlled, which may be relevant for interpreting study results from in vitro and in situ experiments.

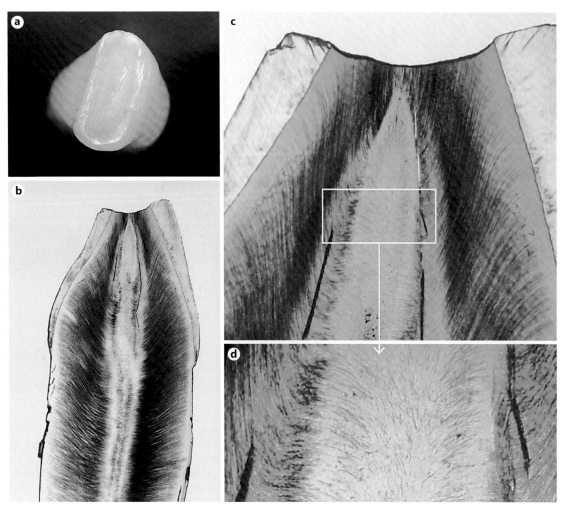

Fig. 6. a Incisor of the lower jaw with occlusal erosive tooth wear extending into dentine. **b, c** The histological section of the incisor of **a** shows involvement of dentine and a partial pulp sclerosis with formation of tertiary dentine (reactionary dentine). The erosive tooth wear caused a moderate irritation of the primary odontoblasts which produced reactionary dentine. The reactionary dentine is characterised by tubules which run without interruption towards the pulp (**d**).

What has rarely been addressed so far is how the pulpo-dentinal complex may react to erosive wear and what kind of tertiary dentine is formed (fig. 6, 7). In principle, odontoblasts survive when mild injuries occur, whereas severe injuries may destroy the odontoblast layer subjacent to the affected dental hard tissue [22]. In the first case, the remaining odontoblasts are forming new (patent) tubules whereas in the second case pulpal cells pro-liferate, forming new reparative (tertiary) dentine. This dentine is often atubular but may also have some tubules. Patent tubules typical for reactionary dentine are responsible for pain patients may suffer when they experience erosive tooth wear.

Normally, the outer ends of the coronal dentinal tubules are closed by enamel, but as soon as dentine is exposed to the oral cavity, pathways from and to the pulp potentially exist.

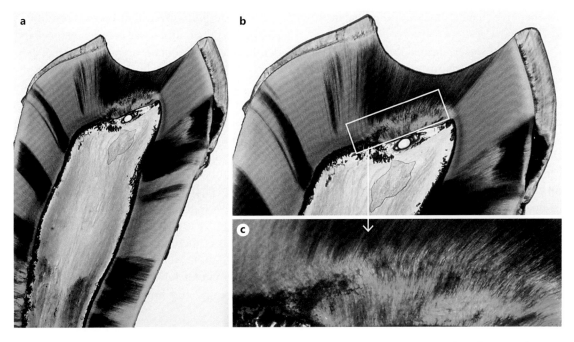

Fig. 7. a Histological section of a primary canine with advanced occlusal erosive wear extending deep into dentine. **b** The enlargement of **a** shows the formation of tertiary dentine with tubules running without interruption through the tertiary dentine. **c** Patent tubules typical for reactionary dentine are responsible for pain patients may suffer when they experience erosive wear.

Mechanical impacts such as curetting or drilling may reduce permeability through creating a smear layer and smear plugs, and several agents, for instance against hypersensitivity, can do so via organic or inorganic precipitation. These protecting layers, however, may not be durable due to various chemical impacts (e.g. acid exposures from intrinsic or extrinsic acid sources).

Lundy and Stanley [23] investigated the reactions of the pulp on dentine exposure. They prepared class V cavities in adult teeth scheduled for extraction for various reasons. The cavities were left unrestored up to several weeks and reactions to mechanical and thermal stimuli as well as histological changes of the pulp were investigated. Within the first days, the teeth became very sensitive and the histological examination revealed severe inflammation including pulpal abscesses. After weeks, however, sensitivity decreased and the histological findings indicated a more chronic stage of inflammation and some healing. Bacterial invasion was also observed to a certain extent. The study indicates that there are pathways from the oral cavity to the pulp and that factors present in saliva can cause reactions of the pulpal tissue. These reactions, however, appear reversible to a certain extent.

What has also been shown is that, similar to caries, a dentinal response to erosion and to other forms of wear is the formation of dentine sclerosis, reparative dentine and dead tracts [24]. This was also found in a study investigating teeth from animals and humans with dentine exposed from attrition. Reparative dentine was found in all permanent human teeth (all caries free and without restorations): bacteria were present in dentinal tubules in 82%, inflammation in 64%, extensive degenerative changes in 29% and pulpal necrosis in 7% [25].

Overall, however, limited knowledge is available about the reactions of the pulpo-dentinal complex to erosive wear. In view of the high prevalence of exposed dentine in the dentition, for example in cases of cupped cusps, cervical lesions or gingival recession, there must be sufficient defence mechanisms against the effects of bacterial invasion into or diffusion of inflammatory factors through the dentine. Clinically, there is no evidence that the exposure of dentine through erosive wear can cause serious damage to the pulp, at least given that the rate of erosive wear and the apposition of reparative dentine are balanced.

In summary, the histology of the eroded dental hard tissues is characterised by surface mineral loss progressing in layers from the natural surface towards the pulp, given that erosive conditions persist. The main difference between enamel and dentine erosion is that the organic portion of dentine is not degraded by clinically relevant acid impacts. The histology of erosive wear needs to be considered when developing preventive, non-invasive and restorative strategies as well as for experimental designs.

Erosive lesions can be easily created experimentally and are in the meantime quite well understood. What warrants further investigation are the histological features of erosive wear in vivo to find out whether the erosive lesions created experimentally are meaningful for the in vivo situation, whether lesions should be created in a manner reflecting more closely the in vivo histology, and how this could be accomplished.

References

1 Berkovitz BKB, Boyde A, Frank RM, Höhling HJ, Moxham BJ, Nalbandian J, Tonge CH: Teeth. Berlin, Springer, 1989.

2 Nikiforuk G: Understanding Dental Caries. Basel, Karger, 1985.

3 Schlueter N, Hara A, Shellis RP, Ganss C: Methods for the measurement and characterization of erosion in enamel and dentine. Caries Res 2011;45:13–23.

4 Meredith N, Sherriff M, Setchell DJ, Swanson SA: Measurement of the microhardness and Young's modulus of human enamel and dentine using an indentation technique. Arch Oral Biol 1996;41:539–545.

5 Addy M, Hunter ML: Can tooth brushing damage your health? Effects on oral and dental tissues. Int Dent J 2003; 53(suppl):177–186.

6 Schlueter N, Hardt M, Lussi A, Engelmann F, Klimek J, Ganss C: Tin-containing fluoride solutions as anti-erosive agents in enamel: an in vitro tin-uptake, tissue loss and scanning electron micrograph study. Eur J Oral Sci 2009;117:427–434.

7 Zentner A, Duschner H: Structural changes of acid etched enamel examined under confocal laser scanning microscope. J Orofac Orthop 1996;57:202–209.

8 Attin T, Koidl U, Buchalla W, Schaller HG, Kielbassa AM, Hellwig E: Correlation of microhardness and wear in differently eroded bovine dental enamel. Arch Oral Biol 1997;42:243–250.

9 Kuroiwa M, Kodaka T, Abe M: Brushing-induced effects with and without a non-fluoride abrasive dentifrice on remineralization of enamel surfaces etched with phosphoric acid. Caries Res 1994; 28:309–314.

10 Rios D, Honorio HM, Magalhaes AC, Silva SM, Delbem AC, Machado MA, Buzalaf MA: Scanning electron microscopic study of the in situ effect of salivary stimulation on erosion and abrasion in human and bovine enamel. Braz Oral Res 2008;22:132–138.

11 Wiegand A, Attin T: Design of erosion/abrasion studies – insights and rational concepts. Caries Res 2011;45:53–59.

12 Mannerberg F: Changes in the enamel surface in cases of erosion. A replica study. Arch Oral Biol 1961;4:59–62.

13 Weatherell JA, Robinson C: The inorganic composition of teeth; in Zipkin I (ed): Biological Mineralization. New York, Wiley, 1973, pp 43–74.

14 Kinney JH, Balooch M, Haupt DL Jr, Marshall SJ, Marshall GWJ: Mineral distribution and dimensional changes in human dentin during demineralisation. J Dent Res 1995;74:1179–1184.

15 Breschi L, Gobbi P, Mazzotti G, Falconi M, Ellis TH, Stangel I: High resolution SEM evaluation of dentin etched with maleic and citric acid. Dent Mater 2002; 18:26–35.

16 Ganss C, Hardt M, Lussi A, Cocks AK, Klimek J, Schlueter N: Mechanism of action of tin-containing fluoride solutions as anti-erosive agents in dentine – an in vitro tin-uptake, tissue loss and SEM study. Eur J Oral Sci 2010;118:376–384.

17 Hara AT, Ando M, Cury JA, Serra MC, Gonzalez-Cabezas C, Zero D: Influence of the organic matrix on root dentine erosion by citric acid. Caries Res 2005; 39:134–138.

18 Ganss C, Klimek J, Starck C: Quantitative analysis of the impact of the organic matrix on the fluoride effect on erosion progression in human dentine using longitudinal microradiography. Arch Oral Biol 2004;49:931–935.

19 Ganss C, Hardt M, Blazek D, Klimek J, Schlueter N: Effects of tooth brushing force on the mineral content and demineralised organic matrix of eroded dentine. Eur J Oral Sci 2009;117:255–260.

20 Klont B, ten Cate JM: Susceptibility of the collagenous matrix from bovine incisor roots to proteolysis after in vitro lesion formation. Caries Res 1991;25: 46–50.

21 Schlueter N, Hardt M, Klimek J, Ganss C: Influence of the digestive enzymes trypsin and pepsin in vitro on the progression of erosion in dentine. Arch Oral Biol 2010;55:294–299.

22 Tziafas D: The future role of a molecular approach to pulp-dentinal regeneration. Caries Res 2004;38:314–320.

23 Lundy T, Stanley HR: Correlation of pulpal histopathology and clinical symptoms in human teeth subjected to experimental irritation. Oral Surg Oral Med Oral Pathol 1969;27:187–201.

24 Stanley HR, Pereira JC, Spiegel E, Broom C, Schultz M: The detection and prevalence of reactive and physiologic sclerotic dentin, reparative dentin and dead tracts beneath various types of dental lesions according to tooth surface and age. J Oral Pathol 1983;12:257–289.

25 Tronstad L, Langeland K: Effect of attrition on subjacent dentin and pulp. J Dent Res 1971;50:17–30.

26 Schlueter N, Klimek J, Ganss C: Randomised in situ study on the efficacy of a tin/chitosan toothpaste on erosive-abrasive enamel loss. Caries Res 2013; 47:574–581.

27 Ganss C, Lussi A, Scharmann I, Weigelt T, Hardt M, Klimek J, Schlueter N: Comparison of calcium analysis, longitudinal microradiography and profilometry for the quantitative assessment of erosion in dentine. Caries Res 2010;43:422–429.

Prof. C. Ganss
Department of Conservative and Preventive Dentistry
Dental Clinic, Justus Liebig University Giessen
Schlangenzahl 14
DE–35392 Giessen (Germany)
E-Mail carolina.ganss@dentist.med.uni-giessen.de

Lussi A, Ganss C (eds): Erosive Tooth Wear. Monogr Oral Sci. Basel, Karger, 2014, vol 25, pp 108–122
DOI: 10.1159/000360749

Dentine Hypersensitivity

Nicola West · Joon Seong · Maria Davies

Periodontology, Clinical Trials Unit, Bristol Dental School, Bristol, UK

Abstract

Dentine hypersensitivity is a common oral pain condition affecting many individuals. The aetiology is multifactorial; however, over recent years the importance of erosion has become more evident. For dentine hypersensitivity to occur, the lesion must first be localised on the tooth surface and then initiated to exposed dentine tubules which are patent to the pulp. The short, sharp pain symptom is thought to be derived from the hydrodynamic pain theory and, although transient, is arresting, affecting quality of life. This episodic pain condition is likely to become a more frequent dental complaint in the future due to the increase in longevity of the dentition and the rise in tooth wear, particularly amongst young adults. Many efficacious treatment regimens are now available, in particular a number of over-the-counter home use products. The basic principles of treatment are altering fluid flow in the dentinal tubules with tubule occlusion or modifying or chemically blocking the pulpal nerve.

© 2014 S. Karger AG, Basel

Dentine hypersensitivity is a common oral pain condition affecting the teeth of many individuals. It is reasonable to surmise that with the increasing life expectancy of the population with a functional natural dentition (with vital or minimally restored teeth [1] prone to tooth wear), dentine hypersensitivity is likely to become a more frequent dental problem. Further, the healthy yet erosive lifestyle, adopted particularly amongst the younger adult population, is leading to a rise in tooth wear and dentine hypersensitivity. This is clearly demonstrated in a recent multicentre European study (7 countries) examining 3,187 young adults attending general dental practices, where 42% of patients aged between 18 and 35 years demonstrated dentine hypersensitivity [2], and about 30% demonstrated tooth wear [3]. Dentine tubules must be patent from the dental pulp to the oral environment to experience pain [4], which is widely thought to result from stimulus-induced tubular fluid flow and consequent nociceptor activation in the pulp/dentine border area [5]. The quality of life of patients is often altered as pain is associated with tangible frequent discomfort [6]. Affected individuals cope by modifying behaviours such as avoiding chilled food and drink and seeking self or professional treatment. The aforementioned study [2] demonstrated that 28% of the population felt dentine hypersensitivity affecting them importantly or very importantly; thus, dentine hypersensitivity is arguably a serious health issue.

Pain Mechanisms

Although much has been learnt about dentine hypersensitivity since it was first documented by Blum [7], clinical evidence-based research, particularly with respect to the pain mechanisms, is lacking and not well understood. Dentine hypersensitivity has been defined as pain arising from exposed dentine, typically in response to chemical, thermal, tactile or osmotic stimuli that cannot be explained as arising from any other form of dental defect or disease [8].

The most widely accepted pain theory is the hydrodynamic theory, first proposed by Gysi [9] and later proven by Brännström [10–12]. This supports the theory that sensitive dentine is based on the stimulus-induced fluid flow in the dentinal tubules and consequent nociceptor activation in the pulp/dentine border area [5, 13]. Intradental myelinated A-β and some A-δ fibres are thought to respond to stimuli that displace the fluid in the dentinal tubules, resulting in the characteristic short, sharp pain of dentine hypersensitivity [5]. Human studies showed that the patency of the dentinal tubules is an important characteristic of sensitive dentine [14], with a significantly positive correlation between the density of tubules and the pain responses induced from exposed cervical dentine surfaces. Further studies of extracted teeth provided compelling evidence for this requirement with sensitive teeth having many more (8×) and wider (2×) tubules at the buccal cervical area compared to non-sensitive teeth [4]. Although number and radius of tubules are relevant to fluid flow and therefore sensitivity, tubule radius is probably more important as fluid flow is proportional to the fourth power of the radius [15]; hence, if the diameter is doubled the tubule fluid flow increases by 16 fold. This explains the concept of why tubular occlusion, of whatever nature, is thought to reduce the pain of dentine hypersensitivity. These features of dentine hypersensitivity lesions clearly have important implications with respect to the possible aetiological factors involved and the development of preventive and management strategies for the condition.

Two other theories that have been proposed to account for the pain of dentine hypersensitivity, the neural theory and the odontoblast transducer theory, are now receiving renewed attention. New evidence suggests that odontoblasts may play a more important role in the dentine sensitivity pain mechanism, the odontoblasts representing a unique mechanosensory system acting as sensor cells [16]. Similarly, there is recent evidence that dental primary afferent neurones express temperature-sensitive transient receptor potential (TRP) channels in response to heat, suggesting that they may directly transduce high, but not low, temperatures [17]. This finding comes as an ever-increasing number of studies aiming to identify the molecular mechanisms by which pain signals are induced and transmitted in dental pulp. A number of growth factors, cytokines and other chemical mediators that sensitise dental afferent neurones have been identified, together with receptors and TRP channels that may be elevated in inflamed pulp and responsible for the pain sensation [18]. Interestingly, as well as a potential role in the direct transduction of heat, evidence exists that several TRP molecules have mechanosensitivity and could be the molecular transducers responsible for the mechanical detection of dentinal fluid movement of the hydrodynamic theory [17]. Similarly, odontoblasts have been shown to express this class of receptors [16]. Identification of these TRP ion channels as potential receptors is starting to provide an insight into the molecular mechanisms underlying all three theories proposed for dentine hypersensitivity.

Prevalence

Epidemiological studies on the prevalence of dentine hypersensitivity have resulted in conflicting data (table 1) [2, 19–50], with figures ranging

Table 1. Summary of prevalence studies on dentine hypersensitivity

Author	Location	Setting	Study type	Volunteer numbers	Volunteers	Single/ multicentre	Prevalence
Jensen [19]	USA	teaching hospital	clinical	3,000	adults	single	30%
Graf and Galasse [20]	Switzerland	practice	clinical	351	aged 7–69 years	single	15%
Flynn et al. [21]	UK	teaching hospital	questionnaire and clinical	369	aged 11–74 years	single	28% (Q) 18% (C)
Fischer et al. [22]	Brazil (urban)	marine dental clinic	questionnaire and clinical	635	aged 13–87 years	single	25% (Q) 17% (C)
Chabanski et al. [23]	UK	teaching hospital	questionnaire	507	periodontology patients	single	84%
Chabanski et al. [24]	UK	teaching hospital	clinical	51	periodontology patients	single	73–98%
Liu et al. [25]	Taiwan	teaching hospital	questionnaire and clinical	780	adult patients	single	32% (Q) 29% (C)
Rees [26]	UK	practice	clinical	3,593	adult patients	multicentre	3.8%
Taani and Awartani [27]	Saudi Arabia	teaching hospital	clinical	295	144 adult patients 151 periodontology patients	single	42% (non-perio.) 60% (perio.)
Rees and Addy [28]	UK	practice	clinical	4,841	adult patients	multicentre	4.1%
Rees et al. [29]	Hong Kong	teaching hospital	clinical	226	periodontology patients	single	68%
Rees and Addy [30]	UK	practice	clinical	5,477	aged 11–90 years	multicentre	2.8%
Udoye [31]	Nigeria	teaching hospital	clinical	220	adult patients	single	16.3%
Bamise et al. [32]	Nigeria	teaching hospital	clinical	2,165	adult patients	single	1.34%
Ye et al. [33]	China (urban)	investigation points on city streets	questionnaire and clinical	2,120	adult population	multicentre	37.9% (Q) 34.1% (C)
Dhaliwal et al. [34]	India (rural)	5 villages	questionnaire and clinical	1,329	general population	multicentre	48.9% (Q) 25% (C)
Bahşi et al. [35]	Turkey	practice	clinical	1,368	patients	single	5.3%
Wang et al. [36]	China (urban and rural)	8 provinces	clinical	6,843	general population	multicentre	34.5%
Que et al. [37]	China (urban)	6 communities in one city	clinical	1,023	general population	single	27.1%
Amarasena et al. [38]	Australia	private practice	observational by clinician	12,692	adult patients	multicentre	9.1%

Table 1. Continued

Author	Location	Setting	Study type	Volunteer numbers	Volunteers	Single/ multicentre	Prevalence
Kehua et al. [39]	China (urban)	6 communities in 1 city	clinical	1,320	general population	multicentre	25.5%
Que et al. [40]	China (urban)	2 districts in 2 cities	questionnaire and clinical	2,640	general population	multicentre	41.7% (Q) 25.5% (C)
Tengrungsun et al. [41]	Thailand	teaching hospital	clinical	420	adult patients	single	30.7%
Irwin and McCusker [42]	UK	practice	questionnaire	250	adult patients	single	**57.2%**
Gillam et al. [43]	UK	practice	questionnaire	277	adult patients	multicentre	52%
Gillam et al. [44]	UK/ South Korea	practice	questionnaire	277 (UK) 280 (Korea)	adult patients	multicentre	52% (UK) 55.4% (Korea)
Clayton et al. [45]	UK	air force	questionnaire	228	military	single	50%
Chi and Milgrom [46]	USA	community health centre	questionnaire	45	homeless 14–28 years old	single	52.6%
Colak et al. [47]	Turkey	university	questionnaire	1,463	university students aged 17–33 years	single	8.4%
Colak et al. [48]	Turkey	teaching hospital	questionnaire and clinical	1,169	adult patients	single	7.6% (C)
Oderinu et al. [49]	Nigeria	university	questionnaire	387	undergraduate students	single	33.8%
Bamise et al. [50]	Nigeria	university	questionnaire (self-diagnosis)	1,019	undergraduate students	single	68.4%
West et al. [2]	Europe	general practice	questionnaire and clinical	3,187	adults 18–35 years	multicentre	41.9%

Search performed on Entrez PubMed using search terms 'prevalence AND dentine hypersensitivity' and 'prevalence AND dentin hypersensitivity'. Only evidence-based articles for which the data could be confirmed are included. In prevalence, Q = Questionnaire; C = clinical; perio. = periodontal.

from 1.34% [32] to 98% [24]. This heterogeneity can be explained by several factors such as the sample population (ethnic origin, study location, periodontal status, dental care regimen), the different diagnostic criteria used to define dentine hypersensitivity and whether the source data is based on clinical evaluation or patient-based questionnaires. The above-mentioned European study [2], showing a dentine hypersensitivity prevalence of 42%, clinically examined patients in general dental practice in 7 European countries from varying economic status and occupation groups from a balanced variety of locations (rural, small town and metropolitan), thus representing an evenly distributed cross-section of the society, although the age range selected was 18–35 years of age. This figure may be considered low in comparison with studies that have reported prevalence figures of 73–98% [24] and 68% [29]. However, the studies by these authors were performed in a university teaching hospital setting where recruitment was drawn from referred patients attending periodontal clinics with known generalised gingival recession and exposed dentine, not giving as good a representation of the true population prevalence.

Dentine hypersensitivity can present from early teenage to old age, but the majority of sufferers range from 20 to 40 years with a peak in incidence at the end of the third decade [26]. After the age of about 40, sensitivity tends to reduce due to reparative processes such as tertiary dentine which will decrease permeability and reduce the hydraulic conductance of dentine. Another complicating factor is the episodic nature of this condition which may evoke or subdue the pain symptoms as the dentine tubules are open or closed [4]. The literature varies as to whether more females present with the condition than men. At least the European study [2], however, showed no difference in prevalence of dentine hypersensitivity in either gender, suggesting overall that as many males as females are susceptible.

Differential Diagnosis

There are a number of other dental conditions which give similar pain symptoms to dentine hypersensitivity. It is therefore essential that a differential diagnosis is performed and dentine hypersensitivity diagnosed after exclusion of the following. Other causes of short, sharp dental pain include:
(1) Chipped teeth causing exposed dentine
(2) Fractured restorations
(3) Pulpal response to caries and to restorative treatment
(4) Lack of care while contouring restorations so the tooth is left in traumatic occlusion
(5) Cracked tooth syndrome, often in heavily restored teeth
(6) Palatogingival groove and other enamel invaginations
(7) Incorrect placement of dentine adhesives in restorative dentistry leading to nanoleakage
(8) Caries
(9) Vital bleaching

Aetiology and Risk Factors

The aetiology of dentine hypersensitivity is based primarily on in vitro and in situ data, case report data and epidemiological surveys – not randomised controlled clinical studies. For dentine hypersensitivity to occur, the dentine surface of a tooth must be exposed (lesion localisation) and a number of dentine tubules in close proximity to each other must be patent from the pulp to the oral environment (lesion initiation) [51]. There is no evidence that there is a differentiation between coronal and radicular dentine hypersensitivity.

Lesion Localisation

Gingival Recession Exposing Dentine
The most common aetiology of exposed root dentine is recession of the gingival marginal tissues. This process is characterised by the displacement of the gingival margin apical to the cement-enamel junction, thereby exposing visible cementum of the root surface, which is then rapidly lost [52]. Epidemiological surveys revealed that gingival recession is a common entity amounting to 60–90% of the adult Western European population [53]. Other causes of recession are dehiscence and fenestration of alveolar bone, soft tissue trauma from for example toothbrushing, periodontitis, orthodontic therapy, oral piercing and self-inflicted injury. These factors are acting synchronously or not, with possible relevance of anatomical, physiological, pathological and traumatic factors needing consideration [54].

There is good evidence demonstrating that periodontal disease and periodontal treatment result in an apical shift of the soft tissue margin

[55] and often result in sensitivity, occurring in approximately half of patients following scaling and root planning [56].

The aetiology of gingival recession in the healthy periodontium is circumstantial and based on clinical observation with epidemiological data [57, 58]. These data associate recession with tooth surfaces that receive the most attention during the brushing cycle, namely the buccal surfaces [59, 60], but overall, the association between tooth-brushing and gingival recession is inconclusive [61]. Recently, there has been an increase in the use of power brushes. Interestingly, their brush head action has not been shown to cause more gingival trauma than manual brushes documented in a Cochrane review [62]. Plaque data suggest an inverse relationship with recession, with plaque scores lower at recession sites [63, 64].

During any brushing cycle, the toothbrush is thought to scratch the gingival tissues to some degree [64, 65], possibly causing recession. Some individuals are known to be more obsessive regarding toothbrushing habits, particularly those with dentine hypersensitivity, regularly brushing 3 or more times a day [66] and for longer periods of time than the average population, again predisposing individuals to more likelihood of permanent trauma and recession. The gingival biotype is rarely mentioned in dentine hypersensitivity studies and reviews, yet places a major role in gingival surgery risk assessment of recession [67, 68].

Loss of Hard Tissue Exposing Dentine
Above the cement-enamel junction, loss of enamel is a necessary prerequisite for dentine exposure. While frank carious lesions with dentine exposure of smooth tooth surface are a rather rare finding today, the development of non-carious cervical lesions is the most important factor for dentine exposure above the gingival margin. This process is usually of multifactorial aetiology, and rarely only due to one of wear phenomenon [69–71].

Toothpaste has the potential to harm the dental hard tissues by virtue of its degree of abrasivity. In situ studies to investigate the effects of abrasion on dentine have shown that dentine is considerably more susceptible than enamel to abrasion alone [72], and that significant differences in dentine wear can be detected between toothpastes with moderate and high RDA [73, 74]. However, careful extrapolation of in vitro data suggests that, in normal use, it would take hundreds of years to remove 1 mm of enamel. Overzealous toothbrushing may be solely responsible for a small percentage of dentine hypersensitivity cases [75]. Toothpaste detergents also chemically 'abrade' dentine, probably by dissolution of the collagen matrix [76]. Toothpastes therefore appear to play a role in potentially localising sites of dentine hypersensitivity by acting synergistically with erosion in removing enamel at the cervical areas [77–79].

Erosion caused by extrinsic acids on hard tooth substrate has been considered to be the most common and important aetiological factor in tooth wear [80, 81]. It is likely that erosive components initiate and localise dentine hypersensitivity, resulting in tissue loss and tubular opening [82]. The exposed dentine surface either has patent dentine tubules or is covered by a smear layer of oral debris such as calcium or toothpaste ingredients. Most acidic soft drinks, citrus fruits and fruit juices, some alcoholic beverages and many herbal teas remove the smear layer [82] after a few minutes of exposure.

In conclusion, lesion localisation and initiation of dentine hypersensitivity can be induced by abrasive and erosion forces. Although erosion is the dominant factor, synergistic action with abrasion is probably the most common occurrence, with both these factors resulting in dentine wear and opening of tubules.

Management Strategies

Prior to advocating treatment regimens it is important to consider changing aetiological causative agents in order to prevent the perpetuation of the condition. The treatment plan would be as follows:

(1) Correct diagnosis based on a history, clinical examination and compatibility with the definition
(2) Differential diagnosis to identify alternative or additional causes of dentinal pain, which if found should be treated first by appropriate methods
(3) Identification of aetiological and predisposing factors, particularly dietary and oral hygiene habits relevant to erosion, abrasion and gingival recession; if tooth wear appears associated with regurgitation or vomiting appropriate referral to medical colleagues is recommended in the first instance
(4) Elimination, reduction or modification of aetiological factors through oral hygiene and dietary advice
(5) Provision/recommendation of proven efficacious treatments based upon individual needs

Two treatment modalities are used in the treatment of dentine hypersensitivity: modification or blocking of the pulpal nerve response and alteration of fluid flow in the tubules.

Modification or Blocking of Pulpal Nerve Response

Desensitising agents such as potassium ions may reduce intradental nerve excitability by diffusing along the tubules and raising the concentration of local extracellular potassium ions, hence blocking intradental nerve function [5]. It is likely that a reservoir of the chemical needs to build up in the tooth to have the desired effect, which may take a couple of weeks. There is much debate on the efficacy of potassium toothpaste; a Cochrane review [83, 84] for potassium nitrate showed weak evidence supporting the efficacy.

Alteration of Fluid Flow in Dentinal Tubules

The most direct approach to desensitising dentine is occlusion of the tubule orifice. The effectiveness of the tubular occluding agents will de-

pend on their resistance to removal, especially in an acid environment. In vitro results often demonstrate occluding properties of treatments but these do not necessarily correlate to the in vivo situation when there must be resistance to the oral challenges of day-to-day activity. Occluding materials can be washed from the tubule or may be acid labile. Currently tubule occlusion is the most favoured mode of treatment, with some treatments giving excellent immediate and long-term results.

A vast array of products are available to treat dentine hypersensitivity, with many new toothpaste products showing good efficacy. It is difficult to prove efficacy of one product over another due to trial design and the subjective nature of the pain condition. A paste with an active agent may be tested against its base paste, a conventional fluoride paste or another paste with an active agent. Further, complicating factors such as the placebo effect, Hawthorne effect, regression to the mode and control product effect compound the interpretation of clinical findings and can hide the true effect of the treatment. Protocols for comparing different agents need to be standardised.

Strontium

Toothpastes containing strontium salts have dominated the market of desensitising pastes for the last 50 years and have therefore been subjected to most methods of testing for efficacy [85]. The theory behind incorporating strontium salts in toothpastes derives from the ability of the salt to have a considerable affinity for dentine owing to the high permeability and possibility for absorption into or onto the organic connective tissues and the odontoblast processes [86]. It has been proposed that strontium combines with dentine to form a strontium apatite complex with a significantly higher radiodensity than hydroxyapatite [87]. Another theory postulated for the therapeutic action of the strontium-based pastes is the possible effect of the abrasive fillers. A clinical study showed that three artificial silica formulations were similar and significantly better than the original strontium chloride and a formalin-based toothpaste in the treatment of dentine hypersensitivity [88]. The resulting strontium acetate/artificial silica (Sr/Si) product has again been shown in studies in vitro and in situ to occlude tubules with an acid-resistant silica/strontium-containing deposit, although the role of the strontium in the substantivity of the deposit cannot as yet be determined [89–95].

Not all RCTs have reported differences in favour of the Sr/Si product compared to a variety of control products, although no studies have reported negative results against controls and some have reached significance in favour [96]. A systematic review on strontium and potassium products showed only minimal evidence for the efficacy of both strontium- and potassium-based toothpastes in relieving symptoms of dentine hypersensitivity [97].

Arginine and Calcium Carbonate
Clinical efficacy for the beneficial effects of arginine and calcium carbonate (A/C) in dentine hypersensitivity initially came from an in-office applied prophylactic paste. The treatment effects were immediate and thought to be due to tubule occlusion by calcium phosphate, with in vitro studies confirming the deposits were calcium and phosphate [98, 99]. Clinical efficacy data first came from RCTs on the A/C prophylactic paste and revealed immediate and 4-week benefits significantly greater than controls [100, 101]. Subsequently, a number of RCTs of varying duration comparing A/C toothpaste with a variety of controls reported, for the most part, superior treatment effects immediately and up to 8 weeks of A/C toothpaste [102–109]. Although more acid labile than the strontium, stannous and calcium sodium phosphosilicate (CSPS) products, pain reduction is maintained by regular application. There are two systematic reviews on arginine, each showing efficacy but on few studies [110, 111].

Stannous Fluoride with and without Sodium Hexametaphosphate
Stannous products have been used for many years, showing good safety records. Evidence from studies in vitro show stannous salt solutions precipitate onto dentine and block tubules and the deposit is water and acid resistant [112]. More recent studies, using stannous fluoride gel, report the same observations [113] and further indicated a protective effect of the dentine smear layer against acid erosion [114]. Consistent with the findings in vitro, clinical studies reported efficacy of stannous fluoride gel or solutions in the treatment of dentine hypersensitivity [115, 116] and the ADA issued a seal of acceptance for a 0.4% stannous fluoride gel in this application. More recently, RCTs have reported that hexametaphosphate-stabilised stannous fluoride toothpaste provided immediate and 4- and 8-week benefits in the treatment of dentine hypersensitivity, which were significantly greater than appropriate control toothpaste products [117–121].

Calcium Sodium Phosphosilicate
CSPS is a bio-glass first used in bone regeneration but more recently formulated into an anhydrous toothpaste product for the treatment of dentine hypersensitivity. CSPS in an aqueous environment is attracted to dentine collagen, reacting to form a deposit or precipitate made up of calcium, phosphate and silica. A number of studies in vitro show that CSPS in solution or toothpaste interacts on the dentine surface and forms a deposit over the dentine and in the tubules [122–125]. This tubule-blocking deposit is water and acid insoluble and mechanically resistant. The deposit has a hydroxyapatite appearance but also contains silica and, when derived from toothpaste vehicle, titanium. A number of RCTs comparing CSPS toothpaste with a variety of controls and extending up to 8 weeks overall showed significantly greater benefits for the CSPS product in the treatment of dentine hypersensitivity [126–128].

Casein Derivatives

The clinical efficacy of casein derivatives has been examined mainly in conjunction with caries, with a systematic review including only one uncontrolled study on dentine hypersensitivity [129]. The finding was that the quantity and quality of clinical trial evidence were insufficient to make conclusions regarding the long-term effectiveness of casein derivatives, specifically CPP-ACP, in treating dentine hypersensitivity.

Oxalates

The mode of action of oxalates has been proposed as tubule occlusion by oxalate ions reacting with calcium ions in the dentinal fluid to form insoluble calcium oxalate crystals deposited in the tubule apertures [130]. This was confirmed by Mongiorgi and Prati [131], with X-ray diffractometer analysis. An in vitro study by Suge et al. [132] evaluated the effects of pre- or post-application of calcium chloride on enhancing the occluding ability of potassium oxalate. However, results showed no significant treatment effect due to calcium-enhanced uptake. In vitro work has shown that while oxalates result in good tubule occlusion, they are acid labile and can be easily washed from the surface of dentine [112]. The oxalate salts commonly used in commercially available products are potassium, citrate, ferric, dipotassium and monohydrogen monopotassium. A systematic review by [133] failed to show substantial significance for oxalate treatment.

Professionally Applied Products in the Management of Dentine Hypersensitivity

A wide range of commercially available products are available for professional treatment. In-office treatments tend to be reserved for individuals who have received preventive advice and have tried products for home use but found them ineffective.

Prophylaxis Paste

With the recent launch of prophylaxis pastes to reduce dentine hypersensitivity, two formulations have shown good efficacy at immediate and long-term relief at pain reduction with dentine tubule occlusion, an arginine-based formulation [100, 101] and a CSPS formulation [134, 135].

Varnishes and Precipitants

A varnish can set by releasing ethanol and taking up moisture. In this way, the insoluble resins in the shape of a sticky-plastic congealing film gradually fall out and adhere. Observation shows that this approach reduces the pain of dentine hypersensitivity for as long as the varnish stays on the tooth and is not particularly effective. However, a calcium/fluoride solution is currently marketed which also contains silica [136], with good anecdotal and clinical evidence for use. Fluoride delivered as a varnish is held in place by the varnish and forms calcium/phosphate precipitates, calcium fluoride and fluorapatite that can block dentine tubules [137]. Clinical studies of the fluoride varnishes have demonstrated that they provide immediate pain relief which lasts for a number of weeks [138, 139]. Varnishes containing chlorhexidine or glutaraldehyde have also been shown to be clinically effective in the treatment of hypersensitivity for a period of up to 12 weeks [140]. Other agents that form precipitates are also commercially available and there is some evidence for the efficacy of these products. Oxalate desensitisers, for example, have been shown to occlude dentine tubules in vitro [141] and reduce dentine hypersensitivity pain scores in vivo over a 4-week period [138]. For all of these products, however, their efficacy is limited to the duration for which they remain on the tooth surface.

Resin-Based Materials

Glass ionomer, resin-reinforced glass ionomer/ compomers, adhesive resin primers and adhesive resin bonding systems have been used successfully for the treatment of dentine hypersensitivity. Treatment can be problematic if there has been little tissue loss and over contouring can lead to plaque retentive sites and gingival inflammation. Further, sufferers of dentine hypersensitivity tend to be meticulous at cleaning their teeth, often using excessive brushing force on frequent occasions. Unless the toothbrushing habits are corrected, materials can be abraded and need replacement. A recent systematic review found little difference between a number of professionally applied products; however, the numbers per group were low with many different controls, weakening the interpretation of the finding [142]. A further systematic review published in 2013 analysed clinical trials of dentine desensitising agents, identifying 5 with satisfactory longer-term results (up to 6 months) [143].

Lasers

Nd:YAG laser irradiation has been advocated for the alleviation of symptoms from dentine hypersensitivity. Lasers work by coagulation of proteins in the dentinal fluid and hence reduce permeability [144]. They are also believed to create an amorphous sealed layer on the dentine surface which appears to be due to partial melt down of the surface [145]. However, there is a possibility that the peripheral tubules are opened, negating any benefit. The Nd:YAG laser has been used with en-couraging results [146, 147]. Other clinical studies do not support this finding [148], with the laser treatment reducing the pain sensation but not significantly different from the placebo treatment.

The GaAlAs laser has been compared to a fluoride varnish in a clinical trial [149] with no significant differences found, and an Er:YAG laser [150] showed some effect compared to the control at low setting. In summary, the clinical results obtained from laser therapy are equivocal and do not seem to justify the high expenditure of the equipment for this purpose. A systematic review by Sgolastra et al. [151] concluded that there was weak evidence for laser treatment with a strong placebo effect.

Conclusion

Clinically, there are many treatment modalities for dentine hypersensitivity which the clinician may find successful in alleviating the pain of dentine hypersensitivity. If one toothpaste is not found to be effective another may be advantageous. Currently, strontium, arginine, stannous and CSPS toothpastes, and strontium and arginine propylaxis pastes, have been proven to be very effective at pain reduction in dentine hypersensitivity with immediate and long-term efficacy.

References

1 Nuttall N, Steele JG, Nunn J, Pine C, Treasure E, Bradnock G, Morris J, Kelly M, Pitts NB, White D: A Guide to the UK Adult Dental Health Survey 1998. London, British Dental Association, 2001, pp 1–6.

2 West NX, Sanz M, Lussi A, Bartlett D, Bouchard P, Bourgeois D: Prevalence of dentine hypersensitivity and study of associated factors: a European population-based cross-sectional study. J Dent 2013;41:841–851.

3 Bartlett DW, Lussi A, West NX, Bouchard P, Sanz M, Bourgeois D: Prevalence of tooth wear on buccal and lingual surfaces and possible risk factors in young European adults. J Dent 2013;41:1007–1013.

4 Absi EG, Addy M, Adams D: Dentine hypersensitivity: a study of the patency of dentinal tubules in sensitive and non-sensitive cervical dentine. J Clin Periodontol 1987;14:280–284.

5 Nähri M, Jyväsjärvi E, Virtannen A: Role of intradental A- and C-type fibres in dental pain mechanisms. Proc Finn Dent Soc 1992;88(suppl 1):507–516.

6 Boiko OV, Baker SR, Gibson BJ, Locker D, Sufi F, Barlow AP, Robinson PG: Construction and validation of the quality of life measure for dentine hypersensitivity (DHEQ). J Clin Periodontol 2010;37:973–980.

7 Anonymous: Artzney Buchlein wider allerlei kranckeyten und gebrechen der tzeen. Leipzig, Michael Blum, 1530.

8   Canadian Advisory Board on Dentine Hypersensitivity: Consensus-based recommendations for the diagnosis and management of dentine hypersensitivity. J Can Dent Assoc 2003;69:221–228.

9   Gysi A: An attempt to explain the sensitiveness of dentin. Br J Dent Sci 1900;43:865–868.

10 Brännström M: A hydrodynamic mechanism in the transmission of pain-produced stimuli through the dentine; in Anderson DJ (ed): Sensory mechanisms in dentine. New York, Pergamon Press, 1963, pp 73–79.

11 Brännström M: The surface of sensitive dentine. Odontol Revy 1965;16:293–299.

12 Brännström M: The sensitivity of dentine. Oral Surg Oral Med Oral Pathol 1966;21:517–526.

13 Matthews B, Andrew D, Wanachantararak S: Biology of the dental pulp with special reference to its vasculature and innervation; in Addy M, Embery G, Edgar WM, Orchardson R (eds): Tooth Wear and Sensitivity. London, Martin Dunitz, 2000, pp 39–51.

14 Nähri M, Kontturi-Nähri V: Sensitivity and surface condition of dentine – an SEM replica study. J Dent Res 1994;73:122.

15 Guyton A: Textbook of Medical Physiology, ed 4. Philadelphia, Saunders, 1971, pp 211–212.

16 Magloire H, Maurin JC, Couble ML, Shibukawa Y, Tsumura M, Thivichon-Prince B, Bleicher F: Topical review. Dental pain and odontoblasts: facts and hypotheses. J Orofac Pain 2010;24:335–349.

17 Chung G, Oh SB: TRP channels in dental pain. Open Pain J 2013;6(suppl 1):31–36.

18 Chung G, Jung SJ, Oh SB: Cellular and molecular mechanisms of dental nociception. J Dent Res 2013;92:948–955.

19 Jensen AL: Hypersensitivity controlled by iontophoresis. Double blind clinical investigation. J Am Dent Assoc 1964,68. 216–225.

20 Graf H, Galasse R: Morbidity, prevalence and intraoral distribution of hypersensitive teeth (abstract No 479). J Dent Res 1977;76:A162.

21 Flynn J, Galloway R, Orchardson R: The incidence of hypersensitive teeth in the West of Scotland. J Dent 1985;13:230–236.

22 Fischer C, Fischer RG, Wennberg A: Prevalence and distribution of cervical dentine hypersensitivity in a population in Rio de Janeiro, Brazil. J Dent 1992;20:272–276.

23 Chabanski MB, Gillam DG, Bulman JS, Newman HN: Prevalence of cervical dentine sensitivity in a population of patients referred to a specialist periodontology department. J Clin Periodontol 1996;23:989–992.

24 Chabanski MB, Gilliam DG, Bulman JS, Newman HN: Clinical evaluation of cervical dentine sensitivity in a population of patients referred to a specialist periodontology department: a pilot study. J Oral Rehabil 1997;24:666–672.

25 Liu HC, Lan WH, Hsieh CC: Prevalence and distribution of cervical dentin hypersensitivity in a population in Taipei, Taiwan. J Endod 1998;24:45–47.

26 Rees JS: The prevalence of dentine hypersensitivity in general dental practice in the UK. J Clin Periodontol 2000;27:860–865.

27 Taani SD, Awartani F: Clinical evaluation of cervical dentin sensitivity (CDS) in patients attending general dental clinics (GDC) and periodontal specialty clinics (PSC). J Clin Periodontol 2002;29:118–122.

28 Rees JS, Addy MA: Cross-sectional study of dentine hypersensitivity. J Clin Periodontol 2002;29:997–1003.

29 Rees JS, Jin JL, Lam S, Kudanowska I, Vowles R: The prevalence of dentine hypersensitivity in a hospital clinic population in Hong Kong. J Dent 2003;31:453–461.

30 Rees JS, Addy M: A cross-sectional study of buccal cervical sensitivity in UK general dental practice and a summary review of prevalence studies. Int J Dent Hyg 2004;2:64–69.

31 Udoye CI: Pattern and distribution of cervical dentine hypersensitivity in a Nigerian tertiary hospital. Odontostomatol Trop 2006;29:19–22.

32 Bamise CT, Olusile AO, Oginni AO, Dosumu OO: The prevalence of dentine hypersensitivity among adult patients attending a Nigerian teaching hospital. Oral Health Prev Dent 2007;5:49–53.

33 Ye W, Feng XP, Li R: The prevalence of dentine hypersensitivity in Chinese adults. J Oral Rehabil 2012;39:182–187.

34 Dhaliwal JS, Palwankar P, Khinda PK, Sodhi SK: Prevalence of dentine hypersensitivity: a cross-sectional study in rural Punjabi Indians. J Indian Soc Periodontol 2012;16:426–429.

35 Bahşi E, Dalli M, Uzgur R, Turkal M, Hamidi MM, Colak H: An analysis of the aetiology, prevalence and clinical features of dentine hypersensitivity in a general dental population. Eur Rev Med Pharmacol Sci 2012;16:1107–1116.

36 Wang Y, Que K, Lin L, Hu D, Li X: The prevalence of dentine hypersensitivity in the general population in China. J Oral Rehabil 2012;39:812–820.

37 Que K, Guo B, Jia Z, Chen Z, Yang J, Gao P: A cross-sectional study: non-carious cervical lesions, cervical dentine hypersensitivity and related risk factors. J Oral Rehabil 2013;40:24–32.

38 Amarasena N, Spencer J, Ou Y, Brennan D: Dentine hypersensitivity in a private practice patient population in Australia. J Oral Rehabil 2011;38:52–60.

39 Kehua Q, Yingying F, Hong S, Menghong W, Deyu H, Xu F: A cross-sectional study of dentine hypersensitivity in China. Int J Dent 2009;59:376–380.

40 Que K, Ruan J, Fan X, Liang X, Hu D: A multi-centre and cross-sectional study of dentine hypersensitivity in China. J Clin Periodontol 2010;37:631–637.

41 Tengrungsun T, Jamornnium Y, Tengrungsun S: Prevalence of dentine hypersensitivity among Thai dental patients at the Faculty of Dentistry, Mahidol University. Southeast Asian J Trop Med Public Health 2012;43:1059–1064.

42 Irwin CR, McCusker PJ: Prevalence of dentine hypersensitivity in a general dental population. J Ir Dent Assoc 1997;43:7–9.

43 Gillam DG, Seo HS, Bulman JS, Newman HN: Perceptions of dentine hypersensitivity in a general practice population. J Oral Rehabil 1999;75:710–714.

44 Gillam DG, Seo HS, Newman HN, Bulman JS: Comparison of dentine hypersensitivity in selected occidental and oriental populations. J Oral Rehabil 2001;28:20–25.

45 Clayton DR, McCarthy D, Gillam DG: A study of the prevalence and distribution of dentine sensitivity in a population of 17- to 58-year-old serving personnel in an RAF base in the Midlands. J Oral Rehabil 2002;29:14–23.

46 Chi D, Milgrom P: The oral health of homeless adolescents and young adults and determinants of oral health: preliminary findings. Spec Care Dentist 2008; 28:237–242.

47 Colak H, Aylikci BU, Hamidi MM, Uzgur R: Prevalence of dentine hypersensitivity among university students in Turkey. Niger J Clin Pract 2012;15:415–419.

48 Colak H, Demirer S, Hamidi M, Uzgur R, Köseoğlu S: Prevalence of dentine hypersensitivity among adult patients attending a dental hospital clinic in Turkey. West Indian Med J 2012;61:174–179.

49 Oderinu OH, Savage KO, Uti OG, Adegbulugbe IC: Prevalence of self-reported hypersensitive teeth among a group of Nigerian undergraduate students. Niger Postgrad Med J 2011;18:205–209.

50 Bamise CT, Kolawole KA, Oloyede EO, Esan TA: Tooth sensitivity experience among residential university students. Int J Dent Hyg 2010;8:95–100.

51 Addy M: Dentine hypersensitivity: New perspectives on an old problem. Int Dent J 2002;52(suppl):367–375.

52 Beveius J, Lindskog S, Hultenby K: The micromorphology in vivo of the buccocervical region of premolar teeth in young adults. A replica study by scanning electron microscopy. Acta Odontol Scand 1994;52:323–334.

53 Susin C, Haas AN, Oppermann RV, Haugejorden O, Albandar JM: Gingival recession: epidemiology and risk indicators in a representative urban Brazilian population. J Periodontol 2004;75:1377–1386.

54 Smith RG: Gingival Recession. Reappraisal of an enigmatic condition and a new index for monitoring. J Clin Periodontol 1997;24:201–205.

55 Serino G, Wennström J, Lindhe J, Eneroth L: The prevalence and distribution of gingival recession in subjects with high standards of oral hygiene. J Clin Periodontol 1994;21:57–63.

56 Von Troil B, Needleman I, Sanz M: A systematic review of the prevalence of root sensitivity following periodontal therapy. J Clin Periodontol 2002; 29(suppl 3):173–177.

57 Kitchin P: The prevalence of tooth root exposure and the relation of the extent of such exposure to the degree of abrasion in different age classes. J Dent Res 1941;20:565–581.

58 Gillette WB, Van House RL: Ill effects of improper oral hygiene procedures. J Am Dent Assoc 1980;10:476–481.

59 Rugg-Gunn AJ, MacGregor IDM: A survey of toothbrushing behaviour in children and young adults. J Periodontol Res 1978;13:382–388.

60 MacGregor IDM, Rugg-Gunn A-J: A survey of toothbrushing sequence in children and young adults. J Periodontol Res 1979;14:225–230.

61 Rajapakse PS, McCraken GI, Gwynnett E, Steen ND, Guentsch A, Heasman PA: Does tooth brushing influence the development and progression of non-inflammatory gingival recession? A systematic review. J Clin Periodontol 2007;34:1046–1061.

62 Robinson PG, Deacon SA, Deery C, Heanue M, Walmsley AD, Worthington HV, Glenny A-M, Shaw BC: Manual versus powered toothbrushing for oral health. Cochrane Database Syst Rev 2005;2:CD002281.

63 Addy M, Mostafa P, Newcombe RG: Dentine hypersensitivity: the distribution of recession, sensitivity and plaque. J Dent 1987;15:242–248.

64 Addy M, Hunter ML: Can toothbrushing damage your health? Effects on oral and dental tissues. Int Dent J 2003;53:177–186.

65 Van der Weijden GA, Timmerman MF, Reijerse E, Snoek CM: Toothbrushing force in relation to plaque removal. J Clin Periodontol 1996;23:724–729.

66 West N: Dentine hypersensitivity: clinical and laboratory studies of toothpastes and their ingredients; thesis, University of Wales College of Medicine, Cardiff, 1985.

67 De Rouck T, Eghbali R, Collys K, De Bruyn H, Cosyn J: The gingival biotype revisited: transparency of the periodontal probe through the gingival margin as a method to discriminate thin from thick gingiva. J Clin Periodontol 2009; 36:428–433.

68 Melsen B, Allais D: Factors of importance for the development of dehiscences during labial movement of mandibular incisors: a retrospective study of adult orthodontic patients. Am J Orthod and Dentofacial Orthop 2005;127:552–561.

69 Addy M: Oral hygiene products: potential for harm to oral and systemic health? Periodontol 2000;48:54–65.

70 Mair LH: Wear in the mouth: the tribology dimension; in Addy M, Embery G, Edgar WM, Orchardson R (eds): Tooth Wear and Sensitivity: Clinical Advances in Restorative Dentistry. London, Dunitz, 2000, pp 181–188.

71 Meurman JH, Sovari R: Interplay of erosion, attrition and abrasion in toothwear and possible approaches to prevention; in Addy M, Embery G, Edgar WM, Orchardson R (eds): Tooth Wear and Sensitivity: Clinical Advances in Restorative Dentistry. London, Dunitz, 2000, pp 171–180.

72 Hooper S, West NX, Pickles M, Joiner A, Newcombe RG, Addy M: Investigation of erosion and abrasion of enamel and dentine: a model in situ using toothpastes of different abrasivity. J Clin Periodontol 2003;30:802–808.

73 Macdonald E, North A, Maggio B, Sufi F, Mason S, Moore C, Addy M, West NX: Clinical study investigating abrasive effects of three toothpastes and water in an in situ model. J Dent 2010;38:509–516.

74 Addy M, Hughes J, Pickles M, Joiner A, Huntington E: Development of a method in situ to study toothpaste abrasion of dentine: comparison of 2 products. J Clin Periodontol 2002;29:896–900.

75 Addy M: Tooth brushing, tooth wear and dentine hypersensitivity – are they associated. Inter Dent J 2005;55:261–267.

76 Moore C, Addy M: Wear of dentine in vitro by toothpaste abrasive and detergents alone and combined. J Clin Periodontol 2005;32:1242–1246.

77 West N, Hooper S, O'Sullivan D, Hughes N, North M, Macdonald E, Davies M, Claydon N: In situ randomised trial investigating abrasive effects of two desensitising toothpastes on dentine with acidic challenge prior to brushing. J Dent 2012;40:77–85.

78 Wiegand A, Kuhn M, Sener B, Roos M, Attin T: Abrasion of eroded dentin caused by toothpaste slurries of different abrasivity and toothbrushes of different filament diameter. J Dent 2009; 37:480–484.

79 Wiegand A, Egert S, Attin T: Toothbrushing before or after an acidic challenge to minimize tooth wear? An in situ/ex vivo study. Am J Dent 2008;21:13–16.

80 Lussi A: Erosive tooth wear – a multifactorial condition of growing concern and increasing knowledge. Monogr Oral Sci 2006;20:1–8.

81 Bartlett DW: The causes of dental erosion. Oral Dis 1997;3:209–211.

82 Absi EG, Addy M, Adams D: Dentine hypersensitivity. The effects of toothbrushing and dietary compounds on dentine in vitro: an SEM study. J Oral Rehabil 1992;19:101–110.

83 Poulsen S, Errboe M, Hovgaard O, Worthington HW: Potassium nitrate toothpaste for dentine hypersensitivity. Cochrane Database Syst Rev 2001; 2:CD001476.

84 Poulsen S, Errboe M, Lescoy Mevil Y, Glenny AM: Potassium containing toothpastes for dentine hypersensitivity. Cochrane Database Syst Rev 2005; 3:CD001476.

85 Kanapka JA: Over the counter dentifrices in the treatment of tooth hypersensitivity: review of clinical studies. Dent Clin North Am 1990;34:545–560.

86 Ross MR: Hypersensitive teeth: effect of strontium chloride in a compatible dentifrice. J Periodontol 1961;32:49–53.

87 Gedalia I, Brayer L, Kalter N, Richter M, Stabholz A: The effect of fluoride and strontium application on dentine: in vivo and in vitro studies. J Periodontol 1978;49:269–272.

88 Addy M, Mostafa P: Dentine hypersensitivity. II. Effects produced by the uptake in vitro of toothpastes onto dentine. J Oral Rehabil 1989;16:35–48.

89 Jackson RJ: Potential treatment modalities for dentine hypersensitivity: home use products; in Addy M, Embery G, Edgar WM, Orchardson R (eds): Tooth Wear and Sensitivity. London, Dunitz, 2000, pp 327–338.

90 Banfield N, Addy M: Dentine hypersensitivity: development and evaluation of a model in situ to study tubule patency. J Clin Periodontol 2004;31: 325–335.

91 Addy M, Mostafa P: Dentine hypersensitivity. I. Effects produced by the uptake in vitro of metal ions, fluoride and formaldehyde onto dentine. J Oral Rehabil 1988;15:575–585.

92 Claydon NCA, Addy M, Macdonald EL, West NX, Maggio B, Barlow A, Parkinson C, Butler A: Development of an in situ methodology for the clinical evaluation of dentine hypersensitivity occlusion ingredients. J Clin Dent 2009;20: 158–166.

93 Parkinson CR, Wilson RJ: A comparative in vitro study investigating the occlusion and mineralization properties of commercial toothpastes in a four-day dentin disc model. J Clin Dent 2011;22:74–81.

94 Parkinson CR, Butler A, Wilson RJ: Development of an acid challenge-based in vitro dentin disc occlusion model. J Clin Dent 2010;21:31–36.

95 Earl JS, Ward MB, Langford RM: Investigation of dentinal tubule occlusion using FIB-SEM milling and EDX. J Clin Dent 2010;21:37–41.

96 Mason S, Hughes N, Sufi F, Bannon L, Maggio B, North M, Holt J: A comparative clinical study investigating the efficacy of a dentifrice containing 8% strontium acetate, 1,040 ppm fluoride in a silica base and a control dentifrice containing 1,450 ppm fluoride in a silica base to provide immediate relief of dentin hypersensitivity. J Clin Dent 2010;21:42–48.

97 Karim BF, Gillam DG: The efficacy of strontium and potassium toothpastes in treating dentine hypersensitivity: a systematic review. J Dent 2013;2013: 573–577.

98 Petrou I, Heu R, Stanick M, Lavender S, Zaidel L, Cummins D, Sullivan RJ, Hsueh C, Gimzewski JK: A breakthrough therapy for dentin hypersensitivity: how dental products containing 8% arginine and calcium carbonate work to deliver effective relief of sensitive teeth. J Clin Dent 2009;20:23–31.

99 Lavender SA, Petrou I, Heu R, Stranick MA, Cummins D, Kilpatrick-Liverman L, Sullivan RJ, Santarpia RP 3rd: Mode of action studies on a new desensitizing dentifrice containing 8% arginine, a high-cleaning calcium carbonate system and 1,450 ppm fluoride. Am J Dent 2010;23:14–19.

100 Hamlin D, Williams KP, Delgado E, Zhang YP, DeVizio W, Mateo LR: Clinical evaluation of the efficacy of a desensitizing paste containing 8.0% arginine and calcium carbonate for the in-office relief of dentin hypersensitivity associated with dental prophylaxis. Am J Dent 2009;22:16–20.

101 Schiff T, Delgado E, Zhang YP, Cummins D, DeVizio W, Mateo LR: Clinical evaluation of the efficacy of a desensitizing paste containing 8.0% arginine and calcium carbonate in providing instant and lasting relief of dentin hypersensitivity. Am J Dent 2009;22:8–15.

102 Ayed F, Ayad N, Delgado E, Zhang YP, DeVizio W, Cummins D, Mateo LR: Comparing the efficacy in providing instant relief of dentin hypersensitivity of a new toothpaste containing 8.0% arginine, calcium carbonate and 1,450 ppm fluoride to a sensitive toothpaste containing 2% potassium ion and 1,450 ppm fluoride and to a control toothpaste with 1,450 ppm fluoride: a three-day clinical study in Mississauga, Canada. J Clin Dent 2009;20:115–122.

103 Nathoo S, Delgado E, Zhang YP, DeVizio W, Cummins D, Mateo LR: Comparing the efficacy in providing instant relief of dentin hypersensitivity of a new toothpaste containing 8.0% arginine, calcium carbonate and 1,450 ppm fluoride relative to a sensitive toothpaste containing 2% potassium ion and 1,450 ppm fluoride and to a control toothpaste with 1,450 ppm fluoride: a three-day clinical study in New Jersey. J Clin Dent 2009;20:123–130.

104 Ayed F, Ayad N, Zhang YP, DeVizio W, Cummins D, Mateo LR: Comparing the efficacy in reducing dentin hypersensitivity of a new toothpaste containing 8.0% arginine, calcium carbonate and 1,450 ppm fluoride to a commercial sensitive toothpaste containing 2% potassium ion: an eight-week clinical study on Canadian adults. J Clin Dent 2009;20:10–16.

105 Docimo R, Montesami L, Maturo P, Costacurta M, Bartolino M, DeVizio W, Zhang YP, Cummins D, Dibart S, Mateo LR: Comparing the efficacy in reducing dentin hypersensitivity of a new toothpaste containing 8.0% arginine, calcium carbonate and 1,450 ppm fluoride to a commercial sensitive toothpaste containing 2% potassium ion: an eight-week clinical study in Rome. J Clin Dent 2009;20:17–22.

106 Docimo R, Montesami L, Maturo P, Costacurta M, Bartolino M, Zhang YP, DeVizio W, Delgado E, Cummins D, Dibart S, Mateo LR: Comparing the efficacy in reducing dentin hypersensitivity of a new toothpaste containing 8.0% arginine, calcium carbonate and 1,450 ppm fluoride to a benchmark commercial sensitive toothpaste containing 2% potassium ion: an eight-week clinical study in Rome. J Clin Dent 2009;20:137–143.

107 Fu Y, Li X, Que K, Wang M, Hu D, Mateo LR, DeVizio W, Zhang YP: Instant dentin hypersensitivity relief of a new desensitizing toothpaste containing 8.0% arginine, a high cleaning calcium carbonate system and 1,450 ppm fluoride: a three-day clinical study in Chengdu, China. Am J Dent 2010;23: 20–27.

108 Que K, Fu Y, Lin L, Hu D, Zhang YP, Panagakos FS, DeVizio W, Mateo LR: Dentin hypersensitivity reduction of a new toothpaste containing 8.0% arginine, a high cleaning calcium carbonate system and 1,450 ppm fluoride: an eight-week clinical study on Chinese adults. Am J Dent 2010;23: 28–35.

109 Schiff T, Delgado E, Zhang YP, DeVizio W, Cummins D, Mateo LR: The clinical effect of a single direct topical application of a dentifrice containing 8.0% arginine, calcium carbonate, and 1,450 ppm fluoride on dentin hypersensitivity: the use of a cotton swab applicator versus the use of a fingertip. J Clin Dent 2009;20:131–136.

110 Yan B, Yi J, Li Y, Chen Y, Shi Z: Arginine-containing toothpastes for dentin hypersensitivity: systematic review and meta-analysis. Quintessence Int 2013; 44:709–723.

111 Sharif M, Iram S, Brunton P: Effectiveness of arginine-containing toothpastes in treating dentine hypersensitivity: a systematic review. J Dent 2013; 41:483–492.

112 Absi EG, Addy M, Adams D: Dentine hypersensitivity: uptake of toothpastes onto dentine and effects of brushing, washing and dietary acid. J Oral Rehabil 1995;22:175–128.

113 von Koppenfels RL, Kozak KM, Duschner H, White DJ, Goetz H, Taylor E, Zoladz JR: Stannous fluoride effects on dentinal tubules (abstract 93). J Dent Res 2005;84.

114 White DJ, Lawless MA, Fatade A, Baig A, von Koppenfels R, Duschner H, Gotz H: Stannous fluoride/sodium hexametaphosphate dentifrice increases resistance to tubule exposure in vitro. J Clin Dent 2007;18:55–59.

115 Blong MA, Volding B, Thrash WJ, Jones DL: Effects of a gel containing 0.4% stannous fluoride on dentinal hypersensitivity. Dent Hyg (Chic) 1985;59:489–492.

116 Snyder RA, Beck FM, Horton JE: The efficacy of a 0.4% stannous fluoride gel on root surface hypersensitivity (abstract 237). J Dent Res 1985;62:201.

117 Thrash WJ, Dodds WJ, Jones DL: The effect of stannous fluoride on dentine hypersensitivity. Int Dent J 1994; 44(suppl 1):107–118.

118 Schiff T, He T, Sagel L, Baker R: Efficacy and safety of a novel stabilized stannous fluoride and sodium hexametaphosphate dentifrice for dental hypersensitivity. J Contemp Dent Pract 2006;7:1–8.

119 Schiff T, Saletta L, Baker RA, Winston JL, He T: Desensitizing effect of a stabilized stannous fluoride/sodium hexametaphosphate dentifrice. Compend Contin Educ Dent 2005;26(suppl 1):35–40.

120 He T, Barker ML, Qaqish J, Sharma N: Fast onset sensitivity relief of a 0.454% stannous fluoride dentifrice. J Clin Dent 2011;22:46–50.

121 He T, Cheng R, Biesbrock AR, Chang A, Sun L: Rapid desensitizing efficacy of a stannous-containing sodium fluoride dentifrice. J Clin Dent 2011;22: 40–45.

122 Layer TM: Development of a fluoridated, daily-use toothpaste containing NovaMin technology for the treatment of dentin hypersensitivity. J Clin Dent 2011;22:59–61.

123 LaTorre G, Greenspan DC: The role of ionic release of NovaMin (calcium sodium silicophosphate) in tubule occlusion: an exploratory in vitro study using radio-labeled isotopes. J Clin Dent 2010;21:72–76.

124 Earl JS, Leary RK, Muller KH, Langford RM, Greenspan DC: Physical and chemical characterization of surface layers formed on dentin following treatment with a fluoridated toothpaste containing NovaMin. J Clin Dent 2011;22:68–73.

125 Earl JS, Topping N, Elle J, Langford RM, Greenspan DC: Physical and chemical characterization of dentin surface following treatment with NovaMin technology. J Clin Dent 2011;22: 62–67.

126 Du Min Q, Bian Z, Jiang H, Greenspan DC, Burwell AK, Zhong J, Tai BJ: Clinical evaluation of a dentifrice containing calcium sodium phosphosilicate (NovaMin) for the treatment of dentin hypersensitivity. Am J Dent 2008;21: 210–214.

127 Pradeep AR, Sharma A: Comparison of the clinical efficacy of a dentifrice containing calcium sodium phosphosilicate with a dentifrice containing potassium nitrate and a placebo on dentinal hypersensitivity. J Periodontol 2010; 81:1167–1173.

128 Litkowski L, Greenspan DC: A clinical study of the effect of calcium sodium phosphosilicate on dentin hypersensitivity – proof of principle. J Clin Dent 2010;21:77–81.

129 Azarpazahooh A, Limeback H: Clinical efficacy of casein derivatives: a systematic review. J Am Dent Assoc 2008;139: 915–924.

130 Greenhill JD, Pashley DH: Effects of desensitizing agents on the hydraulic conductance of human dentine in vitro. J Dent 1981;60:686–698.

131 Mongiorgi R, Prati C: Mineralogical and crystallographical study of calcium oxalate on dentine surfaces in vitro. Arch Oral Biol 1994;39(suppl):152.

132 Suge I, Kawasski A, Ishikawa K, Matsuo I, Ebisu S: Effects of pre- or post-application of calcium chloride on occluding ability of potassium oxalate for the treatment of dentin hypersensitivity. Am J Dent 2005;18:121–125.

133 Cunha-Cruz J, Stout JR, Heaton LJ, Wataha JC: Dentine hypersensitivity and oxalates: a systematic review. J Dent Res 2011;90:304–310.

134 Neuhaus KW, Milleman JL, Milleman KR, Mongiello KA, Simonton TC, Clark CE, Proskin HM, Seemann R: Effectiveness of a calcium sodium phosphosilicate-containing prophylaxis paste in reducing dentine hypersensitivity immediately and 4 weeks after a single application: a double-blind randomized controlled trial. J Clin Periodontol 2013;40:349–357.

135 Milleman JL, Milleman KR, Clark CE, Mongiello KA, Simonton TC, Proskin HM: NUPRO sensodyne prophylaxis paste with NovaMin for the treatment of dentin hypersensitivity: a 4-week clinical study. Am J Dent 2012;25:262–268.

136 Sönmez H, Aras S: SEM investigation of the effects of various fluoride preparations on dentin surface (in Turkish). Ankara Univ Hekim Fak Derg 1989;16:71–76.

137 Petersson LG: The role of fluoride in the preventive management of dentin hypersensitivity and root caries. Clin Oral Investig 2013;17(suppl 1):S63–S71.

138 Merika K, HefitiArthur F, Preshaw PM: Comparison of two topical treatments for dentine sensitivity. Eur J Prosthodont Restor Dent 2006;14:38–41.

139 Ritter AV, Dias WL, Miguez P, Caplan DJ, Swift EJ: Treating cervical dentin hypersensitivity with fluoride varnish: a randomized clinical study. J Am Dent Assoc 2006;137:1013–1020.

140 Sethna GD, Prabhuji ML, Karthikeyan BV: Comparison of two different forms of varnishes in the treatment of dentine hypersensitivity: a subject-blind randomised clinical study. Oral Health Prev Dent 2011;9:143–140.

141 Abdelaziz RR, Mosallam RS, Yousry MM: Tubular occlusion of simulated hypersensitive dentin by the combined use of ozone and desensitizing agents. Acta Odontol Scand 2011;69:395–400.

142 Lin P-Y: Systematic review and network meta-analysis of in-office treatment for dentine hypersensitivity. J Clin Periodontol 2013;40:53–64.

143 Da Rosa WL, Lund RG, Piva E, da Silva AF: The effectiveness of current dentin desensitising agents used to treat dental hypersensitivity: a systematic review. Quintessence Int 2013;44:535–546.

144 Goodis HE, White JM, Marshall GW, Yee K, Fuller N, Gee L, Marshall SJ: Effects of Nd: and Ho:yttrium-aluminium-garnet lasers on human dentine fluid flow and dental pulp-chamber temperature in vitro. Arch Oral Biol 1997;42:845–854.

145 Kumar NG, Mehta DS: Short-term assessment of the Nd:YAG laser with and without sodium fluoride varnish in the treatment of dentin hypersensitivity – a clinical and scanning electron microscopy study. J Periodontol 2005;76:1140–1147.

146 Renton-Harper P, Midda M: Nd:YAG laser treatment of dentinal hypersensitivity. Br Dent J 1992;172:13–26.

147 Lan WH, Liu HC: Treatment of dentine hypersensitivity by Nd:YAG laser. J Clin Laser Med Surg 1996;14:89–92.

148 Lier BB, Rosing CK, Aass AM, Gjermo P: Treatment of dentine hypersensitivity by Nd:YAG laser. J Clin Periodontol 2002;29:501–506.

149 Corona SA, Nascimento TN, Catirse AB, Lizarelli RF, Dinelli W, Palma-Dibb RG: Clinical evaluation of low-level laser therapy and fluoride varnish for treating cervical dentinal hypersensitivity. J Oral Rehabil 2003;30:1183–1189.

150 Schwartz F, Arweiler N, Georg T, Reich E: Desensitising effects of an Er:YAG laser on hypersensitive dentine. J Clin Periodontol 2002;29:211–215.

151 Sgolastra F, Petrucci A, Gatto R, Monaco A: Effectiveness of laser in dentinal hypersensitivity treatment: a systematic review. J Endod 2011;37:297–303.

Prof. N. West
Periodontology, Clinical Trials Unit
Bristol Dental School, Lower Maudlin Street
Bristol BS1 2LY (UK)
E-Mail n.x.west@bristol.ac.uk

West · Seong · Davies

Lussi A, Ganss C (eds): Erosive Tooth Wear. Monogr Oral Sci. Basel, Karger, 2014, vol 25, pp 123–142
DOI: 10.1159/000360355

Methods for Assessment of Dental Erosion

Thomas Attin · Florian Just Wegehaupt

Center for Dental Medicine, Clinic for Preventive Dentistry, Periodontology and Cariology, University of Zurich, Zurich, Switzerland

Abstract

Various assessment techniques have been applied to evaluate the loss of dental hard tissue and the surface-softened zone in enamel induced by erosive challenges. In this chapter, the most frequently adopted techniques for analyzing the erosively altered dental hard tissues are reviewed, such as profilometry, measuring microscope techniques, microradiography, scanning electron microscopy, atom force microscopy, nano- and microhardness tests and iodide permeability test. Moreover, methods for chemical analysis of minerals dissolved from dental hard tissue are discussed. It becomes evident that the complex nature of erosive mineral loss and dissolution might not be comprehended by a single technique, but needs application of different approaches for full understanding.

© 2014 S. Karger AG, Basel

Acid attack leads to an irreversible loss of the outermost enamel and dentine layers and to partial demineralization (softening) of the tooth surface. In enamel, the thickness of the softened layer is estimated to be 2–5 μm [1, 2]. The softened eroded tooth surface is highly susceptible to abrasive wear, and mechanical impacts such as tooth-brushing can easily remove the superficially demineralized dental hard tissue [3–5].

For simulating intra-oral erosion as closely as possible, it is desirable to assess the erosive effects on native tooth surfaces. Most of the methods described below need polished surfaces for precise assessment of the erosively induced defects or for creating reference surfaces, which means that the natural, often fluoridated surface of the tooth has to be removed. However, it should be considered that in the case of intra-oral erosion the outermost surface layers are also continuously removed by the acid attack, so that a 'polished' surface is created. Monitoring the progression of erosive surface alterations at different time points renders it necessary to fix a specimen in the measuring device in a reproducible position. This aspect becomes increasingly more important the smaller the mineral loss is.

In the oral cavity, the contact of the teeth with an acidic substrate is usually limited to a few seconds before clearance by saliva. This means that under natural conditions an early erosive lesion is created with very small loss of mineral and erosive craters in a nanometer scale or even a near-atomic level. Detection of these small surface changes would allow reducing the contact of an acidic substrate with the tooth surface in experiments to a time period resembling intra-oral conditions. Moreover, feasibility to detect these small alterations would enable one to reduce contact of the acid with a tooth to a single and short event instead of long or repeated procedures which are disadvantageous in in situ and in vitro experiments. When erosion is assessed in dentine specimens, it is important to notice that drying may lead to shrinkage of the specimen, rendering difficult the detection of small surface alterations and loss.

It has, however, to be noted that assessment procedures should fulfill intra-assay (coefficient of variation of <10%) and inter-assay precision with time (coefficient of variation of <20%) according to the guidance for bioanalytical methods, as recently described [6, 7]. Moreover, lower limits of quantification should be determined before the application of a method, meaning that only those readings should be considered in the analysis that are higher than the value of the detection limit plus 5 SD [6, 7]. The limit of detection and the precision of a method may depend on the substrate to be analyzed, so that these parameters could not be taken from manufacturers' descriptions, as was exemplarily shown for a calcium assay [8]. Unfortunately, only in few erosion studies are these parameters clearly given for the specific assessment methods applied. Generally, qualitative assessments bear the problem that classification and interpretation of the findings are more or less subjective depending on the investigator. In order to get objective and measurable data, quantitative analyses should be preferred when possible. However, with qualitative determinations (such as scanning electron microscopy, SEM, and confocal laser scanning microscopy, CLSM) changes of tooth structure could be visualized, giving an impression of the different impacts of different substrates on the dental hard tissues.

Due to the lack of fixed intra-oral reference points, it is complicated to monitor the progression of erosive tooth wear accurately on natural tooth surfaces in the oral cavity. Moreover, most of the devices used for detection of mineral loss and changes could only be performed on specially prepared specimens. Therefore, erosive and erosive/abrasive alterations of dental hard tissues are mostly investigated either in in vitro or in situ studies. In the latter, enamel or dentine specimens are extra-orally or sometimes intra-orally subjected to erosive challenges, worn in the oral cavity according to the intra-oral cariogenicity test developed by Koulourides et al. [9–11] and finally assessed in the laboratory for hard tissue loss and surface alterations.

Due to the two patterns – loss and softening of the dental hard tissue – assessments of dental erosions deal with different methodological approaches, namely, to evaluate either surface phenomena only, such as change of surface hardness, or loss of the dental hard tissues per se. Various techniques have been used to investigate these two aspects of dental erosion [12, 13].

In the following, the most established and well-evaluated techniques as well as emerging methods will be described.

Scanning Electron Microscopy and Energy-Dispersive X-Ray Spectroscopy

Using SEM, surface alterations after erosive attacks are qualitatively estimated in some studies [14, 15]. Grading of the severity of surface alteration could be done on individually adopted scales. SEM investigations can be performed on both polished and unpolished native surfaces after gold sputtering. In enamel, acid attacks due to immersion of specimens in erosive solutions lead to a surface etching pattern with exposition of enamel prisms to an extent depending on the severity of the erosive challenge. SEM investigations were also applied for evaluating the efficacy of salivary-acquired pellicle to protect the underlying enamel surface from acidic dissolution [16–

18] or to demonstrate superficially deposited precipitates resulting from mineral dissolution with differently acting acids [19]. In dentine, acid treatments may result in opening of the dentine tubules which could be graded according to its degree [20]. With common SEM, moisture loss of specimens due to necessary preparation of the specimens for the SEM investigation may lead to additional alterations of the eroded surface. To avoid collapse of the fragile eroded enamel surface structure, freeze drying of samples was suggested [21]. Precipitates formed by dissolved enamel mineral may block the enamel surface so that the eroded enamel prism structure might not be seen with SEM. To reduce the risk of artefactual reprecipitation, neutralization of the acid is recommended before removal of samples from the acidic bath. Impregnation of the delicate surface with methacrylate or dentine adhesives allows for fabrication of resin replicas [22]. After complete dissolution of the enamel with HCl, the resin replicas could then be studied with SEM, providing insight into structural surface and subsurface changes.

With environmental SEM (ESEM), no sample preparation is required, reducing the risk for artefacts to a minimum. ESEM also allows for examination of samples without metal or carbon coating, respectively, in low vacuum and in wet conditions. Nevertheless, SEM and ESEM techniques do not provide as much detailed information about surface alterations of eroded samples as other methods used for the evaluation of erosive impact on dental hard tissues.

SEM or ESEM can be coupled with energy-dispersive X-ray spectroscopy and was also used for a microanalysis suitable for analyzing elemental composition of the top few micrometers of a sample surface. An electron beam hitting the surface leads to excitement of atoms resulting in the emission of X-rays, which provides information about the distribution of various elements such as calcium, phosphate, stannous or fluoride with a concentration of about 1 wt%. However, suitability of the method for evaluating erosive processes has not been clearly demonstrated as yet [23].

Both SEM and ESEM are suitable for use with native surfaces. Although both methods only allow subjective qualitative assessment, ESEM is favorable when wet substrates or dentine should be evaluated. For ESEM, specimens do not need to be sputtered. This allows deeper penetration of electrons into the samples, leading to less sharp pictures of the surface. Additionally, a kind of moisture fog may appear above the sample. This leads to the fact that the detector has to be penetrated through the fog, thus approaching the specimen very closely. These conditions allow for lower resolution using an ESEM compared to an SEM.

Measuring Light Microscopy

The use of an optical microscope to measure height differences between eroded and noneroded (reference) areas of enamel samples was firstly reported by Chuenarrom and Benjakul [24] in 2008. For the evaluation of erosive tooth wear, the z-positions (height) of two points on the noneroded area have to be defined as reference height. The two reference points need to be located on both sides of the area to be tested. The depth of the eroded area is determined by focusing on the eroded surface along a distance of about 1.5 mm in steps of 100 μm. The values recorded on one track are averaged.

Measuring with a measuring microscope provides an easy and nondestructive method to determine erosive tooth wear. However, it is not suitable to measure initial erosive wear as the measurement accuracy is determined by the depth of focus of the used objective lens. Therefore, to ensure correct measurement of minor erosive enamel loss, the depth of focus has to be smaller than the expected erosive wear.

Furthermore, an elaborate sample preparation or sample positioning is necessary, as the sample surface has to be absolutely parallel to the focus plan. Otherwise, difference in height between the two reference areas might occur and lead to non-precise values.

Surface 3D Focus Variation Scanning Microscopy

The surface 3D focus variation technique is a relatively new method applied for the characterization of surface damages of solid samples [25].

It has been used in a few recent studies and is based on images taken with difference in focus [26]. For a complete detection of the surface, the optic is moved vertically along the optical axis. A sensor captures a series of 2D data sets during this scanning process. These 2D data are used to construct a 3D image with a vertical resolution of up to 10 nm. With these images topographical measurements can be performed indicating, for example, surface roughness and maximum peak-to-valley distance within the rough surface. Using these values, wear of the eroded surface can be determined. An advantage of the technique is that steep vertical structures can also be captured.

Attenuated Total Reflectance Infrared Spectroscopy

The attenuated total reflectance infrared spectroscopy (ATRIS) is, like other spectroscopic methods, a tool used for the qualitative and quantitative analysis of organic or inorganic compounds of materials [27, 28]. It can thus be used for identifying the occurrence of affected P-O-Ca atomic linkages, which gives an indication of the damage due to an erosive attack [29].

A beam of infrared light is passed through an ATR crystal (e.g. Ge, Si, ZnSe or diamond). This beam is reflected by the crystal surface in contact with the sample. This reflection forms the evanescent (attenuated) wave, which extends into the sample at a depth of 0.5–5 µm depending on the ATRIS system used. The limitation of the penetration depth is one of the advantages of ATRIS compared to other spectroscopic methods and allows higher precision within the respective measured surface layer. The penetration depth depends on wavelength of light, the angle of incidence, and the indices of refraction for the ATR crystal and the specimen analyzed. Using this method, it was recently shown that the erosively induced modification of apatite structures occurs within a surface layer thickness of 700 nm, regardless of the concentration of the applied acid (citric acid) [30]. This observation correlates with other studies having shown that the depth of briefly eroded enamel (1 min in HCl, pH 2.1) amounted to about 500 nm [1].

Optical Specular and Diffuse Reflection Analysis

Optical reflection measurements allow for characterization of etched surfaces and were firstly applied on eroded enamel by Thomas et al. [31]. Specular or mirror-like reflection provided by smooth surfaces follows the law of reflection, reflecting an incoming light beam in a distinct direction. In contrast, diffuse reflection is provided by rough surfaces, resulting in a scattering of the reflected light in a broad range of directions. The reflected light might be recorded by a spectrometer at different wavelengths. With increasing time of erosion, enamel surfaces showed a decrease of specular reflection and an increase of diffuse reflection. This allows for recording enamel surface alterations already after a short duration (0.5–2 min) of an erosive challenge with citric acid (pH 3.6). Thereby, reflection measurements correlate well with calcium loss, surface roughness and hardness measurements. With longer application times of the acid, the reflection reaches steady plateau values, which confines this method to early erosion processes. A direct quantification of the erosive loss is not possible with this method [32].

White Light Interferometry

White light interferometry is another quasi nondestructive method to determine erosive tooth wear, which was described in detail in 2005 [33] and also used in some recent studies. Topography images are taken with an optical interference microscope operating in a vertical scanning interferometry mode. Tooth wear is calculated by subtracting topography images of original (pre-erosion) surfaces (with a reference area resistant against erosive attacks) from topography images taken after the erosive attack. It is important to record baseline topography images, as only this approach guarantees correct determination of erosive tooth loss in reference to the original surface curvature of the samples. The actual determination of the erosive wear is performed by calculating the depth distribution of each pixel in the reference and the test areas. Later, the height of the reference area is set to zero so that the depth of the erosive wear can be identified.

Disadvantageously, a wiping of the etched enamel with a pellet of cotton has to be performed in some cases, as the etching of the enamel will produce a very delicate fibrous surface which tends to scatter and absorb light. This effect can reduce the reflectance of the surface under the detection limit of 2% for the white light interferometer. Wiping the surface leads to better reflection by removing or flattening the fibrous surface. However, this wiping will destroy the 'natural' etched enamel surface, which might influence later reactions of the etched enamel with applied products.

The authors assume that under full control regarding instrumental and systematic errors, a measurement with a precision of 0.01 µm and an accuracy of 0.02 µm could be performed up to an etching depth of 10 µm [33].

Optical Coherence Tomography

Tomography methods are used to generate cross-sectional images of 3D objects which are further analyzed to receive qualitative and quantitative information [34]. Optical coherence tomography (OCT) is of importance in the medical field because it is a noninvasive, nondestructive technique that does not require particular sample preparation and provides rapid screening. The OCT method is based on the principle of light interferometry using broadband light [35, 36]. The optical system focuses the light beam onto the sample and collects backscattered or reflected light back to the interferometer, where the magnitude and the echo time delay of the backscattered light are analyzed. Hence, OCT images show light-scattering intensity from different layers of tissue. Because enamel and dentine have different scattering properties and the optical properties of healthy sound enamel differ from the demineralized tissue, the OCT images can provide information about the enamel thickness, morphology and porosity. For example, demineralized eroded areas of enamel have higher porosity than the healthy hard tissue which causes higher light scattering in the eroded enamel and a reduced depth of light penetration. As a result, demineralized areas appear on the OCT images with increased signal intensity/reflectivity compared to the sound tissue. Analogously, remineralization can be detected as an area with reduced light scattering, i.e. reduced signal intensity compared to the demineralized enamel. OCT was successfully applied for the in vivo quantification of dental erosion in patients with gastroesophageal reflux disease [37]. The authors found a significant difference of loss of enamel thickness in the placebo group (0.8% thickness loss) and patients who were treated with acid-suppressive medication (0.3% thickness loss). Amaechi et al. [38, 39] used OCT for characterization of carious lesions and found a good correlation between the change of tissue reflectivity in OCT images and the fluorescence loss measured by quantitative light-induced fluorescence (QLF) in artificial carious lesions. Nevertheless, due to a limited axial resolution (1 μm highest), a currently used traditional OCT method is applied at the substance loss stage of erosion [40]. In addition, the high refractive index of dental hard tissues determines strong reflection from the tooth surface which can dominate the reflections from the deeper tissue layers and complicate the OCT analysis [41].

To improve the method and to overcome the effect of the surface reflection, different variations of OCT were invented for the quantification of early tooth erosion. Polarization-sensitive OCT, and particularly cross-polarization OCT, allows high-contrast images between sound and demineralized enamel areas, providing more sophisticated erosion quantification. In cross-polarization OCT, the incident light is circularly polarized to partially suppress the surface reflectivity and to reduce the effect of sample orientation/positioning on the signal. The proposed setup could only be applied to the labial surfaces of incisors in vivo; however, there are many hand-held fiber-optic probes under development [42].

In contrast to microradiography, the OCT method provides 3D images of tissues and does not involve ionizing radiation. Disadvantages of the OCT include difficulty in accessing all positions within the oral cavity, relatively high costs and limited penetration depth.

Surface Hardness Measurements

To determine changes of surface hardness of erosively altered dental hard tissues, microhardness and, as a relatively new approach, nanoindentation techniques are often used. With hardness measurements, early stages of enamel and dentine dissolution, which are associated with weakening of the surface, can be determined. The basic method of micro- and nanoindentation involves the indentation of a diamond tip of

known geometrical dimensions for a given load and duration.

For microhardness assessments of eroded tooth surfaces, mostly Knoop or Vickers diamonds are used on previously polished surfaces. Polished surfaces are recommended to produce well-defined indentations. Application of Knoop diamond resulted in a rhomboid indentation and that of Vickers in a tetra-pyramidal one. The lengths of the indentations on the surface are measured under a microscope requiring indentation lengths of about 30–40 μm for precise measurements. Knoop or Vickers hardness numbers are calculated by means of a special formula. In enamel, the length of the indentations is not time dependent and could be recorded immediately. However, in dentine, indentation length changed due to flexibility of the dentine substrate, which was shown for indentations performed with 500 g. In this case, indentations should best be measured 24 h after the indentation has been made [43]. No comparable recommendations are available for dentine indentations conducted with lower forces, although it could be assumed that when applying low forces the time needed to retraction of dentine after loading might be shorter than 24 h. On erosively altered surfaces, the outlines of the indentations are sometimes fuzzy, rendering precise measurements difficult. The hardness measured by indentation is affected not only by the immediate surrounding, but also by changes in the material at a distance of approximately 10 times the dimensions of the indentation. To limit the impact of surrounding material changes, microindentations for determining erosive alterations of the superficial surfaces are performed with low pressure of about 50 g (0.49 N) [44, 45]. Nevertheless, one should be aware that microhardness measurements do not reflect the properties of the surface only. The penetration depth of the Vickers diamond amounted to 1/7 of the indentation length (e.g. with indentations of 35 μm in length, the depth of penetration amounts to 5.0 μm). Penetration depth of the Knoop diamond amounts to 1/30.5 of its indentation length. This means that with the same indentation length and visibility under the assessment microscope the Knoop hardness determination better reflects alterations of the actually outermost layers than the Vickers hardness testing, since Knoop hardness indentations of, for example, 35 μm in length are equivalent to a penetration depth of 1.15 μm. Nevertheless, microhardness measurements such as the Knoop procedure allow discrimination of different erosive potentials of various substances on dental hard tissue, even after short exposures (3 min) to acidic agents [46]. In other studies, immersion periods of at least 20 min were chosen to investigate the impact on surface hardness [47–49]. However it should be noticed that the differences between different aggressive solutions might be less pronounced, since long expositions to different acidic substrates lead to similar depth of the surface softened layer.

By means of the indentations on enamel surfaces, detection of enamel abrasion is also possible by calculating the depth of the indentations. The difference between the depth before and after abrasion provided a direct measurement for the loss of substance by abrasion at this site [50–53]. The main principle behind this method is that the ground of the indentation is not changed and is not removed by the abrasion. Only the surrounding tissue on the surface is removed so that due to the pyramidal geometry the outer contour of the indentation (and thereby its length) is reduced [50, 51]. The substance loss (Δd) is calculated from the change in indentation length (Δl) using the geometrical formula: $\Delta d = 0.032772 \Delta l$. With this procedure, surface loss due to abrasion of previously eroded samples of about 30–100 nm could be determined precisely [54, 55]. Unfortunately, measurements of the amount of substance directly removed by an erosive attack could not be performed with this method, since the acid also removes some substance from the body of the indentation and not only from its surrounding.

In another approach, Schweizer-Hirt et al. [56] visually compared different degrees of disappearance of the indentations after enamel erosion-abrasion, thus estimating substance loss.

The main advantages of microhardness determinations are the relatively low costs and the fact that it is a well-established method and could be combined with measurements of abrasive surface loss.

Surface Profilometry

Irreversible loss of dental hard tissue and surface roughness could be determined using a surface profilometer (surfometer) by scanning specimens with a laser beam or a contact stylus (metal or diamond) with a diameter of about 2–20 μm [4, 57–66]. The contact stylus is loaded with a force of a few millinewtons. By the scanning, a complete map of the specimen topography could be generated. However, the outermost demineralized layer of enamel erosion is very susceptible to mechanical forces so that profilometer measurements can be effected by the tendency of the stylus to penetrate this fragile layer. The tip of the stylus could also be used to render scratches on eroded and noneroded surfaces. By means of atomic force microscopy the depth of the scratch could be quantitatively measured to a nanometer scale in the range of about 10 nm [67, 68].

Application of the laser beam leads to higher resolution compared to the contact stylus (resolution on accuracy in height approx. 10 nm). However, the laser stylus may produce 'overshots' at the sharp edges at the bottom of grooves, which result in artefacts [69]. Moreover, the precision of optical measurement with laser beams is impaired by wet surfaces or measurements under wet conditions due to the reflection of the beam at the surface of the liquids. It should also be noted that dissolution of the enamel due to acid attack leads to surface roughening of about 0.4 μm. Therefore, reliable detection of minimal losses below 1 μm are generally difficult to accomplish with profilometry, although Hooper et al. [70] have demonstrated that profilometry was able to distinguish between different abrasivities of toothpastes creating hard tissue loss of about 0.5 μm. For such precise measurements with low variations, meticulous flattening and polishing of sample surface is an important step.

In studies using surfometry, parts of the surface are protected by nail varnish or adhesive tape prior to the erosive or abrasive attack to produce reference areas allowing comparison between the levels of the untreated and treated surfaces. However, it is also possible to match the baseline scan recorded with the scan conducted after treatment in a computer in order to determine differences in height between these two scans with special software [71, 72]. In this case, it is extremely important to ensure correct repositioning of the sample in the profilometer for the two readings.

When measuring eroded dentine surfaces it has to be respected that dentine and especially eroded dentine is shrinking under ambient conditions. Thus, it was recommended to apply surface profilometry using dentine samples under wet conditions [73]. Moreover, it should be noted that surface profilometry of eroded dentine might interfere with the exposed collagen matrix, thus not reflecting mineral loss of the bulk dentine specimen adequately [74].

Usually, polished surfaces are used in profilometry studies, since native enamel or dentine surfaces show an intrinsic coarseness, rendering detection of small changes due to erosion/abrasion impossible. However, in natural enamel extended depths of at least 50 μm of erosive grooves could also be measured without the need for preparation (polishing) of the surface [58].

Chadwick et al. [75] presented a method to obtain digital surface models using electroconductive replicas generated from silicone impressions of teeth taken at different ages of patients. The replicas were used for surface mapping by means of a computer-controlled probe. Resolution in z-direction is reported to be 1 μm [76]. The resultant maps may be compared using a surface matching and difference detection algorithm. This technique provides readings with good accuracy and reproducibility [77–79]. Erosions of 50 μm in magnitude occurring over a 9-month period were recorded to a precision of about ±15 μm [76].

As summarized, profilometry is a method which may be adopted for surface loss with high precision provided that material loss exceeds about 0.4 μm. The method is also applicable for indirect measurements of intra-oral erosions via replicas.

Iodide Permeability Test

Iodide permeability tests (IPT) were introduced by Bakhos et al. [80] and are based on the principle that defined areas of enamel samples are allowed to soak for a few minutes with potassium iodide which is recovered from the enamel by Millipore prefilter paper discs. The amount of iodide recovered in the discs is determined and provides information about the pore volume of the enamel. It has been shown that (IPT) measurements are closely related to the pore volume of enamel and give sensitive estimations of the early stages of de- and remineralization [81]. Moreover, it has been proven that a linear relationship between IP and calcium loss exists [82]. Changes of enamel structure recorded with IPT have also been shown to correlate well with microhardness testing. This was true for severely eroded samples, in which erosions were performed by immersion in lactate (pH 4.75) for a minimum of 60 min [83]. With shorter exposure periods in the erosive solution, the two methods did not correlate well in this study. Lussi et al. [47] showed that exposure to acidic drinks leads to an increase in IP which was significantly associated with the acidity, pH and mineral contents of the drinks. In contrast to the aforementioned study, Lussi et al. [47] found a correlation between IP and microhardness data for enamel samples immersed in acidic beverages for a period of 20 min.

The IP method has the advantage of low costs, which allows more or less rapid screening of the impact of different erosive substances on enamel.

Chemical Analysis of Minerals Dissolved in the Erosive Agent

Dental enamel consists of 34–39% m/m (g per 100 g) calcium (dry weight) and 16–18% m/m phosphorus [84]. Therefore, determination of dental enamel dissolution by assessing the amount of calcium or phosphate dissolved from the apatite crystals of dental hard tissue could also be regarded as a possible tool for assessing dental erosions. Hence, some authors have applied calcium determination in erosive, acidic solutions after prolonged contact (range 2 min to 24 h) of the solutions with dental hard tissue using calcium-sensitive electrodes, atomic absorption spectrophotometer or the highly sensitive method of inductively coupled plasma mass spectrometry [85–91].

Calcium-sensitive electrodes often need a specific pH of the environment to work precisely. Additionally, calcium complexes formed with certain acids (e.g. citric acid) impair correct measurements of the calcium released from the dental hard tissue. Atomic absorption spectrophotometer requires intensive preparation of the solution to allow for measurement of calcium or phosphate. Both methods additionally need solution volumes exceeding a minimum of 100 µl. Atomic absorption spectrophotometer uses the absorption of light, usually from a hollow-cathode lamp of the element that is being measured, to determine the concentration of gas phase atoms. Since samples are usually liquids or solids, the analyte atoms or ions must be vaporized in a flame or graphite furnace. The atoms absorb ultraviolet or visible light and make transitions to higher electronic energy levels. The analyte concentration is determined from the amount of absorption. Concentration measurements are usually determined from a working curve after calibrating the instrument with standards of known concentration. With the inductively coupled plasma mass spectrometry, the ions are ionized by inductively coupled plasma and quantified by a mass spectrometer. The method is highly sensitive, but susceptible to errors due to contamination.

Recently, the colorimetric Arsenazo III method was described, allowing precise determination of calcium in small volumes of acidic solution (10 µl) by a spectrophotometer [8, 19]. However, this method also could not be applied in all kinds of acids with the same precision. In colorimetric methods, absorbance of light due to the formed colored complex is related to the quantity of the analyte. It should be noted that formation of the colored complex might be impaired by other agents in the solution or by pH.

Determination of phosphorus release during the dissolution process is mostly performed by colorimetric methods such as the ammonium phosphomolybdate method [92, 93]. Another colorimetric method, with 10 times higher sensitivity, is the phosphomolybdate malachite green procedure [94], which has been shown to be suitable for determination of phosphate dissolved from enamel after etching with perchloric acid at a range of 0.025–3.0 mM [95]. Recent studies corroborated this fact showing that, depending on the acid used, the malachite green procedure is a reliable and suitable tool to detect and quantify minimal phosphate contents in small samples of a variety of acidic solutions which have the potential to form erosive lesions [96].

The chemical methods for the assessment of erosive dissolution have the advantage that they allow detection of very small mineral loss using unpolished, native tooth samples. As yet, these methods have only been applied in in vitro experiments.

Microradiography

Microradiography is a tool for quantification of mineral loss based on the attenuation of X-ray irradiation transmitting dental hard tissue. X-ray photons transmitting a dental hard tissue sample can be recorded by photon-counting X-ray detectors, or X-ray sensitive photographic plates or film. The mineral mass can be calculated from the photon counts or gray values of photographic plates or film knowing the appropriate mass attenuation coefficient or by determining photographic density measurements calibrated by an aluminum step wedge [97–99]. For gray value assessment of photographic plates or film densitometers, more recently CCD cameras attached to a microscope are in use.

Microradiography has frequently been used in studies determining mineral changes due to de- and remineralization in the course of caries. The method was used to study these processes in early enamel lesions and less frequently in dentine. For transverse microradiography (TMR) thin sections (50–200 µm) are obtained perpendicular to the sample surface and radiographed with a nickel-filtered Cu Kα line (i.e. at 20 kV, 20 mA) perpendicular to the cut surface. Due to limitations in specimen preparation and alignment, and the geometry of the X-ray beam that spreads radial from a point or line focus rather than parallel, the imaging precision at the sample edge is limited. Usually, the outermost 5–10 µm cannot be exactly reproduced. In early enamel caries with the typical subsurface lesion, mineral loss and changes predominantly occur in the body of the lesion below the pseudo-intact surface layer at a thickness of about 20–50 µm and beyond [100]. TMR is a valid tool for quantitative assessment of the mineral content as a function of depth from the surface of caries and caries-like lesions. From in-depth profiles, the lesion depth and mineral loss integrated over the entire depth (ΔZ) of the lesion can be calculated. Lesion depth is usually defined up to that point, where the mineral content reaches 95% of the mineral content of sound enamel or dentine.

Beyond its original use in caries research, microradiography was adopted for detecting erosive mineral loss. In a TMR-like setup thin enamel or dentine sections can be used to measure erosive mineral loss. In this case, the erosive agent is applied on the cut surface that also contains reference areas not subjected to erosion and X-ray images are taken [101]. Note that in contrast to TMR, as is usually applied in caries research, the erosion is performed on the cut surface of an already prepared tooth slice of 100–200 µm thickness rather than on a specimen's surface that is cut perpendicularly for TMR after an experimental procedure. Hall et al. [101] found a strong correlation between mineral loss determined by either TMR or profilometry even for discrimination of early erosive lesions caused by erosion times of less than 1 h using an orthophosphoric acid-based erosive fluid (pH 3).

Another approach to use TMR for erosive mineral loss determination also depends on the use of reference areas not subjected to an erosive challenge [102, 103]. The erosive challenge is executed on a specimen's surface. Then a slice (50–200 µm) is prepared perpendicular to the surface the same way as for traditional TMR. Thereby, both the depth of the erosive crater and the depth below the bottom of the crater at which mineral content was reduced (surface softening) can be assessed with TMR, giving lesion depth and integrated mineral loss as variables [61, 104, 105]. In these studies, TMR was used to record lesion depths from 20 µm and more. For determination of mineral changes following a small erosive challenge, for example erosive surface softening only, this technique is not sensitive enough due to the fuzziness of the outer 5–10 µm at the edge of the tissue slabs prepared for TMR.

Longitudinal microradiography (LMR) enables the use of thicker specimens (up to 450 µm in thickness) that are usually cut from the tooth comprising the natural enamel surface and some underlying dentine. However, the use of thinner specimens provides better information about the mineral change within the specimen. The specimens are radiographed perpendicular to the surface before (reference) and after treatment(s), and changes in mineral content can be calculated using pixel-by-pixel comparison of gray values of a radiograph after treatment with the gray values of the reference radiograph. In contrast to TMR, LMR cannot be used to determine the mineral profile of a specimen from the surface to depth. Since LMR enables the reuse of specimens, it can be used for longitudinal observations. The mineral loss recorded with LMR consists of both the erosive crater and the loss of mineral in the softened surface zone. LMR is less sensitive to minor changes in mineral content than TMR because of the use of thicker specimens compared to TMR.

Using LMR, erosion progression in both enamel and dentine has also been assessed [106–108]. In these studies, the method has been shown to be suitable to allow for the distinction of different preventive treatment modalities, resulting in detection of different mineral loss. Comparison of LMR in enamel specimens with either profilometry, analysis of dissolved calcium/phosphorus and nanoindentation measurements showed good correlation for the three methods [109, 110]. However, it also became clear that losses below 20 μm should be interpreted with care when using LMR only, since standard deviations were quite high when determining minimal substance loss with LMR.

The main advantage of microradiography is that the method enables one to simultaneously determine surface loss and demineralization of the eroded samples.

Confocal Laser Scanning Microscopy

CLSM is a tool for obtaining high-resolution images, 3D reconstructions and optical sections through 3D specimens. The translucency of teeth allows nondestructive subsurface visualization of their microstructure by CLSM used in reflection mode at a level of about 150–200 μm below the surface [111–113]. Although polished tooth samples are mostly used for CLSM, also unpolished and even wet tooth substrates could be assessed with the method. However, the quality of images obtained from unpolished samples is limited due to reflections and scattering effects caused by the uneven surface. Moreover, surfaces of polished samples could be quite easily aligned parallel to the ground, which is required to obtain images from a defined subsurface level.

In brief, CLSM works as follows: illumination, provided by a gas laser (e.g. Ar/Kr or He/Ar), is focused by an objective lens into a small focal volume within an autofluorescent specimen or a specimen dotted with fluorescent dyes. The laser beam, which could be filtered to select specific wavelengths (often 488 nm) is thereby focused on the focal plane. A mixture of emitted fluorescent light as well as reflected laser light from the illuminated spot is then recollected by the objective lenses and a photon multiplier detector. The focus plane of illumination is the same as the focal plane of detection, which means that they are confocal. Information about the specimen can be collected from different focal planes by raising or lowering the microscopes stage. The computer can generate a 3D picture of a sample by assembling a stack of these 2D images from successive focal planes.

Used in erosion studies, CLSM provides histotomographic images allowing for qualitative assessment and interpretation of hard tissue destruction or mineral dissolution, since light reflection and light scattering of hard tissue samples are influenced by micro-histological changes within a tooth sample [114–116]. Since these images provide only limited information about the exact degree of demineralization, CLSM is mostly combined with other methods (e.g. microhardness, analysis of mineral loss or others). Recently, CLSM was applied also to sections of erosive lesion to measure the depth of erosive loss and of demineralization [117]. This procedure, however, needs some further validation.

The main advantage of CLSM is the high resolution of the system, providing a 3D insight into the erosively altered surface.

Quantitative Light-Induced Fluorescence

QLF was developed as a nondestructive diagnostic method for the longitudinal assessment of early caries lesions [118]. The method applies a xenon gas discharge lamp to illuminate a tooth with filtered blue-violet light to provoke its natural fluorescence. The natural fluorescence is assumed to be caused by fluorophores, which are predominantly located at the dentine-enamel junction and in dentine. Due to higher scattering in carious enamel, less excitation light reaches the fluorescing dentine-enamel junction as well as underlying dentine and less fluorescence from the dentine-enamel junction as well as dentine is able to find its way back through the carious lesion. Therefore, the lesion appears dark in contrast to the surrounding, fluorescing area of the tooth. The area of interest is imaged by a CCD video camera through an optical high-pass filter that blocks the excitation light and allows only the fluorescing light to pass. The averaged difference in fluorescence intensity [ΔF (%)] between the darker fluorescing lesion area and the brighter fluorescing sound area around the lesion is calculated by proprietary software.

As yet, QLF has been applied in only a few studies for monitoring erosive lesions [119–121]. The method was validated in comparison to TMR and was found to be an effective tool for quantification of erosive defects. As already mentioned, the erosive lesion comprises a crater and a softened demineralized surface layer. It could be assumed that the softened surface layer is too thin to create sufficient scattering effects of light. Thus, it is likely that the demineralized surface layer could not account for the loss of fluorescence of the erosive lesion. Therefore, it was hypothesized that the walls of the crater of the erosion are primarily responsible for the dark appearance of the lesion when assessed with QLF. It was assumed that the walls create a shadowing effect and that they hinder release of the fluorescing light due to scattering. With an increase of the depth of the crater these effects might also increase, leading to a more pronounced accentuation of the erosive defect when assessed with QLF. However, the principle behind the reduced fluorescence of erosive lesions is not fully understood and needs to be clarified in further experiments.

Atomic Force Microscopy

Atomic force microscopes (AFM) as well as scanning tunneling microscopes pertain to the family of scanning probe microscopes. In the following, some properties of the instrument are given, as have already been described in detail elsewhere [13, 23, 122]. The main application of AFM is high-resolution imaging of different materials including polymers, ceramics, metals, biomolecules and cells. Different operation modes allow measurement of, among others, surface topography, lateral surface composition and differences in elasticity. Ultra-sharp probes with radii of 4–60 nm are connected to a flexible cantilever and accurate ceramic piezo elements, which allow the sample to be scanned with subnanometer precision. The cantilever deflects in the z-direction due to the surface topography during tip scanning over the surface. A diode laser beam is reflected from the back of the cantilever and is incident on a four-segment photodiode. As the tip moves, the deflection of the cantilever is indicated by the position of the laser on the photodiode, thus constructing a map of the sample surface [23]. The tip can move over the sample in dynamic modes with an oscillating tip moving up and down in either tapping mode (with touching surface contacts) or noncontact mode. In noncontact modes, the tip is placed at the level of the attractive van der Waals forces to detect force gradients. In nondynamic modes, the tip is moved laterally in constant contact with the surface (contact mode). AFM can be used equally well on conducting and insulating materials in ambient conditions, in air or liquids. The resolution is orders of magnitude greater than those with profilometry; however, scan size is limited to at most 0.5 mm × 0.5 mm, taking some 60 min for this size.

AFM was used in erosion studies for qualitative approaches comparing the surface of dental hard tissue and acquired enamel pellicle after exposure to different erosive agents [123–125]. Moreover, substance loss of enamel due to erosion was determined by tapping mode [124] with high resolution. Generally, AFM is able to measure height differences in the order of the size of one atom, rendering the technique suitable for the detection of very early stages of substance loss due to erosive and abrasive attacks. AFM is also suitable to produce images of erosively altered surfaces of dental hard tissues or to measure surface roughness [126].

Nanoindentation

For nanoindentation, an indenter diamond is applied on dental hard tissue with small loads in the order of nanonewtons to millinewtons. Therefore, the indentation depth of the indenter tip could be limited to about 100 nm, allowing for measurements in the outermost softened layer. Mostly, a Berkovich diamond tip is used, resulting in a three-sided pyramidal indentation. The indenter is driven into the sample by applying increasing load to some preset value. The load is gradually decreased until partial or complete relaxation of the sample has occurred. The load and displacement are recorded continuously throughout this process to produce a load displacement curve form from which the nanomechanical properties such as Young's modulus of elasticity, hardness, fracture toughness, time-dependent creep and plastic and elastic energy of the sample could be calculated [127, 128]. Elastic modulus data may be useful in studies of erosion, since it has been shown to be more sensitive than hardness to the presence of underlying hard material. An indentation depth at a force of some 4,500 μN in orange juice-treated enamel was recorded to be in a range of about 200–500 nm. In comparison, water-treated samples showed an indentation depth of 150–350 nm [129]. The nanoindenter could be coupled to the vertical transducer used in combination with AFM, where the cantilever and the laser optical system is replaced by the transducer tip system, allowing for determination of tip displacements with a resolution of 0.2 nm [122, 130]. The tip can be scanned across a substrate, building up an image of the area in contact with the tip. Due to the small size of the tip and the indentations with lengths of about 2 μm, the method should be applicable on unpolished samples and for measurements in tiny defined surface areas. The nanoindentation method is a very sensitive tool, which is able to provide information about material properties. It is less time consuming than AFM, which is used for the mapping of surface topography.

Element Analysis of Solid Samples

In vitro trace element analysis of solid tooth samples is feasible with a variety of methods such as secondary ion mass spectroscopy (SIMS), electron probe microanalysis, laser ablation inductively coupled plasma mass spectroscopy, micro X-ray fluorescence, proton-induced X-ray emission spectroscopy and transmission electron microscopy (TEM) coupled with an X-ray detection system (analytical TEM). However, most of these methods are not described for analyzing dental hard tissue as yet, although they would offer quantitative analysis of elements in very low concentrations in very confined areas of solid samples.

Barbour and Rees [23] described the application of SIMS on erosively altered enamel surfaces giving either topographic images or calcium or magnesium surface maps. These images were able to provide information concerning element loss of the demineralized enamel. The depth of the erosive crater could not be determined with SIMS. Mass spectrometric methods for trace analysis of inorganic materials provide a very sensitive multi-elemental analysis with limits of detection of low ng g^{-1} concentration range [131]. A broad variety of mass spectrometric methods are described in the literature [132] such as SIMS, which allows mono- and multi-elemental trace analysis on solid materials or thin layers. When solid surfaces are bombarded with ions, these ions penetrate into the solid to a certain depth as a function of their energy and mass and the nature and structure of the sample. The bombarded ions transfer their energy to atoms of the solid material. Part of the energy of the primary atoms is returned to the surface and causes sputtering of neutral particles or secondary ions. With SIMS, the secondary ion mass is analyzed in a mass spectrometer where the ions are separated according to their mass-to-charge ratio, giving information about local enrichment or depletion of chemical elements compared to standard reference materials. However, SIMS is only partially quantitative and actual concentrations cannot be measured accurately.

Electron probe microanalysis is another method establishing the chemical composition of very small volumes of solid material which needs to be polished to a plane surface. The method involves bombarding a specimen with a focused high-energy beam of electrons and analyzing the X-ray spectrum emitted from the sample. The X-rays are characteristic of the bombarded elements and allow determination of the quantitative composition of the test samples with wavelength dispersive spectrometers [133]. With sectioned samples, element analysis could be performed in subsurface areas with the electron beam hitting the sectioned surface perpendicular to the natural sample surface. Willershausen and Schulz-Dobrick [134] applied this method for evaluating element distribution in sections of eroded enamel

at a depth of 5–50 µm. Measurements within the first few micrometers of depth of sectioned samples are difficult to perform due to fuzziness at the outermost surface region.

Compared to SEM or TEM equipped with an energy detection system, wavelength dispersive X-ray analyzers in electron probe microanalysis reveals a much higher spectral sensitivity and lower detection limits. Highest lateral resolution (= smallest excited volumes) can be reached with analytical TEM, but this method suffers from the impractical sample preparation of specimens with a maximum thickness of 1 µm and its semi-quantitative results.

In summary, element analysis of solid samples allows very sensitive measurements of early mineral loss depending on the method used. However, suitability for erosion assessment has to be checked for most of these methods in the future.

Ultrasonic Measurement of Enamel Thickness

With ultrasonic pulse-echo measurements the time interval between the transmission of an ultrasound pulse on the enamel surface and the echo produced by the amelodentinal junction is determined. Using these data and the mean longitudinal sound velocity in enamel, the thickness of the enamel layer can be calculated. The method is nondestructive, allowing in vitro as well as in vivo measurements. It shows good correlation between different operators [135]. However, enamel thickness changes of less than 0.33 mm could not be detected precisely with this method [136] and ultrasonic measurements and histological readings of enamel thickness correlated only moderately [137].

The main advantages and the main problems encountered with the described methods are depicted in table 1. Moreover, the methods are judged with respect to the requirements such as their suitability for early erosion or for use with native surfaces. It becomes evident that the com-

Table 1. Survey of the methods described in detail in the text with respect to main advantages and problems as well as to suitability for use with early erosions and with native unpolished surface samples

Method	Advantages	Problems	Suitability for use with early erosions	Suitability for use with native surfaces
SEM and environmental SEM	Applicable for wet samples (ESEM)	Only qualitative assessment	+	++
Measuring microscopy	Allows nondestructive analysis Not time consuming Allows determination of combined erosive/abrasive wear	Low resolution (determined by the depth of focus of objective used) Two reference areas needed	–	–
Surface 3D focus variation scanning microscopy	No special preparation of specimen necessary Provides information about different patterns (roughness, wear) Nondestructive procedure	Time consuming Repetitive measurements of identical regions are difficult	–/+	–/+
ATRIS	Determination of mineral changes throughout the complete surface layer is possible	Sample preparation is demanding Limited quantification of erosive damage	+	–
Optical specular and diffuse reflection analysis	Nondestructive analysis Allows for characterization of early erosive lesions	No quantification of erosive loss	++	+
OCT	Nondestructive analysis Allows for characterization of early erosive lesions	High costs Limited penetration depth	++	+
Surface hardness measurements	Relatively low costs Well-established method Can be combined with determination of surface loss due to abrasion	Measurement of surface hardness is influenced by nondemineralized deeper layers Polished, flat surfaces needed	++	–
Surface profilometry	Applicable for measurement in natural dentition (replica technique)	Time consuming when complete mapping of surfaces Stylus could damage surface	–/+	–/+
IPT	Low costs	Provides only information about increased pore volumes	–/+	+
Chemical analysis of dissolved minerals	Mostly easy and well-established methods	No information about structural changes	+++	++
Microradiography	Determination of both mineral loss and demineralization possible	Limited resolution Demanding sample preparation	–	–
CLSM	High resolution	Only qualitative assessment	++	–/+
QLF	Surface scan is not time consuming	Limited resolution Low experience in erosion studies Exact repositioning of samples for comparative measurements is difficult	–	–
AFM	High resolution Nearly nondestructive	Time-consuming measurement Only limited areas of about 250 × 250 µm could be scanned High costs	+++	+++

Table 1. Continued

Method	Advantages	Problems	Suitability for use with early erosions	Suitability for use with native surfaces
Nanoindentation	Very sensitive Provides also information of material properties	Time-consuming measurements Demanding sample preparation	+++	++
Element analysis of solid samples	Very sensitive (depending on method)	High costs Highly demanding methods	++(+)	++(+)
Ultrasonic measurement	Allows nondestructive analysis without extensive sample preparation	Low resolution	–	–/+

Early erosions: after few minutes of acidic challenge. +++ = Highly suitable; ++ = very suitable; + = suitable; –/+ = limitedly suitable; – = not suitable.

plex nature of erosive mineral loss and dissolution might not be comprehended by a single technique, but needs application of different approaches for full understanding. Especially for determination of early erosion, methods with high resolution providing high accuracy might be helpful to gain more insight into the true nature of erosion development as occurring in the oral cavity.

Acknowledgments

The authors would like to thank Prof. Dr. Wolfgang Buchalla (Department of Operative Dentistry and Periodontology, University of Regensburg), Dr. Andreas Kronz (Department of Geochemistry Geoscience Center, University of Göttingen), Prof. Dr. Adrian Lussi, Ekaterina Rakhmatullina, PhD and Kathy Osann, PhD, MPH for their contribution to parts of the manuscript.

References

1 Wiegand A, Wegehaupt F, Werner C, Attin T: Susceptibility of acid-softened enamel to mechanical wear – ultrasonication versus toothbrushing abrasion. Caries Res 2007;41:56–60.

2 Eisenburger M, Hughes J, West NX, Jandt KD, Addy M: Ultrasonication as a method to study enamel demineralisation during acid erosion. Caries Res 2000;34:289–294.

3 Davis WB, Winter PJ: The effect of abrasion on enamel and dentine and exposure to dietary acid. Br Dent J 1980;148:253–256.

4 Attin T, Koidl U, Buchalla W, Schaller HG, Kielbassa AM, Hellwig E: Correlation of microhardness and wear in differently eroded bovine dental enamel. Arch Oral Biol 1997;42:243–250.

5 Smith BGN, Robb ND: Dental erosion in patients with chronic alcoholism. J Dent 1989;17:219–221.

6 Shah VP, Midha KK, Dighe S, McGilveray IJ, Skelly JP, Yacobi A, Layloff T, Viswanathan CT, Cook CE, McDowall RD: Analytical methods validation: bioavailability, bioequivalence and pharmacokinetic studies. Conference report. Eur J Drug Metab Pharmacokinet 1991;16:249–255.

7 Shah VP, Midha KK, Findlay JW, Hill HM, Hulse JD, McGilveray IJ, McKay G, Miller KJ, Patnaik RN, Powell ML, Tonelli A, Viswanathan CT, Yacobi A: Bioanalytical method validation – a revisit with a decade of progress. Pharm Res 2000;17:1551–1557.

8 Attin T, Becker K, Hannig C, Buchalla W, Hilgers R: Method to detect minimal amounts of calcium dissolved in acidic solutions. Caries Res 2005;39:432–436.

9 Koulourides T, Volker JF: Changes of enamel microhardness in the human mouth. Ala J Med Sci 1964;35:435–437.

10 Koulourides T, Phantumvanit P, Munksgaard EC, Housch T: An intraoral model used for studies of fluoride incorporation in enamel. J Oral Pathol 1974;3:185–196.

11 Koulourides T, Chien MC: The ICT in situ experimental model in dental research. J Dent Res 1992;71:822–827.

12 Grenby TH: Methods of assessing erosion and erosive potential. Eur J Oral Sci 1996;104:207–214.

13 West NX, Jandt KD: Methodologies and instrumentation to measure tooth wear; future perspectives; in Addy M, Embery G, Edgar WM, Orchadson R (eds): Tooth Wear and Sensitivity. London, Martin Dunitz, 2000, pp 105–120.

14 Magalhaes AC, Romanelli AC, Rios D, Comar LP, Navarro RS, Grizzo LT, Aranha AC, Buzalaf MA: Effect of a single application of TiF_4 and NaF varnishes and solutions combined with Nd:YAG laser irradiation on enamel erosion in vitro. Photomed Laser Surg 2011;29: 537–544.

15 Torres CP, Chinelatti MA, Gomes-Silva JM, Rizoli FA, Oliveira MA, Palma-Dibb RG, Borsatto MC: Surface and subsurface erosion of primary enamel by acid beverages over time. Braz Dent J 2010; 21:337–345.

16 Meurman JH, Frank RM: Scanning electron microscopic study of the effect of salivary pellicle on enamel erosion. Caries Res 1991;25:1–6.

17 Hannig M, Balz M: Influence of in vivo formed salivary pellicle on enamel erosion. Caries Res 1999;33:372–379.

18 Hannig M, Balz M: Protective properties of salivary pellicles from two different intraoral sites on enamel erosion. Caries Research 2001;35:142–148.

19 Hannig C, Hamkens A, Becker K, Attin R, Attin T: Erosive effects of different acids on bovine enamel: release of calcium and phosphate in vitro. Arch Oral Biol 2005;50:541–552.

20 Meurman JH, Drysdale T, Frank RM: Experimental erosion of dentin. Scand J Dent Res 1991;99:457–462.

21 Eisenburger M, Shellis RP, Addy M: Scanning electron microscopy of softened enamel. Caries Res 2004;38:67–74.

22 Shellis RP, Hallsworth AS: The use of scanning electron microscopy in studying enamel caries. Scanning Microsc 1987;1:1109–1123.

23 Barbour ME, Rees JS: The laboratory assessment of enamel erosion: a review. J Dent 2004;32:591–602.

24 Chuenarrom C, Benjakul P: Comparison between a profilometer and a measuring microscope for measurement of enamel erosion. J Oral Sci 2008;50:475–479.

25 Vernhes P, Passa R: Optical metrology and scanning electron microscopy of paper damage by writing. Microsc Anal 2008;22:S19–S21.

26 Ren YF, Zhao Q, Malmstrom H, Barnes V, Xu T: Assessing fluoride treatment and resistance of dental enamel to soft drink erosion in vitro: applications of focus variation 3D scanning microscopy and stylus profilometry. J Dent 2009;37:167–176.

27 Harrick NJ: Surface chemistry from spectral analysis of totally internally reflected radiation. J Phys Chem 1960; 64:1110–1114.

28 Fahrenfort J: Attenuated total reflection. A new principle for the production of useful infra-red reflection spectra of organic compounds. Spectrochim Acta 1961;17:698–709.

29 Wang L: Infrared Attenuated Total Reflection Spectroscopy for Monitoring Biological Systems; thesis, Georgia Institute of Technology, 2009.

30 Wang X, Klocke A, Mihailova B, Tosheva L, Bismayer U: New insights into structural alteration of enamel apatite induced by citric acid and sodium fluoride solutions. J Phys Chem B 2008;112:8840–8848.

31 Thomas SS, Mallia RJ, Jose M, Subhash N: Investigation of in vitro dental erosion by optical techniques. Lasers Med Sci 2008;23:319–329.

32 Rakhmatullina E, Bossen A, Hoschele C, Wang X, Beyeler B, Meier C, Lussi A: Application of the specular and diffuse reflection analysis for in vitro diagnostics of dental erosion: correlation with enamel softening, roughness, and calcium release. J Biomed Opt 2011;16:107002.

33 Holme B, Hove LH, Tveit AB: Using white light interferometry to measure etching of dental enamel. Measurement 2005;38:137–147.

34 Fercher AF, Drexler W, Hitzenberger CK, Lasser T: Optical coherence tomography – principles and applications. Rep Prog Phys 2003;66:239–303.

35 Wilder-Smith P, Otis L, Zhang J, Chen Z: Dental OCT; in Drexler W, Fujimoto J (eds): Optical Coherence Tomography: Technology and Applications. Berlin, Springer, 2008, pp 1151–1182.

36 Otis LL, Everett MJ, Sathyam US, Colston BWJ: Optical coherence tomography: a new imaging technology for dentistry. J Am Dent Assoc 2000;131:511–514.

37 Wilder-Smith CH, Wilder-Smith P, Kawakami-Wong H, Voronets J, Osann K, Lussi A: Quantification of dental erosions in patients with GERD using optical coherence tomography before and after double-blind, randomized treatment with esomeprazole or placebo. Am J Gastroenterol 2009;104:2788–2795.

38 Amaechi BT, Higham SM, Podoleanu AG, Rogers JA, Jackson DA: Use of optical coherence tomography for assessment of dental caries: quantitative procedure. J Oral Rehabil 2001;28:1092–1093.

39 Amaechi BT, Podoleanu A, Higham SM, Jackson DA: Correlation of quantitative light-induced fluorescence and optical coherence tomography applied for detection and quantification of early dental caries. J Biomed Opt 2003;8:642–647.

40 Chan KH, Chan AC, Darling CL, Fried D: Methods for monitoring erosion using optical coherence tomography. Proc Soc Photo Opt Instrum Eng 2013;8566: 856606.

41 Kang H, Jiao JJ, Lee C, Le MH, Darling CL, Fried D: Nondestructive assessment of early tooth demineralization using cross-polarization optical coherence tomography. IEEE J Sel Top Quantum Electron 2010;16:870–876.

42 Baumgartner A, Dichtl S, Hitzenberger CK, Sattmann H, Robl B, Moritz A, Fercher AF, Sperr W: Polarization-sensitive optical coherence tomography of dental structures. Caries Res 2000;34: 59–69.

43 Herkströter FM, Witjes M, Ruben J, Arends J: Time dependency of microhardness indentations in human and bovine dentine compared with human enamel. Caries Res 1989;23:342–344.

44 Lussi A, Jaeggi T, Jaeggi-Scharer S: Prediction of the erosive potential of some beverages. Caries Res 1995;29:349–354.

45 Featherstone JD, ten Cate JM, Shariati M, Arends J: Comparison of artificial caries-like lesions by quantitative microradiography and microhardness profiles. Caries Res 1983;17:385–391.

46 Lussi A, Kohler N, Zero D, Schaffner M, Megert B: A comparison of the erosive potential of different beverages in primary and permanent teeth using an in vitro model. Eur J Oral Sci 2000;108:110–114.

47 Lussi A, Jaeggi T, Scharer S: The influence of different factors on in vitro enamel erosion. Caries Res 1993;27:387–393.

48 Lussi A, Jaeggi T, Zero D: The role of diet in the aetiology of dental erosion. Caries Res 2004;38:34–44.

49 Costa CC, Almeida IC, Costa Filho LC: Erosive effect of an antihistamine-containing syrup on primary enamel and its reduction by fluoride dentifrice. Int J Paediatr Dent 2006;16:174–180.

50 Jaeggi T, Lussi A: Toothbrush abrasion of erosively altered enamel after intraoral exposure to saliva: an in situ study. Caries Res 1999;33:455–461.

51 Joiner A, Weader E, Cox TF: The measurement of enamel wear of two toothpastes. Oral Health Prev Dent 2004;2: 383–388.

52 Joiner A, Schwarz A, Philpotts CJ, Cox TF, Huber K, Hannig M: The protective nature of pellicle towards toothpaste abrasion on enamel and dentine. J Dent 2008;36:360–368.

53 Voronets J, Lussi A: Thickness of softened human enamel removed by toothbrush abrasion: an in vitro study. Clin Oral Investig 2010;14:251–256.

54 Joiner A, Pickles MJ, Tanner C, Weader E, Doyle P: An in situ model to study the toothpaste abrasion of enamel. J Clin Periodontol 2004;31:434–438.

55 Lussi A, Jaeggi T, Gerber C, Megert B: Effect of amine/sodium fluoride rinsing on toothbrush abrasion of softened enamel in situ. Caries Res 2004;38:567–571.

56 Schweizer-Hirt CM, Schait A, Schmid R, Imfeld T, Lutz F, Muhlemann HR: Erosion and abrasion of the dental enamel. Experimental study (in German). SSO Schweiz Monatsschr Zahnheilkd 1978; 88:497–529.

57 Hooper S, West NX, Sharif N, Smith S, North M, De'Ath J, Parker DM, Roedig-Penman A, Addy M: A comparison of enamel erosion by a new sports drink compared to two proprietary products: a controlled, crossover study in situ. J Dent 2004;32:541–545.

58 Ganss C, Klimek J, Schwarz N: A comparative profilometric in vitro study of the susceptibility of polished and natural human enamel and dentine surfaces to erosive demineralization. Arch Oral Biol 2000;45:897–902.

59 Cochrane NJ, Cai F, Yuan Y, Reynolds EC: Erosive potential of beverages sold in Australian schools. Aust Dent J 2009; 54:238–244, quiz 277.

60 Cochrane NJ, Yuan Y, Walker GD, Shen P, Chang CH, Reynolds C, Reynolds EC: Erosive potential of sports beverages. Aust Dent J 2012;57:359–364, quiz 398.

61 Ablal MA, Kaur JS, Cooper L, Jarad FD, Milosevic A, Higham SM, Preston AJ: The erosive potential of some alcopops using bovine enamel: an in vitro study. J Dent 2009;37:835–839.

62 Eisenburger M: Degree of mineral loss in softened human enamel after acid erosion measured by chemical analysis. J Dent 2009;37:491–494.

63 Chuenarrom C, Benjakul P: Dental erosion protection by fermented shrimp paste in acidic food. Caries Res 2010;44: 20–23.

64 Chunmuang S, Jitpukdeebodintra S, Chuenarrom C, Benjakul P: Effect of xylitol and fluoride on enamel erosion in vitro. J Oral Sci 2008;49:293–297.

65 Engle K, Hara AT, Matis B, Eckert GJ, Zero DT: Erosion and abrasion of enamel and dentin associated with at-home bleaching: an in vitro study. J Am Dent Assoc 2010;141:546–551.

66 West NX, Hughes JA, Parker DM, Moohan M, Addy M: Development of low erosive carbonated fruit drinks. 2. Evaluation of an experimental carbonated blackcurrant drink compared to a conventional carbonated drink. J Dent 2003; 31:361–365.

67 Beyer M, Reichert J, Sigusch BW, Watts DC, Jandt KD: Morphology and structure of polymer layers protecting dental enamel against erosion. Dent Mater 2012;28:1089–1097.

68 Beyer M, Reichert J, Bossert J, Sigusch BW, Watts DC, Jandt KD: Acids with an equivalent taste lead to different erosion of human dental enamel. Dent Mater 2011;27:1017–1023.

69 Whitehead SA, Shearer AC, Watts DC, Wilson NHF: Comparison of two stylus methods for measuring surface texture. Dent Mater 1999;15:79–86.

70 Hooper S, West NX, Pickles MJ, Joiner A, Newcombe RG, Addy M: Investigation of erosion and abrasion on enamel and dentine: a model in situ using toothpastes of different abrasivity. J Clin Periodontol 2003;30:802–808.

71 Venables MC, Shaw L, Jeukendrup AE, Roedig-Penman A, Finke M, Newcombe RG, Parry J, Smith AJ: Erosive effect of a new sports drink on dental enamel during exercise. Med Sci Sports Exerc 2005; 37:39–44.

72 Attin T, Weiss K, Becker K, Buchalla W, Wiegand A: Impact of modified acidic soft drinks on enamel erosion. Oral Dis 2005;11:7–12.

73 Attin T, Becker K, Roos M, Attin R, Paque F: Impact of storage conditions on profilometry of eroded dental hard tissue. Clin Oral Investig 2009;13:473–478.

74 Ganss C, Hardt M, Blazek D, Klimek J, Schlueter N: Effects of toothbrushing force on the mineral content and demineralized organic matrix of eroded dentine. Eur J Oral Sci 2009;117:255–260.

75 Chadwick RG, Mitchell HL, Cameron I, Hunter B, Tulley M: Development of a novel system for assessing tooth and restoration wear. J Dent 1997;25:41–47.

76 Mitchell HL, Chadwick RG, Ward S, Manton SL: Assessment of a procedure for detecting minute levels of tooth erosion. Med Biol Eng Comput 2003;41: 464–469.

77 Mitchell HL, Chadwick RG: Mathematical shape matching as a tool in tooth wear assessment – development and conduct. J Oral Rehabil 1998;25:921–928.

78 Chadwick RG, Mitchell HL, Ward S: Evaluation of the accuracy and reproducibility of a replication technique for the manufacture of electroconductive replicas for use in quantitative clinical dental wear studies. J Oral Rehabil 2002; 29:540–545.

79 Chadwick RG, Mitchell HL, Ward S: A novel approach to evaluating the reproducibility of a replication technique for the manufacture of electroconductive replicas for use in quantitative clinical dental wear studies. J Oral Rehabil 2004; 31:335–339.

80 Bakhos Y, Brudevold F, Aasenden R: In-vivo estimation of the permeability of surface human enamel. Arch Oral Biol 1977;22:599–603.

81 Brudevold F, Tehrani A, Cruz R: The relationship among the permeability to iodide, pore volume, and intraoral mineralization of abraded enamel. J Dent Res 1982;61:645–648.

82 Bakhos Y, Brudevold F: Effect of initial demineralization on the permeability of human tooth enamel to iodide. Arch Oral Biol 1982;27:193–196.

83 Zero DT, Rahbek I, Fu J, Proskin HM, Featherstone JD: Comparison of the iodide permeability test, the surface microhardness test, and mineral dissolution of bovine enamel following acid challenge. Caries Res 1990;24:181–188.

84 ten Cate JM, Larsen MJ, Pearce EI, Fejerskov O: Chemical interactions between the tooth and oral fluids; in Fejerskov O, Kidd EAM (eds): Dental Caries. The Disease and Its Management. Copenhagen, Blackwell, 2003, pp 49–70.

85 Hannig M, Hess NJ, Hoth-Hannig W, De Vrese M: Influence of salivary pellicle formation time on enamel demineralization – an in situ pilot study. Clin Oral Investig 2003;7:158–161.

86 van Rijkom H, Ruben J, Vieira A, Huysmans MC, Truin GJ, Mulder J: Erosion-inhibiting effect of sodium fluoride and titanium tetrafluoride treatment in vitro. Eur J Oral Sci 2003;111:253–257.

87 Nekrashevych Y, Stosser L: Protective influence of experimentally formed salivary pellicle on enamel erosion. An in vitro study. Caries Res 2003;37:225–231.

88 Mahoney E, Beattie J, Swain M, Kilpatrick N: Preliminary in vitro assessment of erosive potential using the ultra-micro-indentation system. Caries Res 2003;37:218–224.

89 Grenby TH, Phillips A, Desai T, Mistry M: Laboratory studies of the dental properties of soft drinks. Brit J Nutr 1989;62:451–464.

90 Wegehaupt FJ, Sener B, Attin T, Schmidlin PR: Anti-erosive potential of amine fluoride, cerium chloride and laser irradiation application on dentine. Arch Oral Biol 2011;56:1541–1547.

91 Caglar E, Lussi A, Kargul B, Ugur K: Fruit yogurt: any erosive potential regarding teeth? Quintessence Int 2006;37:647–651.

92 Chen PS, Toribara TY, Warner H: Microdetermination of phosphorus. Anal Chem 1956;28:1756–1758.

93 Lowry OH, Roberts NR, Leiner KJ, Wu ML, Farr L: The quantitative histochemistry of the brain. J Biol Chem 1954;207:1–15.

94 Hohenwallner W, Wimmer E: Malachite green micromethod for determination of inorganic phosphate. Clin Chim Acta 1973;45:169–175.

95 Hattab F, Linden LA: Micro-determination of phosphate in enamel biopsy samples using the malachite green method. Acta Odontol Scand 1984;42:85–91.

96 Attin T, Becker K, Hannig C, Buchalla W, Wiegand A: Suitability of a malachite green procedure to detect minimal amounts of phosphate dissolved in acidic solutions. Clin Oral Investig 2005;9:203–207.

97 de Josselin de Jong E, van der Linden AH, ten Bosch JJ: Longitudinal microradiography: a non-destructive automated quantitative method to follow mineral changes in mineralised tissue slices. Phys Med Biol 1987;32:1209–1220.

98 de Josselin de Jong E, van der Linden AH, Borsboom PC, ten Bosch JJ: Determination of mineral changes in human dental enamel by longitudinal microradiography and scanning optical monitoring and their correlation with chemical analysis. Caries Res 1988;22:153–159.

99 Anderson P, Elliott JC: Rates of mineral loss in human enamel during in vitro demineralization perpendicular and parallel to the natural surface. Caries Res 2000;34:33–40.

100 Fejerskov O, Nyvad B, Kidd EAM: Clinical and histological manifestations of dental caries; in Fejerskov O, Kidd EAM (eds): Dental Caries. The Disease and Its Clinical Management. Oxford, Blackwell Munksgaard, 2003, pp 71–98.

101 Hall AF, Sadler JP, Strang R, de Josselin de Jong E, Foye RH, Creanor SL: Application of transverse microradiography for measurement of mineral loss by acid erosion. Adv Dent Res 1997;11:420–425.

102 Amaechi BT, Higham SM, Edgar WM: Use of transverse microradiography to quantify mineral loss by erosion in bovine enamel. Caries Res 1998;32:351–356.

103 Mathews MS, Amaechi BT, Ramalingam K, Ccahuana-Vasquez RA, Chedjieu IP, Mackey AC, Karlinsey RL: In situ remineralisation of eroded enamel lesions by NaF rinses. Arch Oral Biol 2012;57:525–530.

104 Amaechi BT, Higham SM: In vitro remineralisation of eroded enamel lesions by saliva. J Dent 2001;29:371–376.

105 Amaechi BT, Higham SM: Eroded enamel lesion remineralization by saliva as a possible factor in the site-specificity of human dental erosion. Arch Oral Biol 2001;46:697–703.

106 Ganss C, Klimek J, Schaffer U, Spall T: Effectiveness of two fluoridation measures on erosion progression in human enamel and dentine in vitro. Caries Res 2001;35:325–330.

107 Ganss C, Klimek J, Brune V, Schurmann A: Effects of two fluoridation measures on erosion progression in human enamel and dentine in situ. Caries Res 2004;38:561–566.

108 Ganss C, Klimek J, Starck C: Quantitative analysis of the impact of the organic matrix on the fluoride effect on erosion progression in human dentine using longitudinal microradiography. Arch Oral Biol 2004;49:931–935.

109 Buchalla W, Imfeld T, Attin T, Swain MV, Schmidlin PR: Relationship between nanohardness and mineral content of artificial carious enamel lesions. Caries Res 2008;42:157–163.

110 Ganss C, Lussi A, Klimek J: Comparison of calcium/phosphorus analysis, longitudinal microradiography and profilometry for the quantitative assessment of erosive demineralisation. Caries Res 2005;39:178–184.

111 Duschner H, Sonju-Clasen B, Øgaard B: Detection of early caries by confocal laser scanning microscopy; in Stookey GK (ed): Early Detection of Dental Caries. Indianapolis, Indiana University Press, 1996, pp 145–156.

112 Grotz KA, Duschner H, Reichert TE, de Aquiar EG, Gitz H, Wagner W: Histotomography of the odontoblast processes at the dentine-enamel junction of permanent healthy human teeth in the confocal laser scanning microscope. Clin Oral Investig 1998;2:21–25.

113 White DJ, Kozak KM, Zoladz JR, Duschner H, Gotz H: Peroxide interactions with hard tissues: effects on surface hardness and surface/subsurface ultrastructural properties. Compend Contin Educ Dent 2002;23:42–48.

114 Duschner H, Gitz H, Walker H, Lussi A: Erosion of dental enamel visualized by confocal laser scanning microscopy; in Addy M, Embery G, Edgar WM, Orchadson R (eds): Tooth Wear and Sensitivity. London, Martin Dunitz, 2000, pp 67–73.

115 Lussi A, Hellwig E: Erosive potential of oral care products. Caries Res 2001;35(suppl 1):52–56.

116 Zentner A, Duschner H: Structural changes of acid etched enamel examined under confocal laser scanning microscope. J Orofac Orthop 1996;57:202–209.

117 Min JH, Kwon HK, Kim BI: The addition of nano-sized hydroxyapatite to a sports drink to inhibit dental erosion: in vitro study using bovine enamel. J Dent 2011;39:629–635.

118 van der Veen MH, de Josselin de Jong E: Application of quantitative light-induced fluorescence for assessing early caries lesions; in Faller RV (ed): Assessment of Oral Health: Diagnostic Techniques and Validation Criteria. Basel, Karger, 2000, pp 144–162.

119 Pretty IA, Edgar WM, Higham SM: The erosive potential of commercially available mouthrinses on enamel as measured by quantitative light-induced fluorescence (QLF). J Dent 2003; 31:313–319.

120 Pretty IA, Edgar WM, Higham SM: The validation of quantitative light-induced fluorescence to quantify acid erosion of human enamel. Arch Oral Biol 2004;49:285–294.

121 Elton V, Cooper L, Higham SM, Pender N: Validation of enamel erosion in vitro. J Dent 2009;37:336–341.

122 Jandt KD: Atomic force microscopy of biomaterials surfaces and interfaces. Surf Sci 2001;491:303–332.

123 Lippert F, Parker DM, Jandt KD: In vitro demineralization/remineralization cycles at human tooth enamel surfaces investigated by AFM and nanoindentation. J Colloid Interface Sci 2004;280:442–448.

124 Lippert F, Parker DM, Jandt KD: Toothbrush abrasion of surface softened enamel studied with tapping mode AFM and AFM nanoindentation. Caries Res 2004;38:464–472.

125 Finke M, Jandt KD, Parker DM: The early stages of native enamel dissolution studied with atomic force microscopy. J Colloid Interface Sci 2000;232: 156–164.

126 Poggio C, Lombardini M, Vigorelli P, Colombo M, Chiesa M: The role of different toothpastes on preventing dentin erosion: an SEM and AFM study®. Scanning 2013, Epub ahead of print.

127 Oliver WC, Pharr GM: An improved technique for determining hardness and elastic-modulus using load and displacement sensing indentation experiments. J Mater Res 1992;7:1564–1583.

128 Abdullah AZ, Ireland AJ, Sandy JR, Barbour ME: A Nanomechanical investigation of three putative anti-erosion agents: remineralisation and protection against demineralisation. Int J Dent 2012;2012:768126.

129 Finke M, Hughes JA, Parker DM, Jandt KD: Mechanical properties of in situ demineralised human enamel measured by AFM nanoindentation. Surf Sci 2001;491:456–467.

130 Barbour ME, Finke M, Parker DM, Hughes JA, Allen GC, Addy M: The relationship between enamel softening and erosion caused by soft drinks at a range of temperatures. J Dent 2006;34: 207–213.

131 Lodding AR, Fischer PM, Odelius H, Noren JG, Sennerby L, Johansson CB, Chabala JM, Levisetti R: Secondary ion mass spectrometry in the study of biomineralizations and biomaterials. Anal Chim Acta 1990;241:299–314.

132 Becker JS, Dietze HJ: Inorganic trace analysis by mass spectrometry. Spectrochim Acta Part B At Spectrosc 1998; 53:1475–1506.

133 Love G, Scott VD: Electron probe microanalysis using soft X-rays – a review. Part 1. Instrumentation, spectrum processing and detection sensitivity. J Microsc 2001;201:1–32.

134 Willershausen B, Schulz-Dobrick B: In vitro study on dental erosion provoked by various beverages using electron probe microanalysis. Eur J Med Res 2004;9:432–438.

135 Huysmans MC, Thijssen JM: Ultrasonic measurement of enamel thickness: a tool for monitoring dental erosion? J Dent 2000;28:187–191.

136 Louwerse C, Kjaeldgaard M, Huysmans MC: The reproducibility of ultrasonic enamel thickness measurements: an in vitro study. J Dent 2004;32:83–89.

137 Arslantunali Tagtekin D, Oztürk F, Lagerweij M, Hayran O, Stookey GK, Caliskan Yanikoglu F: Thickness measurement of worn molar cusps by ultrasound. Caries Res 2005;39:139–143.

Prof. T. Attin
Center for Dental Medicine, Clinic for Preventive Dentistry
Periodontology and Cariology, University of Zurich
Plattenstrasse 11
CH–8032 Zurich (Switzerland)
E-Mail thomas.attin@zzm.uzh.ch

Lussi A, Ganss C (eds): Erosive Tooth Wear. Monogr Oral Sci. Basel, Karger, 2014, vol 25, pp 143–154
DOI: 10.1159/000359941

Erosion in Relation to Nutrition and the Environment

Michele E. Barbour[a] · Adrian Lussi[b]

[a] School of Oral and Dental Sciences, University of Bristol, Bristol, UK; [b] Department of Preventive, Restorative and Pediatric Dentistry, School of Dental Medicine, University of Bern, Bern, Switzerland

Abstract

When considering the erosive potential of a food or drink, a number of factors must be taken into account. pH is arguably the single most important parameter in determining the rate of erosive tissue dissolution. There is no clear-cut critical pH for erosion as there is for caries. At low pH, it is possible that other factors are sufficiently protective to prevent erosion, but equally erosion can progress in acid of a relatively high pH in the absence of mitigating factors. Calcium and phosphate concentration, in combination with pH, determine the degree of saturation with respect to tooth minerals. Solutions supersaturated with respect to enamel or dentine will not cause them to dissolve, meaning that given sufficient common ion concentrations erosion will not proceed, even if the pH is low. Interestingly, the addition of calcium is more effective than phosphate at reducing erosion in acid solutions. Today, several calcium-enriched soft drinks are on the market, and acidic products with high concentrations of calcium and phosphorus are available (such as yoghurt), which do not soften the dental hard tissues. The greater the buffering capacity of the drink or food, the longer it will take for the saliva to neutralize the acid. A higher buffer capacity of a drink or foodstuff will enhance the processes of dissolution because more release of ions from the tooth mineral is required to render the acid inactive for further demineralization. Temperature is also a significant physical factor; for a given acidic solution, erosion proceeds more rapidly the higher the temperature of that solution. In recent years, a number of interesting potentially erosion-reducing drink and food additives have been investigated.

© 2014 S. Karger AG, Basel

Dental Erosion and Nutrition: Overview

The aim of this chapter is to reveal the main properties of foods and beverages which affect their erosive potential. Many of these properties are chemical in nature (table 1). Numerous in vitro studies and in situ trials have evaluated the erosive potential of different foods and beverages. There is overwhelming evidence that the erosive potential of an acidic drink is not exclusively dependent on its pH value but is also strongly influenced by its mineral content, and many studies suggest the importance of a series of related factors regarding the acid itself such as acid type and concentration, titratable acidity,

Table 1. Chemical factors influencing the erosive potential with respect to food and beverages

pH and buffering capacity of the product
Type of acid (pKa values)
Adhesion of the product to the dental surface
Calcium concentration
Phosphate concentration
Fluoride concentration
Chelating properties of the product

buffering capacity, undissociated acid concentration and presence of potential erosion inhibitors such as some polymers and proteins. The pH value, calcium, phosphate and fluoride content of a drink or foodstuff determine the degree of saturation with respect to the tooth mineral, and this determines the driving force for dissolution. Solutions supersaturated with respect to dental hard tissue will not dissolve it. A solution undersaturated with respect to enamel or dentine is likely to lead to surface demineralization. Temperature is also an important factor; if other factors are equal, erosion will progress more rapidly in a solution at an elevated temperature, so acidic drinks served hot are more erosive than the same drinks at room or refrigerator temperature. The physical motion of the solution must also be taken into account. In an unagitated system, where a moderately small quantity of acid is applied and/or where the solution is static (not stirred or shaken), this dissolution results in a local increase in pH and mineral content in the solution surface layer adjacent to the tooth surface. This layer will then become saturated with respect to enamel (or dentine) and the tissue will not demineralize further. This experimental approach does not adequately address the clinical situation and laboratory studies which use small-volume, static acid aliquots are of limited clinical relevance. An agitated solution (stirring, shaking, etc.) is a better representation of the clinical scenario since the acid solution the patient is consuming will move

about the mouth, over the tooth surfaces, and will be replenished as the patient drinks the beverage over a period of time. This leads to a continued dissolution as long as the acid solution is in contact with the teeth. An increase in agitation (e.g. when a patient is swishing his/her drink in the mouth) will accelerate the dissolution process because the solution on the surface layer adjacent to tooth mineral will be more rapidly renewed. For this reason, it is important that agitation of the acidic solution in laboratory studies is well defined and reproducible.

pH, Buffering Capacity, Undissociated Acids and Chelation

When an excess of an erosive agent is present and agitation of the solution is applied, the pH is the single most decisive factor in determining the relative rates of erosion of different solutions. Many studies compare erosive solutions with only two or three pH values, or a larger number of pH values but with other differing parameters between solutions, making elucidation of the precise relationship between pH and demineralization challenging. For those studies which do compare a range of pH values, the relationship between demineralization and pH may be seen to be linear [1] or non-linear [2], depending on the measurement technique used to quantify the degree of demineralization. What is nevertheless clear is that the pH has a profound effect on the rate of enamel and dentine dissolution. There is no 'critical pH' for erosion as is described for caries, owing in part to the very variable composition of erosive solutions in the mouth (see table 1 in chapter by Lussi and Carvalho, this vol., p. 6).

The relationship between erosion, acid type and buffering capacity is complex. It is clear that in the case of weak (not fully dissociated) acids, the capacity for molecular or ionic dissociation to replenish protons consumed in the dissolution reaction can augment the process of erosion. Simply put: an organic acid has a reservoir of protons which can be released when enamel or dentine dissolves, and this can prolong the conditions which favour tissue dissolution. The impact of buffering appears to be dependent, to some extent, on the pH of the solutions. The most commonly quoted measure of buffering is the titratable acidity. This is doubtless a useful parameter, although the way in which it is discussed in the literature is not always helpful. Units should be standardized (e.g. moles of OH^- required to raise the pH of a test solution to a given value, usually 7) and normalized to volume (i.e. per litre). Unfortunately it has become quite common practice to report titratable acidity along the lines of 'ml 0.5 M NaOH required to raise the pH of 50 ml of solution X to pH 7', which does not lead to easy comparison of figures between studies. It would be useful and chemically correct to use the unit 'mmol/l to pH 5.5', which makes easy comparison possible. It appears that the concentration of undissociated acid is a good indication of erosive dissolution rate in comparison with buffer capacity per se [3]. Further, the amount of drink in the mouth in relation to the amount of saliva present will modify the dissolution process.

Chelation of calcium by certain ions, particularly citrate, has been widely discussed in the erosion literature. The citrate ion is indeed, under certain conditions, capable of chelating metal ions including calcium and this has often been described as a mechanism by which citrate-containing drinks might erode the teeth over and above acid-mediated dissolution. However, although citric acid is one of the most commonly employed acids in in vitro erosion experiments, the effect of chelation isolated from differing pH and degree of saturation has not satisfactorily been addressed. Such experiments would be challenging to design; simple approaches to changing the citrate concentration also involve changing the concentration of undissociated acid and hence titratable acidity and buffering potential, all of which affect erosion. The premise

of significant calcium chelation by drinks of typical pH of around 3 is flawed, given that a citrate ion can only chelate a metal ion if it has at least two ionized carboxyl groups. As discussed elsewhere [see chapter by Shellis et al., this vol., pp. 163–179], at pH 3 the proportion of citrate ions which are appropriately ionized to chelate is less than 3%. At higher pH values the proportion of chelating citrate ions increases; it is around 93% of citrate ions at pH 6 – but at this pH erosion due to acid-mediated dissolution is slow and such solutions are rarely considered a significant clinical erosion risk.

Common Ions: Calcium and Phosphate

The calcium and phosphate contents of a food or drink are important factors for the erosive potential as they influence the concentration gradient within the local environment of the tooth surface. Larsen [4] suggested that erosive potential could be calculated based on the degree of saturation with respect to both hydroxyapatite and fluorapatite by determining the pH, calcium, phosphate and fluoride content of a beverage. The addition of common ions to erosive drinks has yielded some interesting results and provides a practical strategy for reducing erosive potential. Calcium appears to be the most effective ion; phosphate has little or no effect in the absence of calcium [5], which may be due to speciation of the phosphate ion and therefore not all phosphorus is the monophosphate (as opposed to hydrogen- or dihydrogen-phosphate) required to contribute to the degree of saturation. In a programme of work in the late 1990s, it was shown that the erosive potential of a fruit-based drink could be greatly reduced by adding calcium carbonate, although this resulted in a concurrent increase in pH which augmented the effect of the calcium [6–8]. While this was effective, the elevation in pH brought with it a change in taste which limits the appeal of the drink. In terms of adding common ions without

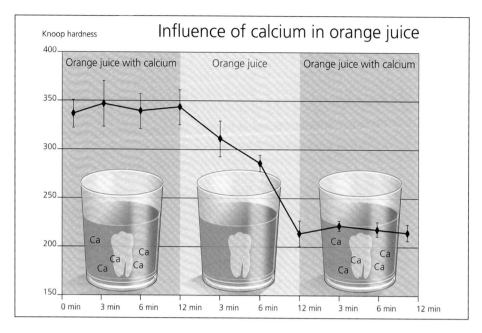

Fig. 1. Impact of a conventional and a Ca-enriched orange juice on softening of enamel.

simultaneously changing pH, supplementation of commercial soft drinks with calcium reduced their erosive potential, and supplementation with a combination of calcium, phosphate and fluoride reduced erosion further still, with three out of four drinks tested [9]. Supplementation of orange juice with calcium citrate or calcium triphosphate was an effective means of reducing erosive potential in vitro [10], as was the addition of calcium glycerophosphate to carbonated drinks, also in vitro [11]. Table 2 shows the pH and calcium concentration of some minimally erosive beverages.

A practical approach to consumer-led control of erosive potential was reported recently by Wegehaupt et al. [12], whereby orange juice was modified by the addition of commercially available dietary supplements containing calcium. The modified juice drink caused wear (erosion + abrasion) comparable to the negative control (water) and much lower than the positive control (unmodified juice). The additions resulted in elevated pH but a taste test incorporated into the study did not reveal any unpalatable effect of these additions.

Today, several Ca-enriched orange juices are on the market, which barely soften the enamel surface (fig. 1). It has to be borne in mind that, with the added mineral, enamel dissolution cannot always be completely prevented, and in some cases the impact on the drink taste is likely to

Table 2. pH and calcium concentration of some minimally erosive beverages (ready to drink)

Available beverage	pH	Added level of calcium mg/l
Ribena really light blackcurrant	3.7–4.0	630
Ribena really light apple	3.7–4.0	440
Ribena really light berry burst	3.7–4.0	400
Ribena really light strawberry	3.7–4.0	400
Ribena really light orange tropical	3.7–4.0	200
Lucozade sport hydroactive citrus	3.7–4.0	370
Orange-flavoured sports drinks	3.8	320
Orange juice (Michel)	3.8	160

prove unacceptable to many consumers. However, the progression of erosion can be retarded, which has some implications for the patient and the clinician, and the taste of some formulations still proves acceptable.

It is, of course, not only drinks which pose an erosion risk, and in recent years acidic candies or sweets have received considerable attention with regard to their propensity to release acids during consumption that can dissolve the dental hard tissues [13–15]. The addition of calcium lactate to fruit-flavoured candies resulted in an elevated calcium concentration in the saliva stimulated by sucking the candy in vivo, thus reducing the erosive potential of the confection [16]. This approach may benefit patient groups in chronic need of dry-mouth treatments which are not erosive [17], as well as the mass market. Yoghurt is an example of a food with a low pH (around 4.0), yet it has hardly any erosive effect due to its high calcium and phosphate content, which render it supersaturated with respect to apatite. A yoghurt or another milk-based food may potentially be erosive if it has a low content of Ca and/or P and a particularly low pH.

Sports drinks have been found to be erosive in vitro [18, 19] and when consumed during strenuous activity when the person is in a state of some dehydration the possible destructive effects may be enhanced further. Sports drinks have been modified in laboratory studies with the intention of reducing their erosive potential. The addition of calcium is the most widely tested approach and this has been shown to reduce the erosion caused by several sports drinks, in some cases in combination with an increase in pH [20, 21]. The addition of calcium and phosphate using the vector of casein phosphopeptide-amorphous calcium phosphate has also been achieved and was effective in reducing erosion in an in vitro model [22, 23]. It should be noted, however, that there is currently little clinical evidence of a link between the consumption of sports drinks and erosion, while data are very convincing for other types of acidic drinks [24]. For further discussion of potential links between sporting activity and erosion, see later in this chapter.

Novel Additives to Reduce Erosion

In recent years, other potentially erosion-reducing drink additives have been investigated. There is some evidence that supplementation of acidic solutions with food polymers such as xanthan and carboxymethylcellulose can confer a modest reduction in hydroxyapatite dissolution in citric acid in vitro [25], although in a later in situ study using enamel as the test substrate, the addition of xanthan gum to a drink containing another erosion-protecting agent did not provide any further benefit over and above the existing protection [26], and the addition of xanthan to orange juice did not reduce its erosive potential when tested on enamel and dentine [27]. Condensed phosphates, as opposed to monophosphate, have been investigated and appear to offer larger erosion-reducing effects when added to acids, both in vitro [25] and in situ [26]. A recent study indicated that a combination of linear polyphosphate and calcium lactate pentahydrate was more effective than either additive alone at reducing erosion of both enamel and dentine in an orange juice in vitro [27], but the finding was not replicated in situ, where the calcium lactate pentahydrate reduced erosion, and the polyphosphate conferred no benefit alone or in combination with the calcium salt [28].

Larger molecules such as certain proteins may be beneficial when added to acidic drinks; the addition of the egg protein ovalbumin reduced hydroxyapatite dissolution in citric acid by 50–75% in an in vitro model, but did not show the same efficacy in malic or lactic acids [29], and was somewhat less effective when the dissolution substrate was enamel [30]. The milk protein casein (as distinct from casein phosphopeptide-calcium phosphate, described above), which contains calcium phosphate, was more effective, reducing hydroxyapatite dissolution [31] and enamel erosion [30] by up to 80%. Recently, phosphoryl oligosaccharides of calcium have been added to a fruit juice and were found to reduce erosive potential while not adversely affecting taste, at least at modest concentrations [32]. Clinical data on the efficacy of these potential erosion-reducing agents are, however, not yet available.

Fluoride

Theoretically, fluoride may offer some protective effect in a drink with a pH higher than that indicated by the saturation curve of fluorapatite at given Ca and PO_4 concentrations. Lussi et al. [33, 34] and Mahoney et al. [35] found an inverse correlation of the erosive potential with the fluoride content of different beverages. Although the title of the manuscript might be seen to suggest otherwise, Larsen and Richards [36] found that the addition of fluoride (as CaF_2) to commercial soft drinks reduced erosion, but only for those drinks with pH >3 and with high total concentrations of fluoride (7–26 mg/l). Supplementation with fluoride is unlikely to prove a useful strategy, however, because the erosive challenge is aggressive and the concentration of fluoride which can be included in a product for consumption is low. Fluoride application direct to the tooth may provide protection against erosion; this is discussed in the chapter by Huysmans et al. [this vol., pp. 230–243].

Properties of Commercial Foods and Drinks

It has long been the desire to predict the erosivity of different beverages and foodstuffs based on their chemical and physical properties. It can be concluded from the above discussion that a ranking for the in vivo erosivity of different acidic foods and drinks based on pH, titratable acidity and/or buffer capacity, Ca, P and F is rather complicated if not impossible. Besides these chemical factors, behavioural factors (such as eating and drinking habits, diets high in acidic fruits and vegetables, excessive consumption of acidic foods and drinks, oral hygiene practices), biological factors (such as saliva flow rate, buffering capacity, acquired pellicle, dental anatomy and anatomy of oral soft tissues, physiological soft tissue movements) and oral hygiene behaviour (toothpaste composition, abrasivity, frequency and duration of use, mouth rinses and other products) also have to be taken into account. Nevertheless, a list of the erosive potential of different products in vitro may help the clinician in judging the erosivity of these products in vivo [see table 3 in chapter by Lussi and Hellwig, this vol., pp. 220–229].

Physical Properties of the Acidic Medium

The physical properties of the erosive medium are also factors to be considered in the erosive process. There appear to be differences in the ability of beverages to adhere to enamel based on their thermodynamic properties, i.e. the thermodynamic work of adhesion [37]. The greater the adhesion of an acidic substance, the longer the likely contact time with the tooth surface, and this may result in a more sustained erosive challenge. It has been shown that displacement of saliva by Cola required 14 mJ/m^2, whereas by Diet Cola the process required 5 mJ/m^2. However, displacement of Cola film by saliva required 45 mJ/m^2, and of Diet Cola by saliva the figure was 52 mJ/m^2. It seems to be more difficult to displace a soft drink film by saliva than it is to displace a salivary film by a soft drink.

The temperature of the acid is also a significant factor. An acidic drink served hot is more erosive than the same drink served cold [38–41]. This, combined with the low pH, explains why some herbal teas can be aggressive erosive agents [42].

As mentioned above, the agitation of an acidic solution also determines, in part, the speed of dissipation of the reaction products of dissolution and this influences the local degree of saturation and thus the rate of dissolution. From a methodological point of view, this means that it is important to select and control agitation in erosion studies carefully and with reference to the clinical situation. From a clinical standpoint, this indicates that those patients prone to habits such as jetting a drink at their teeth through a straw may exhibit localized erosion [43].

Further research is needed to quantify the impact of these physical factors in more detail. This has to be done by using reproducible and standardized methods. For further guidance on methodology in erosion research the reader might consult the paper by Shellis et al. [44].

Professions and Pastimes which Predispose Individuals to Regular, Sustained Acid Contact and the Effect on Dental Erosion

In some cases, an individual's occupation or hobby may affect their vulnerability to dental erosion. Frequent contact with inorganic or organic acids at work or during recreational activities may increase the occurrence and progression of erosion.

In some studies, people working with acids had significantly more teeth with erosive tooth wear than the controls. When battery chargers were compared to automobile mechanics in Ibadan, Nigeria, 41% of the battery chargers' teeth had tooth wear whereas this number was 3% with mechanics [45]. A comparable finding was found in Jordan in the phosphate industry. The acid workers not only showed erosion but also complained in 80% of the cases about dentine hypersensitivity [46]. Acid fumes at work seem to be associated with tooth surface loss with no clinical significant differences between the inorganic and organic acids. Tuominen et al. [47–49] investigated the effect of inorganic and organic acid fumes on teeth. Among 169 workers who participated in one study, 88 were exposed to acid fumes and 81 were controls (not exposed to acid fumes). The

prevalence of tooth surface loss was 63% (workers exposed to inorganic acid) and 50% (workers exposed to organic acid). The corresponding prevalence data for the controls were about 25%. The acid workers had significantly more teeth with erosive defects in the maxilla than the controls. Upper anterior teeth were more often attacked than posterior teeth. The purpose of another study [50] was to evaluate the prevalence and the severity of dental erosion and attrition in relation to exposure of airborne acids in the work environment. Measurements at a German battery factory showed that the workers were exposed to sulphuric acids ($0.4–4.1$ mg/cm^3). Erosion was found only in front teeth while attrition also occurred in posterior teeth. Due to the high level of crown restorations a rather moderate dose-effect relationship was observed. The authors concluded that severe erosion and attrition due to sulphuric acid mists should be recognized as an occupational disease. More recently, a case report was published linking severe erosion in an individual who had worked as a chemical engineer in the chromium plating industry to 20 years' exposure to chromic acid in the workplace [51].

Westergaard et al. [52] examined 425 individuals working at a pharmaceutical and biotechnological enterprise; 202 of these individuals were newly employed by the company and served as a control group. Adjusted for potential confounders, there was no association between history of occupational exposure to proteolytic enzymes and prevalent facial or lingual erosion. With respect to prevalence of class V restorations, the association was significant. This study did not support the hypothesis that occupational exposure to airborne proteolytic enzymes is associated with dental erosion.

Wine tasters are another occupational group at risk of dental erosion. Wine has properties such as low pH (typically in the range 2.95–3.90 for white wine and 3.25–4.11 for red wine [53], for European vintages) and a low content of Ca, which suggests it may present an erosion risk.

Professional wine tasting is very common all over the world. In some countries (e.g. Sweden, Finland) wine tasters are employed by the state to support their state-owned wine shops. Full-time Swedish wine tasters test on average 20–50 different wines, nearly 5 days a week. Wiktorsson et al. [54] investigated the prevalence and severity of tooth erosion in 19 qualified wine tasters in relation to number of years of wine tasting, salivary flow rate and buffer capacity. Salivary flow rate and buffer capacity of unstimulated and stimulated saliva were measured. Data on occupational background and dental and medical histories were collected; 14 subjects had tooth erosion mainly on the labio-cervical surfaces of maxillary incisors and canines. The severity of the erosion tended to increase with years of occupational exposure. Caries activity in all subjects was low. It was concluded that full-time wine tasting is an occupation associated with an increased risk for tooth erosion. Thereafter, the wine tasters employed at the state owned 'Systembolaget' got free dental hygiene prophylactic treatment as erosion was considered to be a work-related condition [pers. commun.]. This conclusion is supported by various case reports [55–57] and in vitro studies [54, 58] of wine-related erosion, as well as more recent studies of incidence in the wine-tasting and related communities. A study comparing erosion incidence in wine makers, who presumably regularly taste or drink their own wine, found significantly more erosion in the wine makers than their spouses [59]. Another study of wine tasters indicated not only that there was a higher incidence of erosion among wine tasters than the control group, but that wine tasters exhibited much more erosion that proceeded as far as dentine, and that the pattern of erosion was different for the two groups [60]. Furthermore, other alcoholic drinks are an erosion risk owing to their composition; cider [61] and carbonated, sweet alcoholic drinks sometimes known as alcopops [62] have also been implicated. The impact of excessive alcohol consumption cannot be ruled out for patients exhibiting signs of alcohol misuse; one has to keep in mind that alcoholics often have regurgitation, which contributes to the clinical presentation of some erosion.

During sports activities dehydration occurs and rehydration and electrolyte replacement is accomplished by sports drinks that have an erosive potential comparable to acidic soft drinks [see chapter by Lussi and Hellwig, this vol., pp. 220–229]. However, for most individuals engaged in physical activity, sports drinks have no performance benefit over water [63]. Probably the greatest benefit of sports drinks to exercising individuals is that they generally increase voluntary fluid consumption [64]. This may be important as during heavy sporting activities only 50% of the rate of fluid loss is compensated for [65]. Dentists should counsel athletes to control the effect of potentially erosive drinks [66].

A few case reports and studies have reported an association between sports activities and erosive tooth wear. The cause could be direct acid exposure or strenuous exercise, which may increase gastroesophageal reflux [67]. Risk groups are swimmers exercising in water with low pH and athletes consuming frequently erosive sports drinks. It has to be kept in mind that sports drinks and occupation may be for some patients a cofactor in the development or increase of dental erosion. However, it is unlikely that one or two isolated factors will be responsible for this multifactorial condition.

In a study with 25 swimmers and 20 cyclists, the latter showed significantly more tooth wear into dentine, but no association between the erosive tooth wear and consumption of sports drinks was found [68]. Professional swimmers train several hours in the water, which should have proper pH regulation. The main disinfection techniques used are gas chlorination and sodium hypochlorite. Where the sodium hypochlorite method is used, very few pools exhibit low pH values [69, 70], but an increased prevalence of dental erosion among intensive swimmers due to low pH gas-chlorinated pool water has been described [71]. The recommended pH for swimming pools is between pH 7.2 and 8.0, and swimming in pH-adjusted pools does not harm the teeth [72]. However, erosion among competitive swimmers was found in 39% of swim team members who trained in a pool with a pH of 2.7, which is an H⁺ concentration 100,000 times higher than that recommended for swimming pools [73].

In a patient complaining of severe dentine hypersensitivity, her case history revealed that she was an active diver over many years with 25 h/week training in chlorinated water and drank 1 litre/day of an acidic soft drink sip-wise. Only later did she admit that she also had regurgitation which was an important factor explaining the clinical appearance of her teeth. Unstimulated saliva flow rate was high (1.2 ml/min) and the buffer capacity as measured with Dentobuff (Vivadent, Schaan, Liechtenstein) was 'medium'. Clinical examination showed severe erosive defects with involvement of dentine on all tooth surfaces (fig. 2–4). A one-bottle dentine adhesive was applied onto the hypersensitive teeth and the eroded parts of the teeth were filled with composite [for treatment procedures, see chapter by Peutzfeldt et al., this vol., pp. 253–261].

Despite the in vitro erosive potential of sports drinks (see above), it is perhaps surprising that most studies have found no association between erosion and the consumption of sports drinks. A sample of athletes in the USA showed usage of sports drinks in 92% and a total prevalence of erosion of 37%. Statistical analysis revealed no association between dental erosion and the use of sports drinks, quantity and frequency of consumption, years of usage and non-sport usage of sports drinks [74]. A more recent study of athletes in Australia found a high prevalence of erosion but could not find any association between erosion and consumption of sports or other soft drinks [66]. An in situ study compared the erosive effect of a commercially available sports drink with that of mineral water over a 10-day

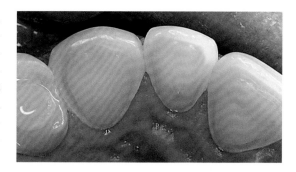

Fig. 2. Severe palatal erosive tooth wear with extensive dentinal exposure. Note the intact enamel along the gingival margin. Patient: aged 38 years, active diver in chlorinated water. Known risk factors: gastroesophageal reflux, acidic soft drinks sip-wise.

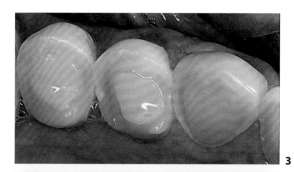

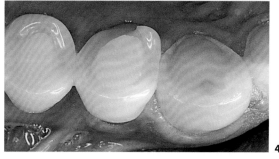

Fig. 3, 4. Severe oral and occlusal erosive tooth wear (same patient as fig. 2). Note the composite fillings rising above the level of the adjacent tooth surfaces.

period on 10 healthy volunteers. Erosion occurred with the sports drink, but to a variable degree between subjects, and the quantity of drink ingested over the study period was described as excessive and unpleasant by the (sedentary) participants [75].

Smoothies are considered a healthy fruit drink as they contain vitamins, fibres and antioxidants. However, an erosive potential exists due to the low pH and the split consumption during the day. Recently, an investigation with an in vitro part followed by an in situ period clearly showed an erosive potential due to the low pH and high titratable acidity. However, the erosive effect was less than citric acid [76].

Conclusion

In summary, it can be said that two very-often-cited parameters, pH and titratable acidity, are not sufficient to derive or define the erosive potential of food and drink. There is no clear-cut critical pH for erosion below which erosion will occur; erosion may be inhibited at low pH if other factors are sufficiently protective, and erosion may proceed at pH above 4 or 5, albeit slowly. The mineral content and degree of saturation with respect to hydroxyapatite and fluorapatite are also important parameters, as are other erosion inhibitors and the temperature of the erosive medium. Chelation by citrate in citric acid-based drinks is unlikely to contribute a great deal to the progression of erosion at typical erosion pH since very little of the citrate is suitably ionized to chelate calcium at these pH values. Besides these factors there are several others such as the composition and flow rate of saliva as well as the temperature and motion of the drink, which have an impact on dental erosion in vivo. All of the above have to be taken into account to explain or even predict to some extent the influence of foods and beverages on dental hard tissue. The influence of all the factors described above in the fluid layer immediately in contact with the tooth surface determines whether erosion can proceed or not. Individuals with lifestyles or professions which predispose them to regular, sustained acid contact may be particularly prone to erosion.

References

1 Barbour ME, Parker DM, Allen GC, Jandt KD: Human enamel dissolution in citric acid as a function of pH in the range 2.30 ≤ pH ≤ 6.30 – a nanoindentation study. Eur J Oral Sci 2003;111:258–262.
2 Meurman JH, Harkonen M, Naveri H, Koskinen J, Torkko H, Rytomaa I, Jarvinen V, Turunen R: Experimental sports drinks with minimal dental erosion effect. Scand J Dent Res 1990;98:120–128.
3 Shellis RP, Barbour ME, Jesani A, Lussi A: Effects of buffering properties and undissociated acid concentration on dissolution of dental enamel in relation to pH and acid type. Caries Res 2013;47:601–611.
4 Larsen MJ: Dissolution of enamel. Scand J Dent Res 1973;81:518–522.
5 Magalhaes AC, Moraes SM, Rios D, Buzalaf MA: Effect of ion supplementation of a commercial soft drink on tooth enamel erosion. Food Addit Contam Part A Chem Anal Control Expo Risk Assess 2009;26:152–156.
6 Hughes JA, West NX, Parker DM, Newcombe RG, Addy M: Development and evaluation of a low erosive blackcurrant juice drink. 3. Final drink and concentrate, formulae comparisons in situ and overview of the concept. J Dent 1999;27:345–350.
7 West NX, Hughes JA, Parker DM, Newcombe RG, Addy M: Development and evaluation of a low erosive blackcurrant juice drink. 2. Comparison with a conventional blackcurrant juice drink and orange juice. J Dent 1999;27:341–344.
8 Hughes JA, West NX, Parker DM, Newcombe RG, Addy M: Development and evaluation of a low erosive blackcurrant juice drink in vitro and in situ. 1. Comparison with orange juice. J Dent 1999;27:285–289.
9 Attin T, Weiss K, Becker K, Buchalla W, Wiegand A: Impact of modified acidic soft drinks on enamel erosion. Oral Dis 2005;11:7–12.
10 Jensdottir T, Bardow A, Holbrook P: Properties and modification of soft drinks in relation to their erosive potential in vitro. J Dent 2005;33:569–575.
11 Barbosa CS, Montagnolli LG, Kato MT, Sampaio FC, Buzalaf MA: Calcium glycerophosphate supplemented to soft drinks reduces bovine enamel erosion. J Appl Oral Sci 2012;20:410–413.
12 Wegehaupt F, Gunthart N, Sener B, Attin T: Prevention of erosive/abrasive enamel wear due to orange juice modified with dietary supplements. Oral Dis 2011;17:508–514.
13 Wagoner SN, Marshall TA, Qian F, Wefel JS: In vitro enamel erosion associated with commercially available original-flavor and sour versions of candies. J Am Dent Assoc 2009;140:906–913.
14 Brand HS, Gambon DL, Van Dop LF, Van Liere LE, Veerman EC: The erosive potential of jawbreakers, a type of hard candy. Int J Dent Hyg 2010;8:308–312.

15 Davies R, Hunter L, Loyn T, Rees J: Sour sweets: a new type of erosive challenge? Br Dent J 2008;204:E3, discussion 84–85.

16 Jensdottir T, Nauntofte B, Buchwald C, Bardow A: Effects of calcium on the erosive potential of acidic candies in saliva. Caries Res 2007;41:68–73.

17 Jensdottir T, Buchwald C, Nauntofte B, Hansen HS, Bardow A: Erosive potential of calcium-modified acidic candies in irradiated dry mouth patients. Oral Health Prev Dent 2010;8:173–178.

18 Sorvari R, Pelttari A, Meurman JH: Surface ultrastructure of rat molar teeth after experimentally induced erosion and attrition. Caries Res 1996;30:163–168.

19 Lussi A, Megert B, Shellis RP, Wang X: Analysis of the erosive effect of different dietary substances and medications. Br J Nutr 2012;107:252–262.

20 Hooper S, West NX, Sharif N, Smith S, North M, De'Ath J, Parker DM, Roedig-Penman A, Addy M: A comparison of enamel erosion by a new sports drink compared to two proprietary products: a controlled, crossover study in situ. J Dent 2004;32:541–545.

21 Venables MC, Shaw L, Jeukendrup AE, Roedig-Penman A, Finke M, Newcombe RG, Parry J, Smith AJ: Erosive effect of a new sports drink on dental enamel during exercise. Med Sci Sports Exerc 2005;37:39–44.

22 Ramalingam L, Messer LB, Reynolds EC: Adding casein phosphopeptide-amorphous calcium phosphate to sports drinks to eliminate in vitro erosion. Pediatr Dent 2005;27:61–67.

23 Manton DJ, Cai F, Yuan Y, Walker GD, Cochrane NJ, Reynolds C, Brearley-Messer LJ, Reynolds EC: Effect of casein phosphopeptide-amorphous calcium phosphate added to acidic beverages on enamel erosion in vitro. Aust Dent J 2010;55:275–279.

24 Li H, Zou Y, Ding G: Dietary factors associated with dental erosion: a meta-analysis. PLoS One 2012;7:e42626.

25 Barbour ME, Shellis RP, Parker DM, Allen GC, Addy M: An investigation of some food-approved polymers as agents to inhibit hydroxyapatite dissolution. Eur J Oral Sci 2005;113:457–461.

26 Hooper SM, Hughes JA, Parker DM, Finke M, Newcombe RG, Addy M, West NX: A clinical study in situ to assess the effect of a food approved polymer on the erosion potential of drinks. J Dent 2007;35:541–546.

27 Scaramucci T, Hara AT, Zero DT, Ferreira SS, Aoki IV, Sobral MA: In vitro evaluation of the erosive potential of orange juice modified by food additives in enamel and dentine. J Dent 2011;39:841–848.

28 Scaramucci T, Sobral MA, Eckert GJ, Zero DT, Hara AT: In situ evaluation of the erosive potential of orange juice modified by food additives. Caries Res 2012;46:55–61.

29 Hemingway CA, Shellis RP, Parker DM, Addy M, Barbour ME: Inhibition of hydroxyapatite dissolution by ovalbumin as a function of pH, calcium concentration, protein concentration and acid type. Caries Res 2008;42:348–353.

30 Hemingway CA, White AJ, Shellis RP, Addy M, Parker DM, Barbour ME: Enamel erosion in dietary acids: inhibition by food proteins in vitro. Caries Res 2010;44:525–530.

31 Barbour ME, Shellis RP, Parker DM, Allen GC, Addy M: Inhibition of hydroxyapatite dissolution by whole casein: the effects of pH, protein concentration, calcium, and ionic strength. Eur J Oral Sci 2008;116:473–478.

32 Mita H, Kitasako Y, Takagaki T, Sadr A, Tagami J: Development and evaluation of a low-erosive apple juice drink with phosphoryl-oligosaccharides of calcium. Dent Mater J 2013;32:212–218.

33 Lussi A, Jaggi T, Scharer S: The influence of different factors on in vitro enamel erosion. Caries Res 1993;27:387–393.

34 Lussi A, Jaeggi T, Jaeggi-Scharer S: Prediction of the erosive potential of some beverages. Caries Res 1995;29:349–354.

35 Mahoney E, Beattie J, Swain M, Kilpatrick N: Preliminary in vitro assessment of erosive potential using the ultra-micro-indentation system. Caries Res 2003;37:218–224.

36 Larsen MJ, Richards A: Fluoride is unable to reduce dental erosion from soft drinks. Caries Res 2002;36:75–80.

37 Ireland AJ, McGuinness N, Sherriff M: An investigation into the ability of soft drinks to adhere to enamel. Caries Res 1995;29:470–476.

38 Barbour ME, Finke M, Parker DM, Hughes JA, Allen GC, Addy M: The relationship between enamel softening and erosion caused by soft drinks at a range of temperatures. J Dent 2006;34:207–213.

39 Eisenburger M, Addy M: Influence of liquid temperature and flow rate on enamel erosion and surface softening. J Oral Rehabil 2003;30:1076–1080.

40 West NX, Hughes JA, Addy M: Erosion of dentine and enamel in vitro by dietary acids: the effect of temperature, acid character, concentration and exposure time. J Oral Rehabil 2000;27:875–880.

41 Amaechi BT, Higham SM, Edgar WM: Factors influencing the development of dental erosion in vitro: enamel type, temperature and exposure time. J Oral Rehabil 1999;26:624–630.

42 Phelan J, Rees JS: The erosive potential of some herbal teas. J Dent 2003;31:241–246.

43 Shellis RP, Finke M, Eisenburger M, Parker DM, Addy M: Relationship between enamel erosion and liquid flow rate. Eur J Oral Sci 2005;113:232–238.

44 Shellis RP, Ganss C, Ren Y, Zero DT, Lussi A: Methodology and models in erosion research: discussion and conclusions. Caries Res 2011;45(suppl 1):69–77.

45 Arowojolu MO: Erosion of tooth enamel surfaces among battery chargers and automobile mechanics in Ibadan: a comparative study. Afr J Med Med Sci 2001;30:5–8.

46 Amin WM, Al-Omoush SA, Hattab FN: Oral health status of workers exposed to acid fumes in phosphate and battery industries in Jordan. Int Dent J 2001;51:169–174.

47 Tuominen M, Tuominen R, Ranta K, Ranta H: Association between acid fumes in the work environment and dental erosion. Scand J Work Environ Health 1989;15:335–338.

48 Tuominen ML, Tuominen RJ, Fubusa F, Mgalula N: Tooth surface loss and exposure to organic and inorganic acid fumes in workplace air. Community Dent Oral Epidemiol 1991;19:217–220.

49 Tuominen M, Tuominen R: Dental erosion and associated factors among factory workers exposed to inorganic acid fumes. Proc Finn Dent Soc 1991;87:359–364.

50 Petersen PE, Gormsen C: Oral conditions among German battery factory workers. Community Dent Oral Epidemiol 1991;19:104–106.

51 Dulgergil CT, Erdemir EO, Ercan E, Erdemir A: An industrial dental erosion by chromic acid: a case report. Eur J Dent 2007;1:119–122.

52 Westergaard J, Larsen IB, Holmen L, Larsen AI, Jorgensen B, Holmstrup P, Suadicani P, Gyntelberg F: Occupational exposure to airborne proteolytic enzymes and lifestyle risk factors for dental erosion – a cross-sectional study. Occup Med (Lond) 2001;51:189–197.

53 Willershausen B, Callaway A, Azrak B, Kloss C, Schulz-Dobrick B: Prolonged in vitro exposure to white wines enhances the erosive damage on human permanent teeth compared with red wines. Nutr Res 2009;29:558–567.

54 Wiktorsson AM, Zimmerman M, Angmar-Mansson B: Erosive tooth wear: prevalence and severity in Swedish winetasters. Eur J Oral Sci 1997;105:544–550.

55 Ferguson MM, Dunbar RJ, Smith JA, Wall JG: Enamel erosion related to winemaking. Occup Med (Lond) 1996; 46:159–162.

56 Chaudhry SI, Harris JL, Challacombe SJ: Dental erosion in a wine merchant: an occupational hazard? Br Dent J 1997; 182:226–228.

57 Gray A, Ferguson MM, Wall JG: Wine tasting and dental erosion. Case report. Aust Dent J 1998;43:32–34.

58 Rees J, Hughes J, Innes C: An in vitro assessment of the erosive potential of some white wines. Eur J Prosthodont Restor Dent 2002;10:37–42.

59 Chikte UM, Naidoo S, Kolze TJ, Grobler SR: Patterns of tooth surface loss among winemakers. SADJ 2005;60:370–374.

60 Mulic A, Tveit AB, Hove LH, Skaare AB: Dental erosive wear among Norwegian wine tasters. Acta Odontol Scand 2011; 69:21–26.

61 Rees JS, Griffiths J: An in vitro assessment of the erosive potential of conventional and white ciders. Eur J Prosthodont Restor Dent 2002;10:167–171.

62 Rees JS, Davis FJ: An in vitro assessment of the erosive potential of some designer drinks. Eur J Prosthodont Restor Dent 2000;8:149–152.

63 Coombes JS, Hamilton KL.: The effectiveness of commercially available sports drinks. Sports Med 2000;29:181–209.

64 Coombes JS: Sports drinks and dental erosion. Am J Dent 2005;18:101–104.

65 Pugh LG, Corbett JL, Johnson RH: Rectal temperatures, weight losses, and sweat rates in marathon running. J Appl Physiol 1967;23:347–352.

66 Sirimaharaj V, Brearley Messer L, Morgan MV: Acidic diet and dental erosion among athletes. Aust Dent J 2002;47: 228–236.

67 Clark CS, Kraus BB, Sinclair J, Castell DO: Gastroesophageal reflux induced by exercise in healthy volunteers. JAMA 1989;261:3599–3601.

68 Milosevic A, Kelly MJ, McLean AN: Sports supplement drinks and dental health in competitive swimmers and cyclists. Br Dent J 1997;182:303–308.

69 Lokin PA, Huysmans MC: Is Dutch swimming pool water erosive? Ned Tijdschr Tandheelkd 2004;111:14–16.

70 Scheper WA, van Nieuw Amerongen A, Eijkman MA: Oral conditions in swimmers. Ned Tijdschr Tandheelkd 2005; 112:147–148.

71 Geurtsen W: Rapid general dental erosion by gas-chlorinated swimming pool water. Review of the literature and case report. Am J Dent 2000;13:291–293.

72 Williams D, Croucher R, Marcenes W, O'Farrell M: The prevalence of dental erosion in the maxillary incisors of 14-year-old schoolchildren living in Tower Hamlets and Hackney, London, UK. Int Dent J 1999;49:211–216.

73 Centerwall BS, Armstrong CW, Funkhouser LS, Elzay RP: Erosion of dental enamel among competitive swimmers at a gas-chlorinated swimming pool. Am J Epidemiol 1986;123:641–647.

74 Mathew T, Casamassimo PS, Hayes JR: Relationship between sports drinks and dental erosion in 304 university athletes in Columbus, Ohio, USA. Caries Res 2002;36:281–287.

75 Hooper SM, Hughes JA, Newcombe RG, Addy M, West NX: A methodology for testing the erosive potential of sports drinks. J Dent 2005;33:343–348.

76 Ali H, Tahmassebi JF: The effects of smoothies on enamel erosion: an in situ study. Int J Paediatr Dent DOI: 10.1111/ipd.12058.

Dr. M.E. Barbour
School of Oral and Dental Sciences
University of Bristol
Lower Maudlin Street
Bristol BS1 2LY (UK)
E-Mail m.e.barbour@bristol.ac.uk

Lussi A, Ganss C (eds): Erosive Tooth Wear. Monogr Oral Sci. Basel, Karger, 2014, vol 25, pp 155–162
DOI: 10.1159/000359942

Oral Hygiene Products, Medications and Drugs – Hidden Aetiological Factors for Dental Erosion

Elmar Hellwig[a] · Adrian Lussi[b]

[a]Department of Operative Dentistry and Periodontology, Center of Dental Medicine, University of Freiburg, Freiburg, Germany; [b]Department of Preventive, Restorative and Pediatric Dentistry, School of Dental Medicine, University of Bern, Bern, Switzerland

Abstract

Acidic or EDTA-containing oral hygiene products and acidic medicines have the potential to soften dental hard tissues. The low pH of oral care products increases the chemical stability of some fluoride compounds and favours the incorporation of fluoride ions in the lattice of hydroxyapatite and the precipitation of calcium fluoride on the tooth surface. This layer has some protective effect against an erosive attack. However, when the pH is too low or when no fluoride is present these protecting effects are replaced by direct softening of the tooth surface. Oral dryness can occur as a consequence of medication such as tranquilizers, antihistamines, antiemetics and antiparkinsonian medicaments or of salivary gland dysfunction. Above all, patients should be aware of the potential demineralization effects of oral hygiene products with low pH. Acetyl salicylic acid taken regularly in the form of multiple chewable tablets or in the form of headache powder, as well as chewing hydrochloric acids tablets for the treatment of stomach disorders, can cause erosion. There is most probably no direct association between asthmatic drugs and erosion on the population level. Consumers and health professionals should be aware of the potential of tooth damage not only by oral hygiene products and salivary substitutes but also by chewable and effervescent tablets. Several paediatric medications show a direct erosive potential in vitro. Clinical proof of the occurrence of erosion after use of these medicaments is still lacking. However, regular and prolonged use of these medicaments might bear the risk of causing erosion. Additionally, it can be assumed that patients suffering from xerostomia should be aware of the potential effects of oral hygiene products with low pH and high titratable acidity.

Erosive tooth wear is caused by different intrinsic and extrinsic acidic sources and may be modified by several factors [see chapter by Lussi and Carvalho, this vol., pp. 1–15]. While much of the literature concerning erosive tooth wear deals with the influence of dietary, environmental and lifestyle factors, only scarce information is available about the contribution of medicaments and/or oral health products to the erosive destruction of dental hard tissues. However, there are some reports in the literature describing acidic medicaments as aetiological factors for the development of erosive lesions. Zero [1], in a review about the aetiology of erosion, mentioned iron tonics, liquid hydrochloric acid, vitamin C, aspirin, acidic oral hygiene products or products with calcium chelators, as well as acidic salivary substitutes and salivary flow stimulants, as potential erosive products.

Oral Hygiene Products

Many oral care products such as toothpastes and fluoride-rinsing solutions exhibit a low pH. This, on the one hand, enhances the chemical stability of some fluoride compounds and, on the other, favours the incorporation of fluoride ions in the lattice of hydroxyapatite, forming fluoridated hydroxyapatite (e.g. in white spot lesions). Furthermore, it favours the precipitation of calcium fluoride on the tooth surface. The formation of the latter on the tooth surface can act as a protection against acid attacks [2–4].

So far, the erosive potential of oral care products has been investigated in only a few studies: an EDTA-containing anticalculus rinsing solution exhibited an erosive effect on enamel after a 2-hour exposure time in vitro. This was explained by the calcium-chelating action of EDTA [5]. In another study, 11 commercially available rinsing solutions were examined for their acid content. The pH values found ranged between 3.4 and 8.3. Also, titration values ('buffer capacity') varied strongly among the solutions tested. Whether or not the solutions were likely to cause erosion was not investigated [6].

Pontefract et al. [7] performed an in situ and in vitro study to measure enamel erosion by low pH mouth rinses. They used an acidified sodium chlorite mouth rinse (pH 3.02), an essential oil mouth rinse (Listerine®, pH 3.59) and a hexetidine mouth rinse (0.1%, pH 3.75). They compared the mouth rinses with orange juice and mineral water and found that all 3 rinses and orange juice led to a progressive enamel loss over time. The acidified sodium chlorite solution produced similar erosion to orange juice and significantly more erosion than the 2 tested rinses and water. The essential oil and the hexetidine mouth rinses produced similar erosion and significantly more mineral loss than water. This was substantiated in their in vitro study. Pretty et al. [8] could also show that Listerine caused erosion. The authors concluded that the patients should avoid using acidic mouth rinses as pre-brushing rinses or following erosive challenges (e.g. vomiting).

In an in vitro model Meurman et al. [9] investigated the erosive effects of commercially available cotton swabs meant for hospital use and compared them to a saliva-stimulating chewing tablet. Disposable cotton swabs are often used for cleaning and moistening the mouth and teeth in bedridden patients or otherwise disabled persons who are not able to take care of their own daily oral hygiene. The authors could demonstrate that disposable cotton swabs with a low pH and a high acid content can cause tooth erosion. Repeated use of such swabs may therefore be detrimental to the teeth. Since bedridden and medically compromised patients often suffer from reduced saliva flow, the erosive effects may be enhanced in these cases. Consequently, those products should be avoided and less erosive products should be used as special mouth-cleaning aids.

Lussi and Jaeggi [10] investigated the erosive potential of various oral care products and compared the results with those of various foodstuffs and beverages. In this in vitro study, they could

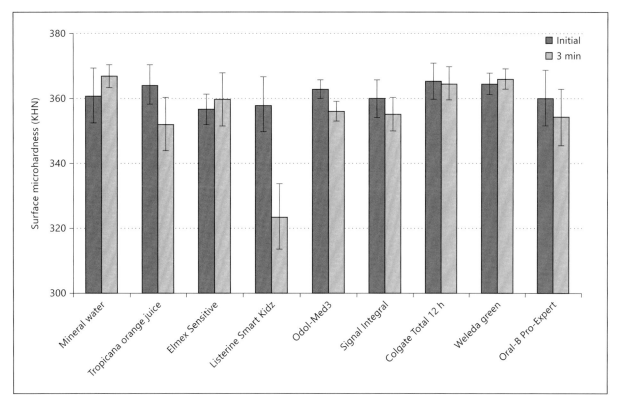

Fig. 1. Initial enamel surface microhardness (dark columns) and after 3 min of immersion in different products (light columns). KHN = Knoop hardness numbers (mean ± SD).

show that among the dental hygiene products only the fluoride-free Weleda toothpaste led to a significant reduction of hardness. They suggested that Weleda softened the tooth surface due to its content of citric acid/citrate and the absence of fluoride in combination with its low pH of 3.7. Although some of the tested products (Elmex® gelée, Meridol® dentifrice, Meridol mouth rinse) had a pH below 5, none of them showed surface softening. Recently, we tested some oral products presently available on the European market in relation to erosive wear on buccal surfaces of molars [Carvalho et al., unpubl. data]. A total of 7 oral products were tested (4 dental rinses and 3 toothpastes) and enamel surface microhardness was determined before (initial) and after 3 min of immersion in the respective product.

Most products presented slight variations on surface microhardness, which were not significant, but 1 product did present some erosive potential. Listerine Smart Kidz rinse caused a significant decrease in enamel microhardness after a 3-min application (fig. 1). Considering the product is targeted towards children (aged 6 years onward according to the manufacturer), whose deciduous teeth may be more susceptible to erosion than the permanent teeth, dentists should be aware of the dangers of excessive use of such products. Interestingly, Weleda toothpaste changed the composition and it has today no erosive potential anymore.

Attin et al. [2] could also demonstrate that the application of a fluoride-containing gel with a pH of 4.75 (Elmex gelée) increased the abrasion resistance of eroded enamel. Lussi and Jaeggi [10] suggested that after topical application of acidic oral hygiene products with a high fluoride content some mineral is dissolved from the enamel surface, thereby increasing the local pH and leading to reprecipitation of fluoridated hydroxyapatite. Moreover, the buffer capacity of saliva and the organic pellicle led to an additional protective effect. It seems that highly concentrated slightly acidic fluoride applications are able to increase abrasion resistance and decrease the development of erosion of enamel and dentine. Wiegand et al. [11] showed that toothbrush abrasion of eroded dentine may be influenced by the fluoride content, by the RDA value and particularly by the buffer capacity of the applied dentifrice or gel.

A different problem arises in patients suffering from xerostomia or oral dryness as a consequence of medication or of salivary gland dysfunction. These individuals sip liquids frequently to eliminate the discomfort associated with reduced saliva. Samarawickrama [12] stated that a properly balanced saliva substitute may become necessary to manage xerostomia when no means of stimulating the saliva are effective. This product should have a neutral pH and contain electrolytes to make the composition similar to natural saliva. Xerostomia and oral dryness is a side effect of a wide variety of drugs such as antidepressants, antihypertensives, antipsychotics and antihistamines [13, 14]. Further, it is one of the most common complaints experienced by patients who undergo radiotherapy of the oral cavity and the head and neck region or who suffer from Sjögren's syndrome. Since the protective effects of saliva (e.g. buffer capacity and oral clearance) is limited in those patients, salivary substitutes or oral hygiene products (mouth rinses, fluoride gels, etc.) with a low pH and a high amount of titratable acid lead to a progressive demineralization of dental hard tissues [15, 16]. Kielbassa et al. [17] found that Biotene® with a pH of 4.15 and Glandosane® with a pH of 4.08

led to mineral loss in enamel and dentine. They concluded that fluoridated saliva substitutes containing mucins, phosphate and calcium are suitable for the relief of symptoms of extensive xerostomia.

Acidic Medicines

If a medicine low in pH and high in titratable acidity is used frequently and/or over a long period of time, it has the potential to produce erosive lesions in teeth. Additionally, some medicines can contribute to increase the danger of erosion when reducing the salivary flow rate and/or buffer capacity of the saliva, e.g. tranquilizers, antihistamines, antiemetics and antiparkinsonian medicaments [13, 14]. Nunn et al. [18] assessed 8 liquid oral medicines and 2 effervescent preparations routinely prescribed for long-term use by paediatric renal patients with respect to pH values and titratable acid. They found that some of the medicines and particularly the 2 effervescent tablets showed low pH values. Titratable acidity for hydralazine hydrochloride solution and Phosphate Sandoz® and Sandoz K® effervescent tablets were critical compared to the other medicaments. They concluded that health professionals need to be aware of the erosive potential of liquid oral medicines and recommend the use of tablets whenever that option exists.

The high popularity of using supplemental vitamin C (L-ascorbic acid), prescribed either professionally or self-prescribed, has increased during the last years. There are different preparations on the market (e.g. chewing tablets, syrup, effervescent vitamin C tablets). Giunta [19] concluded from a case report and from an in vitro test that the pH of saliva can drop while chewing vitamin C tablets, reaching values of <2.0 in the oral cavity. Although the pH level varies from manufacturer to manufacturer, the level of acidity in vitamin C preparations is always high. Since tablets are hard, large and chewable, the time and the area of contact with the teeth may be high. Passon and Jones [20] reported a case of a 58-year-old man who took a 500-mg chewable vitamin C tablet daily over a period of 1 year. This man suffered from severe erosion of the upper and lower left canines and premolars where he held the tablets while he let them slowly dissolve. Consumers should be aware of the potential of tooth damage by chewable tablets and a physician should recommend vitamin C in a form which is safe. This is in accordance with the findings of Meurman and Murtomaa [21] who stated that for individuals with normal salivary flow the consumption of vitamin C preparations should not have erosive effects unless the preparations are left in direct contact with the teeth.

Results from clinical surveys suggest a strong positive correlation between the consumption of vitamin C supplements and the prevalence of erosion [22–24]. Recently, a meta-analysis showed this association between vitamin C and erosion with an odds ratio of 1.16 [25].

Erosion can also result from chronic use of chewable aspirin tablets or headache powder. McCracken and O'Neal [26] reported a 30-year-old female patient with a 3-year history of headache powder use at 6 doses a day, each dose containing 520 mg aspirin. She placed the undissolved powder sublingually to increase the rate of absorption. Oral examination revealed severe erosion on the occlusal surfaces of the mandibular molars and premolars. Rogalla et al. [27] assessed the erosive action of unbuffered and buffered acetyl salicylic acid on tooth hard tissues in vitro. Scanning electron microscopy analysis of the enamel and dentine surfaces showed marked differences in the degree of erosion depending on the duration of exposure and the concentration of acetyl salicylic acid. They suggested that remnants of chewable tablets can stick in deep fissures, thereby exerting a long-lasting erosive effect. Their results are supported by a report published by Grace et al. [28], who showed that tooth erosion can be caused by chewable aspirin tablets. Particular patients with juvenile rheumatic arthritis who took aspirin in the form of multiple chewable tablets per day experienced erosion on the occlusal surface compared to children who swallowed the tablets and had no erosion [29].

Conflicting results concerning the association between asthma and tooth erosion were published [30–32]. Dugmore and Rock [32] in a representative random sample of adolescents in the UK found no association between asthma and tooth erosion. They also reported that 88% of drugs prescribed for asthma had a pH above 5.5. However, some drugs inhaled to combat asthma have a pH low enough to cause erosion, particularly when they come in frequent and/or sustained contact with teeth. When asthma medication is taken from an inhaler, the lips form a seal around the nozzle of the inhaler, covering and protecting the labial surfaces of the incisors and canine teeth. Consequently, it is unlikely that any acidic medicaments would spread to the labial surfaces of the teeth subsequent to inhalation [32]. The authors listed a number of factors leading to erosion in asthmatic patients. The acidic nature of the medication is able to act directly on the teeth. Prolonged use of β_2-adrenoreceptor stimulants such as salbutamol, salmeterol or terbutaline leads to decreased salivary flow, thus reducing the modifying and protective effects of saliva. Drugs used as bronchodilators act to relax smooth muscle. This may affect the oesophageal sphincter in addition to the bronchus and thereby potentiate the gastroesophageal reflux, which is a recognized aetiological factor in tooth erosion. The patients might increase their consumption of acidic drinks in an attempt to compensate for reduced saliva flow, increased dry mouth and the taste of drugs. The authors concluded that it is difficult to support an association between such drugs and the erosion on the population level. They also stated that most asthma inhalation medicaments are not acidic and pose no threat to the dentition. There seems to be no clear evidence of an association between decreased salivary flow rate due to asthma medication and tooth erosion. The proportion of drugs used that may promote gastroesophageal reflux is low and unlikely to have a significant influence on tooth erosion prevalence, and they could not approve the thesis that asthmatic children consume more potentially erosive drinks than non-asthmatics. Sivasithamparam et al. [33] in a case control study from South East Queensland supported their conclusions. They also found no differences between asthmatics and other patients concerning citrus fruit and acidic soft drink consumption. Although Sivasithamparam et al. [33] found that gastroesophageal reflux does not appear to contribute in a side-specific manner to erosion in asthmatics, Al-Dlaigan et al. [30] observed that the higher prevalence of erosion in their sample of asthmatic patients was associated with reflux. This is interesting, because the systematic review by Tolia and Vandenplas [34] showed that the prevalence of gastroesophageal reflux disease in asthmatic children (pooled weighted average prevalence of 23.4%) is greater than in healthy controls. This is also true in adults, where the prevalence of gastroesophageal reflux disease in those suffering from asthma is as high as 59.2% [35]. Although it is still not known whether there is an actual causality association between both conditions, dentists should consider the likelihood of erosive lesions in asthmatic patients to be related with a possible reflux disease.

HCl tablets are used in order to treat stomach disorders and have also been cited as a cause of enamel erosion. Maron [36] described the case of severe enamel erosion caused after chewing hydrochloric acid tablets over a 5-year period. He concluded that dentists must be aware that highly erosive acids are obtainable without prescription, and that the misuse of acidic medicine might be responsible for severe erosive destruction of tooth hard tissues. In the reported case, a woman chewed the hydrochloric acid tablets rather than swallowing them.

Maguire et al. [37] assessed 97 paediatric medicines according to their erosive potential. All formulations exhibited prolonged oral clearance and were identified as being used regularly and long term by children and also by older people. They found that 75% of the formulations had an endogenous pH of <5.5. Moreover, effervescent preparations and nutrition and blood preparations were significant predictors of higher titratable acidity. Also, Arora et al. [38] could show that some paediatric medicines given regularly and long term to children exhibit an erosive potential. Costa et al. [39] in a pH cycling experiment could observe that an antihistamine-containing syrup (Claritin D) caused erosive changes of primary enamel. However, the use of fluoride dentifrice was able to diminish the erosive effect. Neves et al. [40] determined titratable acids and viscosity of 23 paediatric medicines available on the Brazilian market. They found that only 2 of the medicines were not acidic. The sample consisted of antihistamines, antitussives, bronchodilators and mucolytics. Dietary medicines are usually viscous syrups that adhere to the tooth surface and therefore have a prolonged oral clearance. This might lead to a higher likelihood of erosion. However, information on the relation between viscosity and erosion of dental hard tissues is rare, and Valinoti et al. [41] found that in patients with erosion high viscosity medicines might even protect the tooth surface from further erosion. A recent study showed that increasing the viscosity of soft drinks reduced enamel erosion [42].

Lussi et al. [43] evaluated different dietary substances in medications containing acetylsalicylic acid, vitamin C, tartaric acid and citric acid monohydrate. They concluded that a wide range of medications exhibit an erosive potential depending mainly on low pH, buffer capacity, fluoride and calcium concentrations [see chapter by Lussi and Hellwig, this vol. pp. 220–229].

Also, Babu et al. [44] investigated the endogenous erosive potential of 8 of the most commonly used paediatric liquid medicaments in primary teeth. In the very basic in vitro study using SEM pictures they found that paracetamol, amoxicillin, erythromycin, salbutamol and multivitamin preparations showed a particular erosive effect.

Clinical proof of the occurrence of erosion after use of these medicaments is still lacking. However, regular and prolonged use of these medicaments might bear the risk of causing erosion.

References

1 Zero DT: Etiology of dental erosion: extrinsic factors. Eur J Oral Sci 1996;104: 162–177.
2 Attin T, Deifuss H, Hellwig E: Influence of acidified fluoride gel on abrasion resistance of eroded enamel. Caries Res 1999;33:135–139.
3 Ganss C, Klimek J, Schäfer U, Spall T: Effectiveness of two fluoridation measures on erosion progression in human enamel and dentine in vitro. Caries Res 2001;35:325–330.
4 Lussi A, Jaeggi T, Schaffner M: Prevention and minimally invasive treatment of erosions. Oral Health Prev Dent 2004; 2:321–325.
5 Rytömaa I, Meurman JH, Franssila S, Torkko H: Oral hygiene products may cause dental erosion. Proc Finn Dent Soc 1989;85:161–166.
6 Bhatti SA, Walsh TF, Douglas CW: Ethanol and pH levels of proprietary mouthrinses. Community Dent Health 1994; 11:71–74.
7 Pontefract H, Hughes J, Kemp K, et al: The erosive effects of some mouthrinses on enamel: a study in situ. J Clin Periodontol 2001;28:319–324.
8 Pretty IA, Edgar WM, Higham SM: The erosive potential of commercially available mouthrinses on enamel as measured by quantitative light-induced fluorescence (QLF). J Dent 2003;31: 313–319.
9 Meurman JH, Sorvari R, Pelttari A, Rytomaa I, Franssila S, Kroon L: Hospital mouth-cleaning aids may cause dental erosion. Spec Care Dentist 1996;16:247–250.
10 Lussi A, Jaeggi T: The erosive potential of various oral care products compared to foodstuffs and beverages. Schweiz Monatsschr Zahnmed 2001;111:274–281.

11 Wiegand A, Wolmershäuser S, Hellwig E, Attin T: Influence of buffering effects of dentifrices and fluoride gels on abrasion on eroded dentine. Arch Oral Biol 2004;49:259–265.
12 Samarawickrama DY: Saliva substitutes: how effective and safe are they? Oral Dis 2002;8:177–179.
13 Atkinson JC, Wu AJ: Salivary gland dysfunction: causes, symptoms, treatment. Am Dent Assoc 1994;125:409–416.
14 Cassolato SF, Turnbull RS: Xerostomia: clinical aspects and treatment. Gerodontology 2003;20:64–77.
15 Meyer-Lueckel H, Kielbassa AM: Use of saliva substitutes in patients with xerostomia. Schweiz Monatsschr Zahnmed 2002;112:1037–1058.
16 Kielbassa AM, Shohadai SP: Die Auswirkungen von Speichelersatzmitteln auf die Läsionstiefe von demineralisiertem Schmelz. Dtsch Zahnärzt Z 1999;54: 757–763.
17 Kielbassa AM, Shohadai SP, Schulte-Monting J: Effect of saliva substitutes on mineral content of demineralized and sound dental enamel. Support Care Cancer 2001;9:40–47.
18 Nunn JH, Ng SK, Sharkey I, Coulthard M: The dental implications of chronic use of acidic medicines in medically compromised children. Pharm World Sci 2001;23:118–119.
19 Giunta JL: Dental erosion resulting from chewable vitamin C tablets. J Am Dent Assoc 1983;107:253–256.
20 Passon JC, Jones GK: Atypical dental erosion: a case report. Gerodontics 1986; 2:77–79.
21 Meurman JH, Murtomaa H: Effect of effervescent vitamin C preparations on bovine teeth and on some clinical and salivary parameters in man. Scand J Dent Res 1986;94:491–499.

22 O'Sullivan EA, Curzon ME: A comparison of acidic dietary factors in children with and without dental erosion. ASDC J Dent Child 2000;67:186–192.
23 Al-Malik MI, Holt RD, Bedi R: The relationship between erosion, caries and rampant caries and dietary habits in preschool children in Saudi Arabia. Int J Paediatr Dent 2001;11:430–439.
24 Al-Dlaigan YH, Shaw L, Smith A: Dental erosion in a group of British 14-year-old school children. II. Influence of dietary intake. Br Dent J 2001;190: 258–261.
25 Li H, Zou Y, Ding G: Dietary factors associated with dental erosion: a meta-analysis. PlosOne 2012;7:e42626.
26 McCracken M, O'Neal SJ: Dental erosion and aspirin headache powders: a clinical report. J Prosthodont 2000;9: 95–98.
27 Rogalla K, Finger W, Hannig M: Influence of buffered and unbuffered acetylsalicylic acid on dental enamel and dentine in human teeth: an in vitro pilot study. Methods Find Exp Clin Pharmacol 1992;14:339–346.
28 Grace EG, Sarlani E, Kaplan S: Tooth erosion caused by chewing aspirin. J Am Dent Assoc 2004;135:911–914.
29 Sullivan RE, Kramer WS: Introgenic erosion of teeth. J Dent Child 1983;56: 92–196.
30 Al-Dlaigan YH, Shaw L, Smith AJ: Is there a relationship between asthma and dental erosion? A case control study. Int J Paediatr Dent 2002;12:189–200.
31 Shaw L, al-Dlaigan YH, Smith A: Childhood asthma and dental erosion. ASDC J Dent Child 2000;67:102–106.
32 Dugmore CR, Rock WP: Asthma and tooth erosion: is there an association? Int J Paediatr Dent 2003;13:417–424.

33 Sivasithamparam K, Young WG, Jirattanasopa V, Priest J, Khan F, Harbrow D, Daley TJ, Sullivan RE, Kramer WS: Dental erosion in asthma: a case-control study from South East Queensland. Aust Dent J 2002;47:298–303.

34 Tolia V, Vandenplas Y: Systematic review: the extra-oesophageal symptoms of gastro-oesophageal reflux disease in children. Aliment Pharmacol Ther 2009; 29:258–272.

35 Havemann et al: The association between gastro-esophageal reflux disease and asthma: a systematic review. Gut 2007;56:1654–1664.

36 Maron FS: Enamel erosion resulting from hydrochloric acid tablets. J Am Dent Assoc 1996;127:781–784.

37 Maguire A, Baqir W, Nunn JH: Are sugar-free medicines more erosive than sugar-containing medicines? An in vitro study of paediatric medicines with prolonged oral clearance used regularly and long term by children. Int J Paediatr Dent 2007;17:231–238.

38 Arora R, Mukherjee U, Arora V: Erosive potential of sugar-free and sugar-containing pediatric medicines given regularly and long term to children. Indian J Pediatr 2012;79:759–763.

39 Costa CC, Almeida IC, da Costa Filho LC, Oshima HM: Morphology evaluation of primary enamel exposed to antihistamine and fluoride dentifrice – an in vitro study. Gen Dent 2006;54:21–27.

40 Neves BG, Farah A, Lucas E, de Sousa VP, Maia LC: Are paediatric medicines risk factors for dental caries and dental erosion? Community Dent Health 2010; 27:46–51.

41 Valinoti AC, Pierro VS, Da Silva EM, Maia LC: In vitro alterations in dental enamel exposed to acidic medicines. Int J Paediatr Dent. 2011;21:141–150.

42 Aykut-Yetkiner A, Wiegand A, Ronay V, Attin R, Becker K, Attin T: In vitro evaluation of the erosive potential of viscosity-modified soft acidic drinks on enamel. Clin Oral Investig, Epub ahead of print.

43 Lussi A, Megert B, Shellis RP, Wang X: Analysis of the erosive effect of different dietary substances and medications. Br J Nutr 2012;107:252–262.

44 Babu KL, Rai K, Hedge AM: Pediatric liquid medicaments – do they erode the teeth surface? An in vitro study. Part I. J Clin Pediatr Dent 2008;32:189–194.

Prof. E. Hellwig
Department of Operative Dentistry and Periodontology
Center of Dental Medicine, University of Freiburg
Hugstetter Strasse 55
DE–79106 Freiburg (Germany)
E-Mail elmar.hellwig@uniklinik-freiburg.de

Lussi A, Ganss C (eds): Erosive Tooth Wear. Monogr Oral Sci. Basel, Karger, 2014, vol 25, pp 163–179
DOI: 10.1159/000359943

Understanding the Chemistry of Dental Erosion

R. Peter Shellis[a, b] · John D.B. Featherstone[c] · Adrian Lussi[b]

[a]School of Oral and Dental Sciences, University of Bristol, Bristol, UK; [b]Department of Preventive, Restorative and Paediatric Dentistry, School of Dental Medicine, University of Bern, Bern, Switzerland; [c]Department of Preventive and Restorative Dental Sciences, University of California at San Francisco, San Francisco, Calif., USA

Abstract

Dental erosion is caused by repeated short episodes of exposure to acids. Dental minerals are calcium-deficient, carbonated hydroxyapatites containing impurity ions such as Na^+, Mg^{2+} and Cl^-. The rate of dissolution, which is crucial to the progression of erosion, is influenced by solubility and also by other factors. After outlining principles of solubility and acid dissolution, this chapter describes the factors related to the dental tissues on the one hand and to the erosive solution on the other. The impurities in the dental mineral introduce crystal strain and increase solubility, so dentine mineral is more soluble than enamel mineral and both are more soluble than hydroxyapatite. The considerable differences in structure and porosity between dentine and enamel influence interactions of the tissues with acid solutions, so the relative rates of dissolution do not necessarily reflect the respective solubilities. The rate of dissolution is further influenced strongly by physical factors (temperature, flow rate) and chemical factors (degree of saturation, presence of inhibitors, buffering, pH, fluoride). Temperature and flow rate, as determined by the method of consumption of a product, strongly influence erosion in vivo. The net effect of the solution factors determines the overall erosive potential of different products. Prospects for remineralization of erosive lesions are evaluated.

© 2014 S. Karger AG, Basel

Our objective is to provide a model for the chemical understanding of dental erosion. A true understanding of the mechanisms involved makes it possible to readily interpret observations both in research and in the clinic, and provides a sound basis for preventive interventions and therapy for patients. The chemistry behind erosion is the key to assimilating the information in this monograph and putting it into practice in the real world.

A fundamental property of any solid is its solubility, which determines whether it will dissolve in a given solution. Erosion is caused by numerous brief episodes of exposure to acid, so the *rate of dissolution* is crucial and this is influenced by many factors besides solubility. Some of these are properties of the solution, while others are related to the structure of the dental tissues and how this influences interactions with the solution.

Therefore, the first objective of this review is to outline basic concepts of solubility and to explain how this influences interactions between solid and solution. The second objective is to describe the factors which influence the kinetics of dissolution, both those associated with the nature of the tissues and those associated with erosive solutions.

Solubility and Dissolution

The minerals in enamel and dentine are imperfect forms of a calcium phosphate, hydroxyapatite (HAp): $Ca_{10}(PO_4)_6(OH)_2$ [1]. As such, they are crystalline solids made up of the ions Ca^{2+}, PO_4^{3-} and OH^-, together with various 'impurity' ions which, as will be explained later, affect the chemical properties of the mineral.

When any solid is immersed in a solution the interface between the two phases becomes a site for continuous exchange of the components of the solid (in this case, Ca^{2+}, PO_4^{3-} and OH^- ions). Ions leave the surface to dissolve in the solution *(dissolution)* and leave the solution to attach to the solid surface *(crystal growth)*. When the rate at which ions enter the solution equals that at which they attach to the crystal surface, the solid and solution are in a state of equilibrium and there is no net change to the solid. At equilibrium, the solution is said to be *saturated* with respect to the solid and the concentration of solid dissolved in the solution is a measure of the *solubility* of the solid. However, this is a definition of limited usefulness because the equilibrium concentration varies markedly with pH and the concentrations of background ions. Instead, the *chemical activity* of the solid at equilibrium is used to define solubility. The chemical activity of ionic solids is defined by the *ion activity product (I)* which for HAp is:

$$I_{HAp} = (Ca^{2+})^{10}(PO_4^{3-})^6(OH^-)^2 \qquad (1)$$

Here, the round brackets denote ion activities, which are proportional to their concentra-tions. *I* for any ionic solid is thus given by the product of all the ion activities each raised to a power equal to the number of that ion in each formula unit.

The value of the ion activity product in a solution in equilibrium with a solid is called the *solubility product*, K_S. It can be determined by equilibrating samples of the solid with solutions (e.g. water, dilute acids or buffer solutions), and then analysing the ion concentrations and computing the value of *I*. Unlike the solubility defined as concentration, the solubility product is constant for a given temperature. It can be used to calculate solubilities as concentrations for any set of conditions (as in fig. 3). It can also be used to predict the probable fate of the relevant solid in solutions of interest. If a solution has a value of *I* which is less than K_S, it is said to be *undersaturated* and the solid will tend to dissolve until the ion concentrations, and hence *I*, have increased to where the solution is saturated. If *I* is greater than K_S the solution is said to be *supersaturated* and the solid will tend to precipitate, causing loss of ions from solution until *I* has been reduced to the point where the solution has again reached saturation. The phrase 'tend to' is used instead of 'will' because for a variety of reasons dissolution/precipitation reactions can be inhibited, as will be explained later. However, it is always true that dissolution does not occur in a supersaturated solution or precipitation in an undersaturated solution.

There are problems in defining and measuring the solubility products of dental minerals. As the minerals are heterogeneous they present a range of solubilities [2]. It has proved difficult to determine solubility products defined on the basis of the actual mineral composition [3–5]. Therefore, solubility products are defined in terms of HAp composition [2, 6–9], which can be interpreted as reflecting the influence of impurities and crystal imperfections on HAp solubility. There are also practical difficulties associated with failure to achieve true equilibrium, owing to the tendency

Table 1. Acid composition of different beverages

Beverage	pH	Phosphoric	Citric	D-isocitric	Malic	Other
Apple juice	3.0–3.4		0.05–2	0.01	7.4	lactic: 0.17 formic: 0.02
Cola beverage	2.2–2.6	3.3	9			carbonic: 4–6
Grapefruit juice (fresh)	3.2–3.4		13.9	0.19	0.44	
Orange juice (fresh)	3.4–3.7		7.6–11.9	0.1	1.2–2.9	
Red wine	3.4–3.7				0.3–5.1	lactic: 2.25–2.4 tartaric: 1.0–1.5
White wine	3.4–3.7		0.14		3.5	lactic: 1.7 tartaric: 0.5–1.5

Acid composition values are in grams/litre.

Table 2. Dissociation constants for acids relevant to erosion

Acid	pK_{a1}	pK_{a2}	pK_{a3}	$pK_{Ca}(1)$	$pK_{Ca}(2)$	$pK_{Ca}(3)$
Carbonic	6.35	10.31		1.11	3.22	
Phosphoric	2.15	7.20	12.35	0.56	2.42	6.46
Acetic	4.76			1.18		
Lactic	3.86			1.45		
Malic	3.46	5.10		1.02	2.66	
Oxalic	1.25	4.27		1.84	3.19[2]	
Tartaric	3.04	4.37		0.92[1]	2.80	
Citric	3.13	4.74	6.42	1.10	3.09	4.48

$pK_{a1-3} = -\log_{10}$ acid dissociation constants. $pK_{Ca}(1-3) = -\log_{10}$ dissociation constants for complex of Ca^{2+} with anions with 1, 2 or 3 negative charges. Larger values indicate stronger binding of anion to H^+ or Ca^{2+}. Values for 25°C, zero ionic strength, unless indicated [101, 102].
[1] Temperature not stated; ionic strength 0.2.
[2] 18°C; zero ionic strength.

of the surface of the crystal to acquire a composition different from the interior and for the surface layer to control the solubility [10]. However, non-equilibrium studies, which investigate whether demineralization of dental tissues occurs as predicted by different solubility products [5, 9, 11, 12], allow hypotheses on solubility to be tested and a reasonable general picture of solubility relationships of dental minerals has been built up.

In erosion the H^+ ions responsible for demineralization are supplied by a variety of acids (tables 1, 2). The only strong acid (i.e. one which is fully dissociated at all pH) that is involved in erosion is HCl. All the other acids are weak acids, which dissociate progressively as pH rises. For instance, citric acid, which is tribasic (contains three groups which can dissociate to produce a hydrogen ion), dissociates in three steps:

$$H_3Citrate^0 \rightleftharpoons H_2Citrate^- + H^+ \ (pK_{a1} = 3.13) \quad (2a)$$

$$H_2Citrate^- \rightleftharpoons HCitrate^{2-} + H^+ \ (pK_{a2} = 4.74) \quad (2b)$$

$$HCitrate^{2-} \rightleftharpoons Citrate^{3-} + H^+ \ (pK_{a3} = 6.42) \quad (2c)$$

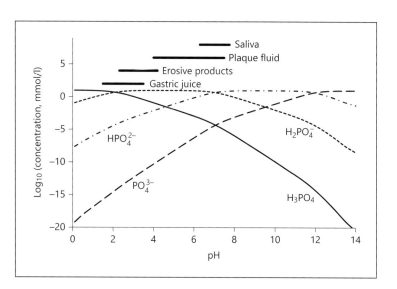

Fig. 1. Dissociation of phosphoric acid (tribasic). Calculated for 10 mmol/l total acid, 25°C. The approximate pH ranges for fluids relevant to erosion and caries are shown at the top. As pH rises, the concentrations of successive anions increase to a maximum (in this case to almost 100% of the total), and then decrease as they in turn dissociate to generate the succeeding anion. The PO_4^{3-} ion is the end product of dissociation and makes up almost 100% of total phosphate at pH >13. At pH typical for erosion, in contrast, its concentration is extremely low.

Here, 'Citrate' stands for $^-OOC-CH_2-(OH)C(COO^-)-CH_2-COO^-$. The superscript symbol after 'Citrate' gives the number of negative charges on the anion. The undissociated acid and its derivative anions will in the following be referred to as 'species'.

The extent of dissociation, and hence the balance between the species present at a given pH, is determined by the acid dissociation constants (K_a). These are shown after the above equations and in table 2 as the negative logarithms (pK_a). The dissociation of another tribasic acid (phosphoric) is illustrated in figure 1, which shows the successive rise and fall in the concentration of the different anions, and how this is related to the pK_a values. From figure 1, it is clear that, although the concentration of any species can fall to very low levels, it is never zero. In other words, all species are present at all pH values, even if in minute concentrations.

The pK_a is a measure of the affinity of the dissociating anion at each step for H^+ ions. Thus, citric acid ($H_3Citrate^0$) is a stronger acid than $H_2Citrate^-$ because the pK_a controlling its dissociation is smaller (3.13 vs. 4.74). Whereas HCl acts simply as a source of H^+ ions, equations 2a–c show that, over a more or less wide range of pH, weak acids can either release or take up H^+ ions, depending on whether acid or base is added. Hence weak acids act as *buffers* which can resist pH change. The buffering power of a weak acid reaches a maximum at a pH which equals a pK_a.

In solution, cations and anions can associate with each other to form *ion pairs*, e.g. those of Ca^{2+} with F^- (CaF^+) or OH^- ($CaOH^+$), which are maintained by simple electrostatic attraction. More stable *complexes* involve formation of chemical bonds. A particular form of complex occurs if the anion can form two or more co-ordinate bonds with a cation, resulting in the formation of a ring: a phenomenon known as *chelation* [13]. This requires two features on the chelating anion: the presence of at least two ionized or polar groups, and a molecular structure which allows these charged groups to co-ordinate with the cation. Chelation is therefore a phenomenon associated mainly with polybasic acids. The acetate and formate anions, which have only one ionized group, can form an ion pair with Ca^{2+} but do not chelate. The remaining acids in tables 1 and 2 can form anions with

Shellis · Featherstone · Lussi

more than one negative charge, and so can form more than one stable complexes with Ca^{2+}. The co-ordinating groups on the anions include alcoholic OH groups, which are weakly acidic (pK$_a$ = 16–18; lactic, malic, tartaric and citric acids) as well as carboxyl or phosphate groups. Examples of chelation by citrate anions are shown in figure 2. Table 2 provides (as negative logarithms, pK$_{Ca}$) the dissociation constants for the complexes of Ca^{2+} with the acids found in erosive products: the larger the value of pK$_{Ca}$, the more stable the complex. It can be seen that the stability of the Ca complexes increase with the charge on the anion. The chelating effect by acids found in erosive products will, however, be weak compared with that of an efficient chelator, EDTA, which has pK$_{Ca}$ values up to 11.0 [14].

The roles of buffering and chelation in erosion are discussed later.

Enamel and Dentine: Minerals and Tissue Structure

As noted above, the minerals of dental tissues are imperfect forms of HAp. The imperfections arise from the incorporation into the crystals of 'impurity' ions from tissue fluids as the mineral crystals form during hard tissue formation. These ions replace ions in the crystal structure of HAp. The major substitutions are: CO_3^{2-} for PO_4^{3-} or OH^-; Na^+ and Mg^{2+} for Ca^{2+}. Because the impurity ions differ from the native HAp ions in size, charge or both, they have the effect of introducing strain in the crystal structure of the HAp and this in turn increases the solubility [15–17].

Synthetic HAp formed in the presence of carbonate and sodium can be described as calcium-deficient carbonated HAp [18]. A simplified formula that helps to illustrate the composition is:

$$Ca_{10-x}Na_x(PO_4)_{6-y}(CO_3)_z(OH)_{2-u}F_u \qquad (3)$$

This type of mineral is calcium-deficient because some of the calcium is replaced by sodium.

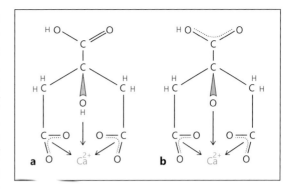

Fig. 2. Schematic representation of citrate ion chelating a calcium ion. **a** The situation where 2 of the COOH groups have lost the hydrogen and are negatively charged, thereby able to form coordinate bonds (represented by arrows) with the positively charged calcium ion. **b** In the basic pH range, the complex is stabilized further by formation of coordinate bond with the polar alcoholic OH on the C2 carbon. Modified from Bell [13].

Table 3. Major inorganic constituents of enamel and dentine

Constituent	Enamel	Dentine
Ca	36.6	26.9
P	17.7	13.2
CO$_3$	3.2	4.6
Na	0.7	0.6
Mg	0.4	0.8
Cl	0.4	0.06
K	0.04	0.02

Values are % dry weight [1].

The Na^+/Ca^{2+} substitution helps to rectify the imbalance of electric charge associated with the CO_3^{2-}/PO_4^{3-} substitution. Carbonate replaces some of the phosphate but not on a one-to-one basis: hence the phosphate is designated as 6-y and the carbonate as z.

The concentrations of the major constituents of enamel and dentine are shown in table 3. On the basis of the chemical composition and work on synthetic carbonated HAp noted above, Verbeeck [1] suggested the following average composition for enamel mineral:

$$[Ca_{8.9}Na_{0.3}Mg_{0.14}K_{0.01}\square_{0.65}][(PO_4)_{5.1}(HPO_4)_{0.4}$$
$$(CO_3)_{0.5}][(OH)_{1.08}(CO_3)_{0.05}Cl_{0.1}\square_{0.77}] \qquad (4)$$

This formula takes into account evidence that about 10% of the CO_3^{2-} substitutes for OH^- rather than PO_4^{3-} [19]. The symbol $\square$ indicates vacancies in the crystal lattice where ions are missing. Fluoride is not included because of its low concentration in bulk enamel (<1% substitution for OH^-).

Table 3 shows that dentine contains more carbonate and magnesium in relation to calcium and phosphorus than enamel. The values in table 3 are average values for the tissues. It is well known that in enamel there are gradients in several constituents with depth. Calcium and phosphorus (i.e. total mineral) decrease from the enamel surface to the enamel-dentine junction, while carbonate and magnesium increase [20–22]. For dentine, an increase in Mg concentration with depth has been reported but information on other gradients is lacking [1].

Enamel mineral exists as well-formed crystals approximately 70 nm wide and 25 nm thick [23]. The true length is often difficult to determine in electron micrographs, but lengths of up to 1,000 nm have been reported. Crystals of dentine mineral are much smaller and have the form of thin plates about 30 nm wide and 3 nm thick [24]. The mineral of enamel is also much better crystallized.

Figure 3, based on various experimental data [5, 8, 9], shows that enamel is somewhat more soluble than HAp, while dentine is considerably more soluble. The greater solubility of dentine compared with that of enamel is correlated with the higher concentration of impurities and the lower crystallinity. On available evidence the small crystal size of dentine would be only poorly correlated with solubility [17] but the greater surface area/volume ratio could enhance interaction with acid and hence the dissolution rate. Within enamel, the solubility increases with depth from the surface [5, 11], in accordance with the gradients in

impurity ion concentrations. In addition, the prism junctions are sites of raised solubility [5].

A fourth mineral – fluorapatite (FAp): $Ca_{10}(PO_4)_6(F)_2$ – is included in figure 3. In this mineral, OH^-, as found in HAp, is replaced by F^-, which is a slightly smaller ion with the same charge. Unlike the solubility-increasing substitutions in dental minerals, this substitution reduces solubility when fluoride is present, as figure 3 shows. The difference in solubility depends on the fluoride concentration in solution: we have chosen to calculate the solubilities for the minimum and maximum fluoride concentrations for the products studied by Lussi et al. [25].

As figure 3 shows, the solubility of all four minerals is strongly dependent on pH. This is due to the fact that as pH falls, the concentration of PO_4^{3-} falls (fig. 1), as does the OH^- concentration. As these changes would reduce the value of I_{HAp} (equation 1) and also I_{FAp}, more mineral has to dissolve in order to achieve saturation.

In enamel and dentine, the mineral forms a composite material in association with an organic matrix, composed of protein and lipid, and water [26, 27]. The overall compositions of the two tissues are shown in table 4, in terms of relative volumes. Clearly, dentine is considerably more porous than enamel, having about 7 times the water content.

The organic phase of enamel consists of approximately equal parts of protein and lipid and forms a coating on the crystals. Most of the water and organic matrix are distributed between the closely packed crystals within the prisms to form a system of extremely narrow pores. Larger pores are located at the prism boundaries, but make up only a small fraction of the total porosity. The overall porosity also increases with depth, in conformity with the fall in mineral concentration.

The great majority (90%) of the organic matrix of dentine consists of fibres of type I collagen. In the developing tooth the fibres act as a scaffold for mineralization, which involves deposition of the small mineral crystals both within and between the fibres, as in bone and other calcified collage-

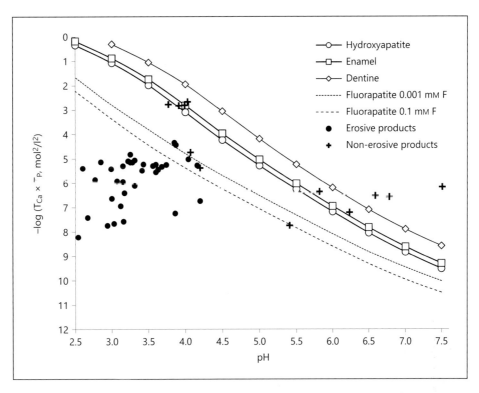

Fig. 3. Diagram showing the relative solubilities of the dental tissues, HAp and FAp. Each curve represents concentrations at which solution saturated with respect to the respective solid. It is assumed that solid is dissolving in strong acid (e.g. HCl), Ca/P ratio 5/3, at 37°C. Calculations performed using following solubility products: HAp $10^{-117.26}$ [99]; FAp 10^{-121} [100]; enamel $10^{-115.54}$ [8]; dentine 10^{-110} [9]. Points represent products studied for erosive potential by Lussi et al. [25]. Solid circles: erosive products, causing surface softening of enamel after a 2-min exposure; crosses: non-erosive products. Points on or close to solubility lines represent solutions that are saturated with respect to that solid. Points above and below the lines represent solutions that are respectively super- or undersaturated with respect to that solid. The vertical distance from the solubility line indicates approximately the degree of super- or undersaturation (it should be remembered that the y-axis is a logarithmic scale, so concentration changes 10-fold for each change in 1 unit on this axis).

Table 4. Composition of enamel and dentine by volume

Constituent	Enamel, vol%	Dentine, vol%
Mineral	91.0	49.5
Organic material (protein and lipid)	5.3	29.0
Water	3.4	21.4

Calculated from published density distribution [103], water contents [104] and organic content [1]. Lipid content assumed to be 1% w/w in both tissues [105]. Mineral contents by difference. These volume fractions give density of dentine mineral as 3.07 g/ml and of enamel mineral as 3.12 g/ml.

nous tissues [28]. The proportion of intrafibrillar mineral has been estimated at 25–80% [29–31]. In dentine the tubules probably account for much of the porosity. As the tubules increase in density and size towards the pulp [32] there is a corresponding increase in porosity. The remaining porosity is presumably distributed evenly throughout the intertubular dentine, where the average porosity is about 15 vol%. For a review of the pore structure of enamel and dentine see [33].

The third dental tissue – cementum – is important when considering erosion of exposed root surfaces. Its composition has been little studied but from the available information it probably has similar physical and chemical properties to dentine. On exposed root surfaces, just apical to the limit of the enamel, cementum is acellular, and so would have a lower porosity than dentine.

Reactions between Erosive Solutions and Dental Tissues

When HAp is exposed to an erosive solution it dissolves according to the reaction:

$$Ca_{10}(PO_4)_6(OH)_2 + (2 + 3x+2y+z)H^+ \rightarrow 10Ca^{2+} + xH_3PO_4^0 + yH_2PO_4^- + zHPO_4^{2-} + 2H_2O \quad (5)$$

$$(x + y + z = 6)$$

The proportions of the different phosphate anions depend on pH, as shown in figure 1. The PO_4^{3-} ion is omitted on the right-hand side because at low pH its concentration is extremely small (fig. 1). The equations for dissolution of dental mineral are a little more complex. For enamel mineral (formula 4) the acid-base reactions are:

$$1.08\ OH^- + 1.08\ H^+ \rightarrow 1.08\ H_2O \quad (6a)$$

$$5.1\ PO_4^{3-} + 0.4\ HPO_4^{2-} + (3x + 2y + z - 0.4)H^+ \rightarrow xH_3PO_4^{3-} + yH_2PO_4^- + zHPO_4^{2-} \quad (6b)$$

$$(x + y + z = 5.5)$$

$$0.55\ CO_3^{2-} + 1.1\ H^+ \rightarrow 1.1\ CO_2\ (gas) + 1.1\ H_2O \quad (6c)$$

The overall reaction is then:

$$[Ca_{8.9}Na_{0.3}Mg_{0.14}K_{0.01}\square_{0.65}][(PO_4)_{5.1}(HPO_4)_{0.4}$$
$$(CO_3)_{0.5}][(OH)_{1.08}(CO_3)_{0.05}Cl_{0.1}\square_{0.77}] + (1.78 + 3x+2y+z)H^+ \rightarrow 8.9\ Ca^{2+} + 0.3\ Na^+ + 0.14\ Mg^{2+} + 0.01\ K^+ + 0.1\ Cl^- + xH_3PO_4^{3-} + yH_2PO_4^- + zHPO_4^{2-} + 1.1\ CO_2\ (gas) + 2.18\ H_2O \quad (6d)$$

On exposure of enamel to an erosive solution, only the initial dissolution occurs at the tissue surface. Thereafter, demineralization occurs within the near-surface enamel, through diffusion of the solution into the enamel, accompanied by partial dissolution of crystals [34]. This creates a 'softened layer' at the tooth surface. Demineralization at the prism junctions, which are sites of raised solubility [5], occurs in advance of demineralization within the prisms [35]. If the erosive challenge continues, the rate of mineral loss reaches a steady state: presumably, advance of demineralization into the tissue is balanced by total loss of mineral from the surface [36]. The softened layer is never more than a few micrometres thick. An acid solution, as it diffuses into the narrow enamel pores, starts to dissolve mineral. This consumes H^+ ions, so that the pH rises and the OH^- ion concentration rises. At the same time calcium and phosphate ions are released into the solution, and the overall result is that the ion activity product for HAp rises (see equation 1). Because of the low solubility of the mineral, the solution soon becomes saturated with respect to the enamel mineral, so that dissolution ceases within a short distance from the surface.

Erosive demineralization of dentine also occurs beneath the tissue surface but, in contrast to enamel erosion, demineralization leaves intact a surface layer of insoluble collagenous matrix. As erosion proceeds, the thickness of the demineralized layer, and thus the diffusion distance between the surface and the demineralization front, increases so the net rate of mineral loss decreases with time [36, 37]. There is evidence that the intrafibrillar mineral is dissolved more slowly than the interfibrillar mineral [38, 39], as would be expected by the intimate association of collagen with the crystals, which would inhibit diffusion. Nevertheless, the eroded matrix appears to be completely demineralized and to have a relatively sharp boundary with the underlying unaffected dentine [38] [see also fig. 2 in chapter by Shellis and Addy, this vol., pp. 32–45] (see also fig. 3, 4 in chapter by Ganss et al., this vol., pp. 99–107). The demineralized dentine at the surface is eventually removed by subsequent abrasion and possibly by enzymic hydrolysis, but it is rather durable and so persists for some time [34].

Although enamel is less soluble than dentine, the steady-state enamel dissolution rate and the initial dentine dissolution rate, normalized using the respective volume fractions of mineral, were found to be equal at low pH (2.45) and enamel dissolved more slowly only at higher pH (3.2, 3.9) [36]. These variations were attributed to the presence of insoluble matrix in dentine, which would inhibit transport of H^+ ions and mineral-ion end products of dissolution. Removal of the matrix greatly accelerates dentine erosion [37]. These observations show that the solubilities of the minerals are not by themselves an infallible guide to relative rates of dissolution.

Physical Factors Controlling the Rate of Dissolution

The temperature and the flow rate of the test solution in relation to the substrate are important variables which need to be controlled in experimental models. In vivo, these factors have a strong impact on how the mode of consumption of acidic products affects the risk of erosion.

Temperature
Most chemical reactions depend on temperature, and it has been shown that the erosion rate of enamel in acid solutions or fruit drinks increases with increasing temperature [40, 41].

Flow Rate
The erosion rates of both enamel and dentine depend on the velocity of the solution flowing over the solid surface [40, 42, 43]. This indicates that erosion is controlled by the rate at which end products of dissolution are cleared from the solid into the solution. The thin layer of solution adjacent to any solid/solution interface is relatively static and transport across it is diffusion controlled. Increasing the flow rate reduces the thickness of this 'diffusion layer' and hence increases the rate of transport between the solid and the bulk solution. In the case of dental tissues, the thin salivary pellicle usually present at the surface acts as a further diffusion barrier.

Solution Factors Controlling the Rate of Dissolution

Undersaturation of the solution is a necessary precondition for the dissolution of solid to occur and supersaturation is necessary for crystal growth. The degree of undersaturation or supersaturation can be quantified and measures how far the solution composition is from equilibrium. In general, as the degree of undersaturation or supersaturation increases, the rate of dissolution or growth will also increase up to a certain point and will then level off and remain constant despite further change in saturation [44]. Solutions which lack calcium, phosphate or both (as in many erosive products) are said to be unsaturated. In such solutions, dissolution would proceed at the maximum rate.

However, the calculated degree of saturation does not necessarily predict with certainty whether dissolution or crystal growth will occur, or the rate at which they proceed. This is illustrated by figure 3, in which data from a study on erosive potential against enamel of a wide variety of acidic products [25] are plotted in relation to solubilities of relevant solids [see table 3 in chapter by Lussi and Hellwig, this vol., pp. 220–229]. Erosive products, which caused softening of enamel after 2 min of exposure, were all undersaturated with respect to enamel, the data points being clustered below the solubility line for this tissue. These were mostly soft drinks and fruit juices. All products that were supersaturated with respect to enamel were non-erosive: these included yoghurts which, although having a low pH, contain enough calcium and phosphate to cause slight supersaturation. Note that 6 of the 8 non-erosive products were still undersaturated with respect to dentine mineral, so would probably be erosive towards that tissue. However, a small number of products seemed to be non-erosive, even though analysis suggested that they were slightly undersaturated. There can be various reasons for this anomalous result:

(1) Analytical or computational uncertainties can result in the calculated degree of saturation being less than it actually is; this is a particular problem in near-saturated solutions.

(2) If the solution in which a specimen is immersed is only slightly undersaturated with respect to the mineral, demineralization might be so limited as to be undetectable by most modern methods. Slight dissolution would raise the pH and the concentrations of calcium and phosphate ions in the diffusion layer adjacent to the tooth surface, so this layer would quickly become saturated and demineralization would cease [34]. Such an effect would be enhanced by inefficient stirring. Indeed, where the erosive solution is completely static, even erosion in plain citric acid solution (pH 3.2) is almost completely eliminated [42].

(3) Erosive products might contain inhibitory substances, which adsorb to the solid surface and hinder or prevent exchange between the solid and the solution. Dissolution and growth of crystals occur primarily at certain specific sites on the surface, so the concentration of adsorbed inhibitor required to interfere with these processes need not be very high, provided that the specific dissolution/growth sites are blocked [45].

(4) Most erosive products contain fluoride in low concentrations (1–100 µmol/l in the products shown in fig. 3). Since fluoride inhibits demineralization of dental tissues (see next section), it could help to prevent erosion.

It is probable that, especially in biological situations, inhibitors modify the rate of dissolution even if they do not prevent erosion altogether. In the oral cavity, inhibitors include a variety of macromolecules such as statherin [46, 47] and ions such as pyrophosphate [48] and Mg^{2+} ions [49], in addition to inhibitors which may occur in erosive products. Several food-approved substances have been shown to be effective inhibitors with a persistent effect [50] and could reduce the erosive potential of drinks.

High concentrations of Ca or high Ca/P ratio in solution can reduce, and even prevent, softening of enamel in undersaturated solutions [51]. The addition of calcium also reduces the rate of dissolution of enamel in unsaturated citric acid solutions containing no phosphate [52]. Barbour et al. [51] suggested that high Ca concentrations in solution blocked the release of Ca^{2+} ions from the crystal surfaces. Alternatively, an increased calcium concentration in the diffusion layer or in the intercrystalline solution within the softened enamel could increase saturation, so that dissolution would slow down or cease. The finding that the addition of calcium reduces erosion has led to the development of low-erosive drinks [52, 53]. As the calcium is added in the form $CaCO_3$ [54], the pH of the drink is also increased so erosion is reduced by much more than would be expected from the relatively low calcium concentration used. However, raised temperature and high flow rate have virtually no effect on the low erosivity [41, 42]. This suggests that there might be additional inhibition from other components of the soft drink.

Buffering and pH are considered important factors in erosion kinetics, in two respects. First, the more effective the buffering of a product, the longer an erosive challenge will last, because the product will better resist the neutralizing effect of saliva. There is scope for experimental study of this aspect of erosion, because it has not been quantified. Second, buffering is an important factor in relation to erosive potential, at least against enamel, as several multivariate analyses of data on various products have shown [see chapter by Lussi and Hellwig, this vol., pp. 220–229]. Buffering has been assessed in two ways: the *buffer capacity*, which is a measure of buffering at the pH of the solution, and the *titratable acidity*, which measures the total buffering between the starting pH and a defined higher pH value. Both can be assessed by titration: buffer capacity from the slope of the titration curve at the solution pH, and titratable acidity from the amount of base required to raise the pH to some value of interest. Titratable acidity is usually measured to pH 5.5 or pH 7.0. The former pH is more appropriate for erosion research [55], essentially because the region between pH 5.5 and pH 7.0 is of little relevance to the erosion process. Titratable acidity is the total concentration of all acid species which dissociate to supply H^+ ions between the initial and final pH values. It is therefore unfortunate that many papers report titratable acidity simply as the volume of base added to raise the pH by the required amount. To enable comparison between studies, it is essential, first, to specify the end pH of titration and, second, to express the results as the concentration of titratable acid. This is easily derived as follows. If V_{base} = the volume of base added (ml), V_{sample} = the volume of sample (ml) and C_{base} = the concentration of base used for titration (mmol/l), then titratable acidity (TA, mmol/l) is given by: $TA = (C_{base} \cdot V_{base})/V_{sample}$.

Experimental studies using defined acid solutions confirm that the rate of erosive dissolution of enamel increases with increasing buffering [56, 57], although the response to buffering is strongly acid- and pH-dependent. However, the difference between acids disappears if dissolution is considered as a function of the *undissociated acid concentration*, and the variation with pH is then small [57]. This result agrees with earlier work which identified undissociated acid as an important factor in caries [58, 59] and confirms an earlier suggestion [60] that the same is true for enamel erosion. The significance of undissociated acid is that this species is uncharged and should therefore diffuse more readily into the near-surface enamel, where dissolution occurs, and thus provide a mobile source of H^+ ions which helps to maintain the undersaturated conditions which support dissolution. As titratable acidity is related more directly than the buffer capacity to the concentration of undissociated acid, it is the more appropriate measure of buffering to use in studies of erosive potential [57].

Work to date suggests that buffering and undissociated acid concentration have little or no effect on the dissolution of *dentine* [9, 37] and this would be an interesting area for further research.

Some previous studies have suggested that erosion rate is high at low pH and falls rapidly towards pH 5 in a logarithmic fashion [61, 62]. However, it is difficult to separate the effects of pH and undissociated acid concentration in these data because the pH was adjusted by varying the acid concentration. As the pH of many soft drinks, especially fruit-based drinks, is adjusted in the same way, assessing the independent role of pH in erosive potential is a problem. However, all studies agree that erosion increases as pH falls. This is probably due to adsorption of increasing amounts of H^+ ions to surface anionic groups, which weakens the binding of Ca^{2+} ions and leads to their release into the solution. This process is termed *proton-promoted dissolution* [45]. The pH has been identified as a significant factor in erosive potential against enamel [see chapter by Barbour and Lussi, this vol., pp. 143–154].

Binding of a chelating anion to surface Ca^{2+} ions also enhances dissolution by weakening bonds within the surface: a process known as *li-*

gand-promoted dissolution [45]. The extent to which this phenomenon enhances the erosive effect of organic acids has yet to be quantified. At pH 3 the proportion of chelating anions makes up less than 3% of citric, malic or tartaric acids but rises to 93% or more at pH 6. Therefore, any contribution of chelation to erosion will be small at low pH but could increase at higher pH. In general, erosion rates are very low in liquids with pH >5 [61, 62] and products containing citrate or other chelating anions tend to have a low pH. However, there is qualitative evidence that high citrate concentrations promote erosion at pH 4–6 [63]. Further, some chelating anions may be used at approximately neutral pH in medicinal products (e.g. magnesium citrate) or as food additives (various tartrates). Therefore, experimental studies to evaluate the possible erosion risk from such products, and the importance of chelation in erosion, would be useful.

Several of the solution properties discussed here have been found to play a practical role in the erosive potential, as determined experimentally in studies such as Lussi et al. [25].

Fluoride and Erosion

Fluoride incorporated into HAp reduces the dissolution rate in acids [64], but the effect is less than that of fluoride dissolved at relatively low concentrations in the acid solution [65]. F^- ions from solution replace OH^- groups at the crystal surface, thereby locally converting the surface composition to that of FAp and stabilizing adjacent Ca^{2+} ions [66]. Solubility of any solid is controlled by the properties of the surface, even if this differs from those of the interior, because diffusion of ions into the crystal lattice is negligible at ordinary temperatures. Therefore, if the solution concentration of fluoride is high enough to allow fluoride adsorption over the entire crystal surface, the mineral will behave as though it was composed of FAp or a very similar complex, as

deduced for fluorhydroxyapatites (FHAp), in which there is partial F^-/OH^- substitution [67] and for carbonated HAp equilibrated with fluoride-containing solutions [68, 69]. Even if the crystal surfaces are not entirely covered by an FAp layer the rate of dissolution is still reduced according to the proportion of the crystal surfaces which have become fluoridated [70, 71].

Experimental models of dissolution have mostly used conditions relevant to caries: buffers or partly saturated solutions with relatively high pH (≥4). Under these conditions, dissolution is inhibited by low fluoride concentrations. Thus, formation of in vitro caries under realistic conditions is inhibited and even prevented by fluoride at concentrations <5 mg/l [72, 73]. The objective of using fluoride to prevent caries is therefore to maintain low fluoride concentrations in the milieu of the tooth and the strategy for achieving this is to form intra-oral reservoirs by frequent application of topical fluoride. These reservoirs include the oral mucosa, deposits on the tooth surfaces of calcium fluoride-like mineral (alkali-soluble fluoride) and dental plaque itself [74, 75]. In erosion research, great attention has been paid to alkali-soluble fluoride as being closest to the actual site of erosion.

The main impediment to the success of this strategy in relation to dental erosion is that the challenge to tooth integrity is very much greater: the pH is much lower (fig. 1) and the tooth environment is either unsaturated or is much more undersaturated than plaque fluid. Consequently, higher fluoride concentrations are needed to inhibit erosion. Equilibration of erosive drinks (pH 2.45–3.84) with calcium fluoride increased the fluoride concentration to 3.8–26 mg/l but this resulted in only 6–46% inhibition of erosion (3 solutions actually showing an increase in erosion). Larsen and Richards [76] calculated that these drinks would remove any deposits of alkali-soluble fluoride from the tooth surfaces so quickly that they could not act as fluoride reservoirs and would not reduce erosion. This view seems to be unduly pessimistic, partly because the retention of alkali-soluble fluoride is much better under oral conditions than in vitro [77]. Nevertheless, the calculations of Larsen and Richards [76] surely indicate the reason for the relatively poor performance of conventional fluorides, which has led recent research to explore prevention using high fluoride concentrations, varnishes and tin or titanium fluorides [78].

Crystal growth and precipitation are also markedly influenced by dissolved fluoride. This is attributed to the formation of less soluble FHAp, which increases the driving force for precipitation, or to accelerated transformation of intermediates such as octacalcium phosphate [79]. Crystal growth in the presence of fluoride will result in deposition of fluoridated mineral, probably FHAp, which is less soluble than the original mineral [64], so that the overall stability of the solid will tend to increase. This effect of fluoride is obviously important in efforts to remineralize caries and erosive lesions [80].

Remineralization of Eroded Dental Tissues

In principle, the mineral lost during erosion can be replaced by subsequent exposure to a supersaturated solution, which can drive regrowth of crystals or precipitation of new mineral, i.e. *remineralization*. It should be noted that supersaturation with respect to one of the dental minerals will not result in reformation of that mineral, as that owes its composition and solubility properties to having been formed in tissue fluid and not in the oral environment. Instead, the likely result would be deposition of HAp or, in the presence of fluoride, less soluble fluoridated minerals. Complete remineralization would not only restore the mechanical strength of the damaged tissue but also improve resistance to subsequent acid challenges.

Numerous experimental studies have shown that some degree of remineralization of both enamel and dentine is possible, mostly in relation

to caries [80]. However, most of the evidence comes from in vitro studies and in general these have used synthetic remineralizing solutions which will give the maximum effect. In vivo, the medium for remineralization is saliva, which contains inhibitors of precipitation and growth of calcium phosphates. Inclusion of salivary proteins in remineralization models influences the outcome considerably [81].

In relation to caries, even partial remineralization is valuable because it helps to preserve the relatively intact surface layer, thereby maintaining mechanical strength and preventing cavitation. In contrast, erosive lesions are vulnerable to further damage (by abrasion or enzymic hydrolysis) immediately they are formed. The aim of remineralizing erosive lesions is therefore to restore mechanical strength as quickly as possible to avoid such damage and the evidence shows that this is at present far from being achieved. In vitro, it is possible to restore resistance of enamel to mechanical forces by several hours exposure to artificial saliva [82–86]. In vivo, remineralization of both enamel and dentine only partly restores resistance to abrasion and improvements take hours to weeks of exposure to saliva [see chapter by Wiegand and Schlueter, this vol., pp. 215–219 and chapter by Lussi and Carvalho, this vol., pp. 1–15].

The main impediments to effective remineralization in vivo are likely to be the low supersaturation of saliva [87] and the presence of inhibitors of calcium phosphate precipitation: both limit the amount and rate of crystal growth. Erosive lesions, especially of enamel, are highly accessible to saliva and adsorption of inhibitory proteins to the partly dissolved mineral enhances the inhibition of crystal growth. Part of the difficulty of remineralizing erosive dentine lesions may be the retention of soluble phosphoproteins which are inhibitory in solution [88] and need to be extracted in order to achieve remineralization [89, 90]. These phosphoproteins are not removed during demineralization with organic acids [89, 90] and this could account for poor remineralization, although lesions created using acetic and lactic acids can be partly remineralized [84].

In one in vitro study the mineral deposited on remineralized enamel was in the form of crystals randomly distributed on the specimen surface [83]. This is not an ideal form of remineralization, as it is much less effective than regrowth of partly dissolved crystals in promoting recovery of mechanical strength. Recovery of mechanical strength of demineralized dentine probably requires regrowth of crystals within the matrix collagen fibres [91] but it is unlikely that this has

been achieved in remineralization experiments. Electron microscopy shows that mineral is deposited in scattered islands throughout the tissue [89, 90]. This result, suggesting that remineralization involves de novo precipitation of crystals rather than deposition within the matrix fibres, is supported by the finding that removal of collagen does not affect remineralization in vitro [84].

Fluoride, and other agents such as casein phosphopeptide-amorphous calcium phosphate have proved to have variable effects on enamel remineralization [92–98].

References

1 Verbeeck RMH: Minerals in human enamel and dentine; in Driessens FCM, Wöltgens JHM (eds): Tooth Development and Caries. Boca Raton, CRC Press, 1986, pp 95–152.

2 Patel PR, Brown WE: Thermodynamic solubility product of human tooth enamel: powdered sample. J Dent Res 1975;54:728–736.

3 Moreno EC, Aoba T: Solubility of human enamel mineral. J Biol Buccale 1990;18:195–201.

4 Moreno EC, Aoba T: Comparative solubility study of human dental enamel, dentin, and hydroxyapatite. Calcif Tissue Int 1991;49:6–13.

5 Shellis RP: A scanning electron-microscopic study of solubility variations in human enamel and dentine. Arch Oral Biol 1996;41:473–484.

6 Moreno EC, Zahradnik RT: Chemistry of enamel subsurface demineralization in vitro. J Dent Res 1974;53:226–235.

7 Larsen MJ, Jensen SJ: The hydroxyapatite solubility product of human dental enamel as a function of pH in the range 4.6–7.6 at 20 degrees C. Arch Oral Biol 1989;34:957–961.

8 Shellis RP, Wahab FK, Heywood BR: The hydroxyapatite ion activity product in acid solutions equilibrated with human enamel at 37°C. Caries Res 1993; 27:365–372.

9 Shellis RP: Formation of caries-like lesions in vitro on the root surfaces of human teeth in solutions simulating plaque fluid. Caries Res 2010;44:380–389.

10 Driessens FCM, Verbeeck RMH: Evidence for intermediate metastable states during equilibration of bone and dental tissues. Z Naturforsch C 1980;35:262–267.

11 Theuns HM, Driessens FC, van Dijk JW, Groeneveld A: Experimental evidence for a gradient in the solubility and in the rate of dissolution of human enamel. Caries Res 1986;20:24–31.

12 ten Cate JM, Damen JJ, Buijs MJ: Inhibition of dentin demineralization by fluoride in vitro. Caries Res 1998;32:141–147.

13 Bell CF: Principles and applications of metal chelation. Oxford, Oxford University Press, 1977.

14 Sillén LG, Martell AE, Bjerrum J (eds): Stability Constants of Metal-Ion Complexes. London, Chemistry Society, 1964.

15 Featherstone JDB, Mayer I, Driessens FCM, Verbeeck RMH, Heijligers HJM: Synthetic apatites containing Na, Mg, and CO3 and their comparison with tooth enamel mineral. Calcif Tissue Int 1983;35:169–171.

16 Featherstone JDB, Shields CP, Khademazad B, Oldershaw MD: Acid reactivity of carbonated apatites with strontium and fluoride substitutions. J Dent Res 1983;62:1049–1053.

17 Baig AA, Fox JL, Young RA, Wang Z, Hsu J, Higuchi WI, Chhetry A, Zhuang H, Otsuka M: Relationships among carbonated apatite solubility, crystallite size, and microstrain parameters. Calcif Tissue Int 1999;64:437–449.

18 Elliott JC: Structure and Chemistry of the Apatites and Other Calcium Orthophosphates. Studies in Inorganic Chemistry 18. London, Elsevier, 1994.

19 Elliott JC, Holcomb DW, Young RA: Infrared determination of the degree of substitution of hydroxyl by carbonate ions in human dental enamel. Calcif Tissue Int 1985;37:372–375.

20 Weatherell JA, Robinson C, Hiller CR: Distribution of carbonate in thin sections of dental enamel. Caries Res 1968; 2:1–9.

21 Weatherell JA, Robinson C, Hallsworth AS: Variations in the chemical composition of human enamel. J Dent Res 1974; 53:180–192.

22 Robinson C, Weatherell JA, Hallsworth AS: Distribution of magnesium in mature human enamel. Caries Res 1981;15: 70–77.

23 Daculsi G, Kérébel B: High-resolution electron microscope study of human enamel crystallites: size, shape, and growth. J Ultrastruct Res 1978;65:163–172.

24 Daculsi G, Kérébel B, Verbaere A: Méthode de mesure des cristaux d'apatite de la dentine humaine en microscopie électronique à transmission de haute resolution. C R Acad Sci Hebd Seances Acad Sci D 1978;286: 1439–1442.

25 Lussi A, Megert B, Shellis RP, Wang X: Analysis of the erosive effect of different dietary substances and medications. Brit J Nutr 2012;107:252–262.

26 Linde A: Dentine: structure, chemistry and formation; in Thylstrup A, Leach SA, Qvist V (eds): Dentine and Dentine Reactions in the Oral Cavity. Oxford, IRL Press, 1983, pp 17–26.

27 Simmer JP, Hu JC: Dental enamel formation and its impact on clinical dentistry. J Dent Educ 2001;65:896–905.

28 Landis WJ: Mineral characterization in calcifying tissues: atomic, molecular and macromolecular perspectives. Conn Tissue Res 1996;34:239–246.

29 Shellis RP: Structural organization of calcospherites in normal and rachitic human dentine. Arch Oral Biol 1983;28: 85–95.

30 Katz EP, Wachtel E, Yamauchi M, Mechanic GL: The structure of mineralized collagen fibrils. Conn Tissue Res 1989; 21:149–154.

31 Kinney JH, Habelitz S, Marshall SJ, Marshall GW: The importance of intrafibrillar mineralization of collagen on the mechanical properties of dentin. J Dent Res 2003;82:957–961.

32 Garberoglio R, Brännström M: Scanning electron microscopic investigation of human dentinal tubules. Arch Oral Biol 1976;21:355–362.

33 Shellis RP: Transport processes in enamel and dentine; in Addy M, Embery G, Edgar WM, Orchardson R (eds): Tooth Wear and Sensitivity. London, Martin Dunitz, 2000, pp 19–27.

34 Lussi A, Schlueter N, Rakhmatullina E, Ganss C: Dental erosion – an overview with emphasis on chemical and histopathological aspects. Caries Res 2011; 45(suppl 1):2–12.

35 Eisenburger M, Shellis RP, Addy M: Scanning electron microscopy of softened enamel. Caries Res 2004;38:67–74.

36 Shellis RP, Barbour ME, Jones SB, Addy M: Effects of pH and acid concentration on erosive dissolution of enamel, dentine and compressed hydroxyapatite. Eur J Oral Sci 2010;118:475–482.

37 Hara AT, Ando M, Cury JA, Serra MC, González-Cabezas C, Zero DT: Influence of the organic matrix on root dentine erosion by citric acid. Caries Res 2005; 39:134–138.

38 Selvig KA: Ultrastructural changes in human dentine exposed to a weak acid. Arch Oral Biol 1968;13:719–734.

39 Balooch M, Habelitz S, Kinney JL, Marshall SJ, Marshall GW: Mechanical properties of mineralized collagen fibrils as influenced by demineralization. J Struct Biol 2008;162:404–410.

40 Eisenburger M, Addy M: Influence of liquid temperature and flow rate on enamel erosion and surface softening. J Oral Rehabil 2003;30:1076–1080.

41 Barbour ME, Finke M, Parker DM, Hughes JA, Allen GC, Addy M: The relationship between enamel softening and erosion caused by soft drinks at a range of temperatures. J Dent 2006;34:207–213.

42 Shellis RP, Finke M, Eisenburger M, Parker DM, Addy M: Relationship between enamel erosion and flow rate. Eur J Oral Sci 2005;113:232–238.

43 Wiegand A, Stock A, Attin R, Werner C, Attin T: Impact of the acid flow rate on dentin erosion. J Dent 2007;35:21–27.

44 Blum AE, Lasaga AC: Monte Carlo simulations of surface reaction rate laws; in Stumm W (ed): Aquatic Surface Chemistry. Chemical Processes at the Particle Water Interface. New York, Wiley, 1987, pp 255–292.

45 Stumm W: Chemistry of the Solid-Water Interface. New York, Wiley, 1992.

46 Moreno EC, Varughese K, Hay DI: Effect of human salivary proteins on the precipitation kinetics of calcium phosphate. Calcif Tissue Int 1979;28:7–16.

47 Johnsson M, Richardson CF, Bergey EJ, Levine MJ, Nancollas GH: The effects of human salivary cystatins and statherin on hydroxyapatite crystallization. Arch Oral Biol 1991;36:631–636.

48 Hausmann E, Bisaz S, Russel RG, Fleisch H: The concentration of inorganic pyrophosphate in human saliva and dental calculus. Arch Oral Biol 1970;15:1389–1392.

49 Johnsson MS-A, Nancollas GH: The role of brushite and octacalcium phosphate in apatite formation. Crit Rev Oral Biol Med 1992;3:61–82.

50 Barbour ME, Shellis RP, Parker DM, Allen GC, Addy M: An investigation of some food-approved polymers as agents to inhibit hydroxyapatite dissolution. Eur J Oral Sci 2005;113:457–461.

51 Barbour ME, Parker DM, Allen GC, Jandt KD: Enamel dissolution in citric acid as a function of calcium and phosphate concentrations and degree of saturation with respect to hydroxyapatite. Eur J Oral Sci 2003;111:421–433.

52 Hughes JA, West NX, Parker DM, Newcombe RG, Addy M: Development and evaluation of a low erosive blackcurrant juice drink in vitro and in situ. 1. Comparison with orange juice. J Dent 1999; 27:285–289.

53 Hughes JA, West NX, Parker DM, Newcombe RG, Addy M: Development and evaluation of a low erosive blackcurrant juice drink in vitro and in situ. 3. Final drink and concentrate, formulae comparisons in situ and overview of the concept. J Dent 1999;27:345–350.

54 Venables MC, Shaw L, Jeukendrup AE, Roedig-Penman A, Finke M, Newcombe RG, Parry J, Smith AJ: Erosive effect of a new sports drink on dental enamel during exercise. Med Sci Sports Exerc 2005; 37:39–44.

55 Barbour ME, Lussi A, Shellis RP: Screening and prediction of erosive potential. Caries Res 2011;45(suppl 1):24–32.

56 Barbour ME, Shellis RP: An investigation using atomic force microscopy nanoindentation of dental enamel demineralisation as a function of undissociated acid concentration and differential buffer capacity. Phys Med Biol 2007;52: 899–910.

57 Shellis RP, Barbour ME, Jesani A, Lussi A: Effects of buffering properties and undissociated acid concentration on dissolution of dental enamel, in relation to pH and acid type. Caries Res 2013;47: 601–611.

58 Gray JA: Kinetics of enamel dissolution during formation of incipient caries-like lesions. Arch Oral Biol 1961;11:397–421.

59 Featherstone JDB, Rodgers BE: Effect of acetic, lactic and other organic acids on the formation of artificial carious lesions. Caries Res 1981;15:377–385.

60 Featherstone JD, Lussi A: Understanding the chemistry of dental erosion; in Lussi A (ed): Dental Erosion. Monogr Oral Sci 20. Basel, Karger, 2006, pp 66–76.

61 Davis WB, Winter PJ: The effect of abrasion on enamel and dentine after exposure to dietary acid. Br Dent J 1980;148: 253–256.

62 Larsen MJ, Nyvad B: Enamel erosion by some soft drinks and orange juices relative to their pH, buffering effect and contents of calcium phosphate. Caries Res 1999;33:81–87.

63 West NX, Hughes JA, Addy M: The effect of pH on the erosion of dentine and enamel by dietary acids in vitro. J Oral Rehabil 2001;28:860–864.

64 Okazaki M, Moriwaki Y, Aoba T, Doi Y, Takahashi J: Dissolution rate behavior of fluoridated apatite pellets. J Dent Res 1981;60:1907–1911.

65 Wong L, Cutress TW, Duncan JF: The influence of incorporated and adsorbed fluoride on the dissolution of powdered and pelletized hydroxyapatite in fluoridated and non-fluoridated acid buffers. J Dent Res 1987;66:1735–1741.

66 de Leeuw N: Resisting the onset of hydroxyapatite dissolution through the incorporation of fluoride. J Phys Chem B 2004;108:1809–1811.

67 Brown WE, Gregory TM, Chow LC: Effects of fluoride on enamel solubility and cariostasis. Caries Res 1977; 11(suppl 1):118–141.

68 Zhuang H, Baig AA, Fox JL, Wang Z, Colby SJ, Chhettry A, Higuchi WI: Metastable equilibrium solubility behavior of carbonated apatites in the presence of solution fluoride. J Colloid Interface Sci 2000;222:90–96.

69 Papangkorn K, Yan G, Heslop DD, Moribe K, Baig AA, Otsuka M, Higuchi WI: Influence of crystallite microstrain on surface complexes governing the metastable equilibrium solubility behavior of carbonated apatites. J Colloid Interface Sci 2008;320:96–109.

70 Christoffersen MR, Christoffersen J, Arends J: Kinetics of dissolution of calcium hydroxyapatite. VII. The effect of fluoride ions. J Cryst Growth 1984;67:107–114.

71 Arends J, Christoffersen J: Nature and role of loosely bound fluoride in dental caries. J Dent Res 1990;69:601–605.

72 ten Cate JM, Duijsters PPE: Influence of fluoride in solution on tooth demineralization. Caries Res 1983a;17:193–199 and 1983b;17:513–519.

73 Margolis HC, Moreno EC, Murphy BJ: Effect of low levels of fluoride in solution on enamel demineralization in vitro. J Dent Res 1986;65:23–29.

74 Vogel GL: Oral fluoride reservoirs and the prevention of dental caries; in Buzalaf MAR (ed): Fluoride and the Oral Environment. Monogr Oral Sci 22. Basel, Karger, 2011, pp 146–157.

75 Duckworth RM: Pharmacokinetics in the oral cavity: fluoride and other active ingredients; in van Loveren C (ed): Toothpastes. Monogr Oral Sci 23. Basel, Karger, 2013, pp 125–139.

76 Larsen MJ, Richards A: Fluoride is unable to reduce dental erosion from soft drinks. Caries Res 2002;36:75–80.

77 Ganss C, Schlueter N, Klimek J: Retention of KOH-soluble fluoride on enamel and dentine under erosive conditions – a comparison of in vitro and in situ results. Arch Oral Biol 2007;52:9–14.

78 Magalhães AC, Wiegand A, Rios D, Buzalaf MAR: Fluoride in dental erosion; in Buzalaf MAR (ed): Fluoride and the Oral Environment. Monogr Oral Sci 22. Basel, Karger, 2011, pp 158–170.

79 Aoba T: The effect of fluoride on apatite structure and growth. Crit Rev Oral Biol Med 1997;8:136–153.

80 ten Cate JM, Featherstone JDB: Mechanistic aspects of the interactions between fluoride and dental enamel. Crit Rev Oral Biol 1991;2:283–296.

81 Fujikawa H, Matsuyama K, Uchiyama A, Nakashima S, Ujiie T: Influence of salivary macromolecules and fluoride on enamel lesion remineralization in vitro. Caries Res 2008;42:37–45.

82 Attin T, Buchalla W, Gollner, Hellwig E: Use of variable remineralization periods to improve the abrasion resistance of previously eroded enamel. Caries Res 2000;34:48–52.

83 Eisenburger M, Addy M, Hughes JA, Shellis RP: Effect of time on the remineralization of enamel after citric acid erosion. Caries Res 2001;35:211–215.

84 Klont B, ten Cate JM: Remineralization of bovine root incisor root lesions in vitro: the role of the collagenous matrix. Caries Res 1991;25:39–45.

85 Mukai Y, ten Cate JM: Remineralization of advanced root dentin lesions in vitro. Caries Res 2002;36:275–80.

86 Hara AT, Karlinsey RL, Zero DT: Dentine remineralization by simulated saliva formulations with different Ca and Pi contents. Caries Res 2008;42:51–56.

87 Larsen MJ, Fejerskov O: Chemical and structural challenges in remineralization of dental enamel lesions. Scand J Dent Res 1989;97:285–296.

88 Lussi A, Crenshaw MA, Linde A: Induction and inhibition of hydroxyapatite formation by rat dentine phosphoprotein in vitro. Arch Oral Biol 1988;33:685–691.

89 Clarkson BH, Feagin FF, McCurdy SP, Sheetz JH, Speirs RL: Effects of phosphoprotein moieties on the remineralization of human root caries. Caries Res 1991;25:166–173.

90 Clarkson BH, Chang SR, Holland GR: Phosphoprotein analysis of sequential extracts of human dentin and the determination of the subsequent remineralization potential of these dentin matrices. Caries Res 1998;32:357–364.

91 Bertassoni LE, Habelitz S, Kinney JH, Marshall SJ, Marshall GW: Biomechanical perspective on the remineralization of dentin. Caries Res 2009;43:70–77.

92 Ganss C, Schlueter N, Friedrich D, Klimek J: Efficacy of waiting periods and topical fluoride treatment on toothbrush abrasion of eroded enamel in situ. Caries Res 2007;41:146–151.

93 Maggio B, Guibert RG, Mason SC, Karwal R, Rees GD, Kelly S, Zero DT: Evaluation of mouthrinse and dentifrice regimens in an in situ erosion remineralization model. J Dent 2010; 38(suppl 3):S37–S44.

94 Willershausen B, Schulz-Dobrick B, Gleissner C: In vitro evaluation of enamel remineralization by a casein phosphopeptide-amorphous calcium phosphate paste. Oral Health Prev Dent 2009;7:13–21.

95 Srinavasan N, Kavitha M, Loganathan SC: Comparison of the remineralization potential of CPP-ACP and CPP-ACP with 900 ppm fluoride on eroded human enamel: an in situ study. Arch Oral Biol 2010;55:541–544.

96 Wang X, Megert B, Hellwig E, Neuhaus KW, Lussi A: Preventing erosion with novel agents. J Dent 2011;39:163–170.

97 Mathews MS, Amaechi BT, Ramalingam K, Ccahuana-Vasquez RA, Chedieu IP, Mackey AC, Karlinsey RL: In situ remineralization of eroded enamel lesions by NaF rinse. Arch Oral Biol 2012;57:525–530.

98 Wegehaupt FJ, Tauböck TT, Stillhard A, Schmidlin PR, Attin T: Influence of extra- and intra-oral application of CPP-ACP and fluoride on re-hardening of eroded enamel. Acta Odontol Scand 2012;70:177–183.

99 McDowell H, Gregory TM, Brown WE: Solubility study of $Ca_5(PO_4)_3OH$ in the system $Ca(OH)_2$-H_3PO_4-H_2O at 5, 15, 25 and 37°C. J Res Natl Bur Stand A Phys Chem 1977;81A:273–281.

100 Moreno EC, Kresak M, Zahradnik RT: Physicochemical aspects of fluoride-apatite systems relevant to the study of dental caries. Caries Res 1977; 11(suppl 1):142–171.

101 Martell AE, Smith RM: Critical Stability Constants. Other Organic Ligands. New York, Plenum Press, 1976.

102 Smith RM, Martell AE: Critical Stability Constants. Inorganic Complexes. New York, Plenum Press, 1976.

103 Manly RS, Hodge HC: Density and refractive index studies of dental hard tissues. II. Density distribution curves. J Dent Res 1939;18:203–211.

104 Dibdin GH, Poole DFG: Surface area and pore size analysis for human enamel and dentine by water vapour sorption. Arch Oral Biol 1982;27:235–241.

105 Odutuga AA, Prout RES: Lipid analysis of human enamel and dentine. Arch Oral Biol 1974;19:729–731.

Dr. R.P. Shellis, PhD
Department of Preventive, Restorative and Pediatric Dentistry
School of Dental Medicine, University of Bern
Freiburgstrasse 7
CH–3010 Bern (Switzerland)
E-Mail peter.shellis@btinternet.com

Lussi A, Ganss C (eds): Erosive Tooth Wear. Monogr Oral Sci. Basel, Karger, 2014, vol 25, pp 180–196
DOI: 10.1159/000360369

Intrinsic Causes of Erosion

Rebecca Moazzez · David Bartlett

Department of Prosthodontics, King's College London Dental Institute, London, UK

Abstract

Gastric juice entering the mouth causes dental erosion. Common causes for the migration of gastric juice through the lower and upper oesophageal sphincters are reflux disease, laryngopharyngeal reflux, eating disorders, chronic alcoholism and pregnancy. Gastroesophageal reflux is a common condition affecting up to 65% of the Western population at some point in their lifetime. A typical clinical sign of acidic gastric juice entering the mouth is palatal dental erosion. As the condition becomes more chronic it becomes more widespread. There have been relatively few randomised studies investigating the aetiology of acids causing erosion. Of the few that have reported their findings, it appears that gastric acids have the potential to induce moderate-to-severe erosion. This literature review reports the conditions associated with the movement of gastric juice and dental erosion using medical and dental sources.   © 2014 S. Karger AG, Basel

Gastric juice travelling up through the oesophagus and entering the mouth may cause intrinsic dental erosion. The pH and titratability of gastric juice is significantly greater than dietary acids and so the level of destruction is normally more severe. The acid reaches the mouth either through vomiting or by regurgitation. Vomiting disorders such as anorexia and bulimia nervosa have long been recognised as factors in the development of dental erosion, partly when associated with eating disorders. On the other hand, regurgitation, defined as involuntary movement of the gastric contents from the stomach into the mouth, has also been acknowledged as a common cause of severe dental erosion. There are a number of medical conditions associated with the movement of gastric acid from the stomach to the mouth including rumination, chronic alcoholism, vomiting caused by eating disorders or pregnancy. An underlying common feature of most of these conditions is gastroesophageal reflux disease (GERD). This is the term used to describe the retrograde movement of the stomach contents past the lower oesophageal sphincter (LOS). In a systematic review Dent et al. [1] reported that approximately 10–20% of the population suffer from GERD based on weekly reports of heartburn or regurgitation. The acidity nature of gastric contents regurgitated into the mouth has the potential to cause severe destruction of teeth [2]. Although dietary acids have also been associated with dental erosion the wear caused by the gastric contents is often severe and widespread.

Early erosion results in softening of the surface enamel and is seen as loss of enamel from the palatal surfaces of the upper incisors, but as the erosion progresses the palatal cusps and surfaces of the premolars and molars also become involved.

Finally, more generalised erosion on the occlusal surfaces of molars and the facial surfaces of all teeth produces loss of tooth tissue and in extreme circumstances can result in the total obliteration of the crowns of teeth by gastric acids. The consequences of intrinsic erosion are often severe and require extensive restorative management to replace the lost tooth tissue. Under these circumstances, the treatment which may be required to restore the worn dentition is both expensive and clinically challenging [3, 4].

Diagnosis of the wear is a very important part of the overall care plan so that preventive measures can be put in place. A thorough history and a comprehensive clinical examination are needed to assess the most likely cause of wear [5]. However, with some it is difficult to make an accurate diagnosis and be certain of the aetiology of the wear [6].

The association of gastric causes with the development of palatal tooth wear has been investigated by a number of researchers. One study investigated a randomly selected group of Swiss adults and diagnosed the cause of tooth wear. In this population, although severe palatal erosion was rare, multiple regression analysis showed that vomiting was associated with its development [7]. Other studies have also investigated groups of patients presenting with palatal erosion and found associations with gastric causes [6, 8]. The association with palatal erosion and gastric acid has also been supported by the observations of Scandinavian researchers in a number of studies [9–11] as well as studies from the UK [12, 13] and the USA [14–16]. Overall there is significant support for the assertion that regurgitated or vomited gastric contents cause dental erosion [see also chapter by Schlueter and Tveit, this vol., pp. 74–98].

Gastroesophageal Reflux

Anatomy and Physiology of the Oesophagus
The human oesophagus is a hollow muscular tube about 25 cm long bounded by a muscular sphincter at each end. The LOS and upper oesophageal sphincters (UOS) are physical barriers to the retrograde movement of the gastric contents to the mouth and pulmonary system. The upper part of the oesophagus, including the UOS, is composed of striated muscle. The LOS is not an anatomical but a physiological sphincter and involves the diaphragm and muscle folds. At the gastroesophageal junction, there is an abrupt change from squamous to simple columnar epithelial cells with gastric glands and pits but the precise location of the squamocolumnar junction in relation to the LOS is variable [17]. This junction is an important site as premalignant changes to the epithelium, called Barrett's oesophagitis, have been associated with reflux disease [18].

The main function of the oesophagus is to control the passage of solids and fluids from the mouth to the stomach in a coordinated manner, clearing regurgitated material and preventing gastroesophageal reflux. In normal swallowing, the pharynx pumps and propels a bolus from the oropharynx, across a relaxed UOS, into the oesophagus. Following that, oesophageal peristalsis drives the bolus into the stomach through a relaxed LOS [19]. In healthy subjects, primary peristalsis is a series of coordinated propulsive contractions passing down the oesophagus at a speed of 2–5 cm/s to reach the stomach [20].

The main role of the LOS is to prevent the stomach contents from passing into the oesophagus. The LOS is not a tight sphincter and movement of the gastric contents into the distal oesophagus can occur [21]. Transient relaxations of the LOS (TRLOS), an incompetent LOS and abnormalities of the muscular function of the oesophagus, which are termed motility disorders and can result in the loss of peristaltic activity in the oesophageal body, are some of the reasons for lack of clearance of gastric contents in the oesophagus [22]. The most common symptoms associated with gastroesophageal reflux include heartburn, regurgitation, dysphagia and chest pain [23, 24].

Table 1. Manifestations of gastroesophageal reflux disease

Oesophageal (typical) signs and symptoms of reflux	
Heartburn	Radiates along the oesophagus[1]
Regurgitation	Stomach contents passing into the mouth[1]
Dysphagia	Difficulty in swallowing
Extra-oesophageal (atypical) symptoms of reflux	
Cardiac	Non-cardiac chest pain, sino-atrial block
Pulmonary	Chronic cough, asthma, micro-aspiration, pneumonia
ENT	Sore throat, hoarseness, alteration of voice laryngitis, pharyngitis, globus[1]

[1] Associated with dental erosion [8–10, 30].

Gastroesophageal reflux occurs when LOS pressure is lower than intragastric pressure. The LOS is tonically closed at rest, maintaining an average pressure of about 20 mm Hg, and serves to prevent gastroesophageal reflux. Under normal circumstances a small amount of reflux occurs when LOS pressures are low and during TRLOS, and when increases in intra-abdominal pressure or intragastric pressure overcome the resting LOS pressure. The TRLOS is independent of a swallow. Transient relaxation of the sphincter that is independent of a swallow can also occur with pharyngeal stimulation. However, these relaxations are different from the regular TRLOS and do not appear to be associated with reflux. Their relaxation is less pronounced and they do not involve inhibition of the diaphragm. In both patients and normal subjects, the TRLOS in the face of normal LOS pressure is the most common mechanism of reflux, accounting for virtually all episodes in normal subjects and about two thirds in GERD patients. The acid load to the oesophagus is greater in GERD patients, in part because more TRLOSs are associated with reflux even though the number of TRLOS is more or less similar. In addition, the duration of the relaxation with a TRLOS is longer than that with a swallow. The physiological reasons for these phenomena are unknown [25].

Gastroesophageal Reflux Disease

Gastroesophageal reflux is a physiological phenomenon and gastric contents entering the oesophagus are cleared by a combination of peristalsis, which removes the bulk of the fluid, followed by neutralization of any acid by saliva [26]. A certain number of gastroesophageal reflux episodes are within the physiological range of normality but GERD is a pathological condition [27]. GERD develops when the reflux of stomach contents causes troublesome symptoms and/or complaints [28]. GERD has been reported to be most prevalent in Western countries, but less so in Middle-Eastern countries and even lesser so in the Far East [28]. In a systematic review Dent et al. [1] reported that approximately 10–20% of the population suffer from GERD based on weekly reports of heartburn or regurgitation. The manifestations of GERD are many and can be categorised into oesophageal (typical) and extra-oesophageal (atypical). The oesophageal symptoms include heartburn, regurgitation, belching, bloating, globus and dysphagia [29, 30]. Heartburn and regurgitation are the two most common symptoms and have been defined as 'characteristic symptoms of the typical reflux syndrome' by 44 members of the global consensus group which achieved 95% agreement [27] (table 1).

The least frequent symptom of GERD is dysphagia, and is often only reported in patients with long-standing disease [31]. Dysphagia is the result of oesophagitis, dysmotility and stricture formation closing the oesophageal lumen and so resisting the passage of food into the stomach.

The extra-oesophageal (atypical) manifestations are many and can be broadly catogorised into cardiac, pulmonary, ENT and dental.

Heartburn
Heartburn is a substernal burning radiating pain along the length of the oesophagus often passing to the throat. Heartburn has been recognised as a classic symptom of GERD [32]. Nebel et al. [33], in a study of hospitalised, non-hospitalised and control subjects, reported that 14% of hospitalised patients, 15% of outpatients and 7% of normal individuals complained of daily heartburn. A survey in the UK showed that nearly half of the participants complained of having heartburn at least once a month. It also revealed that 29% took medication at least once a month [34]. In previous studies 11% of adolescents examined reported suffering from heartburn once a week and 31.6% had the symptom on a monthly basis [35, 36].

Regurgitation
Regurgitation can be defined as 'the sudden, effortless return of gastric or oesophageal contents into the pharynx and implies UOS relaxation or insufficiency'. Regurgitation can also be the perception of flow of these fluids into the mouth or hypopharynx. Regurgitation should be distinguished from vomiting, which is the propulsion of the stomach contents coordinated by the vomiting centre in the brain [37]. Once past the UOS, the regurgitated material can either enter the oral cavity or be aspirated by the pulmonary system. The UOS therefore has an important role in the prevention of high reflux. The prevalence of regurgitation in the studies reported above was slightly lower than heartburn on a weekly basis but similar to the monthly reported basis [35, 36].

Cardiac
Severe chest pain is a distressing and worrying symptom for patients and can present clinicians with a difficult differential diagnosis with heart disease. Gastroesophageal reflux can present as chest pain and is a common cause of non-cardiac chest pain [8, 9, 31].

Chronic Cough
Chronic cough linked to GERD can be the sole presentation of GERD [38]. Micro-aspiration of refluxate has been demonstrated to cause symptoms after acid enters the pulmonary system [39–42].

Gastroesophageal Reflux Disease-Related Asthma
Asthma has long been recognised as a debilitating complication of GERD. The complex pathology of asthma seems to overlap with GERD-related asthma [43–45].

Laryngeal
A variety of extra-oesophageal reflux symptoms have been linked to the larynx. Examples include oedema with erythema, laryngeal stenosis [46, 47] and vocal cord ulcers [30, 48]. The presence of refluxed gastric contents above the UOS is believed to cause the inflammation.

Chronic Hoarseness
As distinct from chronic cough, some patients present with chronic hoarseness with no discernible cause. It is uncertain whether vocal cord irritation occurs by the direct action of acid or by chronic throat clearing and coughing resulting from oesophageal acid stimulating a vagally mediated reflex.

Globus
The sensation of a persistent painless lump or ball in the throat on swallowing without dysphagia (difficulty in swallowing) is termed globus and is derived from the Greek for ball. The literature suggests that there may be an association between globus and GERD [49].

Table 2. Common factors related to reflux

Mechanisms involved with reflux
Reduced lower oesophageal sphincter pressure and change in oesophageal motility, reduced salivary flow rate, increase in abdominal pressure (obesity, pregnancy) [52]

Factors precipitating reflux
Diet – onions, fatty foods, chocolate, peppermint, spicy foods and pickles [38]; alcohol – reduces LOS tone, delays gastric emptying and increasing GOR [44] – it is also an irritant of the oesophageal mucosa
Posture – bending or lying down increases GOR [38, 52]
Exercise – heartburn and nausea can occur as a result of strenuous exercise [53, 54]
Alcohol – reduces the LOS tone [55]

Pathophysiology of Reflux

In health, the pH of the oesophagus varies between 5 and 7. GERD is defined internationally by gastroenterologists as episodes during which the pH in the oesophagus falls below 4 (table 2). In healthy subjects, brief episodes of physiological reflux occurs which are effectively cleared by oesophageal peristalsis followed by salivary neutralisation and this occurs mainly after food intake (postprandial periods) [50]. In most healthy individuals, dietary excess and alcohol consumption usually late at night can cause some discomfort from reflux and is normally termed 'indigestion'. A useful term is that the symptoms interfere with the 'quality of life'. Three mechanisms by which the LOS permits gastroesophageal reflux have been suggested: transient inappropriate or spontaneous LOS relaxation, transient increase in intra-abdominal pressure and spontaneous free reflux associated with low resting pressure of the LOS; however, the predominant reflux mechanism is the TRLOS [51]. For patients with GERD the pH within the oesophagus drops below 4 for long periods of time and the symptoms are more exaggerated and prolonged.

Some lifestyle and dietary factors are known to provoke reflux. For many people who have infrequent symptoms dietary excess can produce symptoms which are time limited and do not interfere with the subject's quality of life, but for those with GERD the symptoms are prolonged and require little provocation.

Some of these factors are listed above in table 2.

Diagnosis of Gastroesophageal Reflux Disease – pH Monitoring

Persistent and prolonged heartburn and regurgitation are the most common and typical symptoms of GERD and their presence is often a good indication of the presence of GERD. However, even in the absence of these symptoms GERD cannot be excluded. GERD can be divided into three categories on the basis of the presence of reflux symptoms and oesophageal mucosal breaks on endoscopy: (1) symptomatic – typical GERD symptoms with oesophageal mucosal breaks, (2) silent – mucosal breaks without symptoms and (3) non-erosive reflux disease – typical symptoms but no mucosal breaks [56].

Many patients, particularly when the condition first manifests, self-medicate and do not seek specialist advice. However, if the condition becomes more chronic and uncomfortable they tend to seek medical intervention. Self-medication can involve purchasing over-the-counter antireflux medication without any special tests or medical intervention. In more persistent cases further investigation is warranted. Diagnosis in clinical practice is based on symptoms and response to antireflux medication [56]. If there is diagnostic uncertainty or insufficient therapeutic effect on the symptoms specialist opinion is sought. The most commonly used techniques used to investigate GERD are endoscopy followed by 24-hour ambulatory pH monitoring measuring a drop in oesophageal pH below 4 [57].

Endoscopy allows the visual examination of the oesophagus. It is undertaken to directly examine the presence of diaphragmatic herniation, inflammation or ulceration around the distal oesophagus using an endoscope. A positive finding implies that reflux is occurring although it remains a subjective opinion. The presence or absence of inflammation does not necessarily imply that reflux is occurring. Endoscopy also does not provide any information about the efficiency of peristalsis or quantify oesophageal motility with any certainty. Ambulatory pH monitoring involves passing electrodes attached to narrow catheters into the oesophagus via the nose to a position 5 cm above the LOS. The data recorded by the pH electrodes are stored digitally and analysed using internationally recognised criteria. The patients normally have the test over 24 h and are allowed home to follow a near-normal day. The ambulatory test attempts to replicate normality and provide the clinician with a quantitative assessment of the reflux disease [20]. The specificity and sensitivity of the 24-hour pH test is around 80%, whereas for endoscopy it is much less [58].

The drawbacks of the test, however, are that it can be uncomfortable and embarrassing, leading to altered behaviour and therefore reducing reflux episodes and symptoms in cases of infrequent reflux episodes not occurring during the 24-hour period [59], and the lack of assessment of non-acidic reflux [57]. Two innovative methods of diagnosis that may address some of these limitations are wireless pH monitoring and electrical impedance recording. Wireless pH monitoring involves a radiotelemetric capsule being attached to the oesophageal mucosa and the pH data transmitted wirelessly over several days [59]. It allows

more reliable diagnosis of reflux and is much better tolerated by patients. However, it is expensive and not available in all centres [59]. A recent study compared the traditional 24-hour pH test to a wireless system (Bravo; Given Imaging, Yoqneam, Israel) and concluded that wireless pH monitoring had an important clinical impact on the diagnosis and management of patients with typical reflux symptoms and is a very useful diagnostic tool for patients with false-negative results or intermittent symptoms and those sensitive to catheterization [59]. Impedance recording on the other hand is based on the measurement of electrical impedance (pressure changes) between closely arranged electrodes mounted on a thin intraluminal probe. The electrical impedance drops when a liquid passes and rises when air passes. It is therefore capable of detecting acidic, non-acidic and gas reflux. A recent debate concluded that the combination of pH monitoring and impedance has the ability to detect all forms of reflux and correlate them to symptoms and, therefore, at present it has a role in patients with refractory symptoms or those suffering from atypical symptoms of GERD. However, improvements are needed in the software and hardware and more studies are needed looking at outcomes of treatment diagnosed using this combined method [60].

Attempts have been made to simplify the diagnosis of GERD and employ less invasive methods. Examples of these are the use of standardised questionnaires or the detection of pepsin in saliva and sputum. The diamond study compared symptom-based diagnosis using the RDQ (Reflux Disease Questionnaire), a standardised questionnaire, and found the sensitivity and specificity to pH monitoring to be 62 and 67%, respectively [61]. A more conservative and less invasive method of diagnosis which has interested researchers involves the detection of pepsin in the sputum or saliva. Pepsin is a proteolytic enzyme that digests dietary proteins and is released by the chief cells of the stomach as its precursor pepsinogen. Acids convert pepsinogen into pepsin and therefore pepsin operates at a pH of 1–3 but can remain active up to pH 6.5 and is not irreversibly denatured below pH 8. It can stay in a 'dormant' phase and be reactivated at a pH of 6 or below [62]. The presence of pepsin in the oesophagus and more proximal organs indicates the presence of refluxate in those regions [63]. Results of studies evaluating pepsin as a diagnostic tool are conflicting at present but further work is underway in the validation of this method.

Laryngopharyngeal Reflux
When reflux contents travel beyond the UOS and into the laryngopharyngeal space a specific term, namely laryngopharyngeal reflux disease (LPR), is used. It is a condition which, unlike gastroesophageal reflux, is always thought to be beyond normal physiological boundaries [64]. Research on the prevalence of LPR is lacking but evidence so far suggests that LPR is more prevalent in those suffering from GERD [62]. The interesting concept is that some individuals may suffer from LPR but have none of the typical GERD symptoms. Identification of this group can be challenging at times. Reulbach et al. [65] reported that 35% of patients recruited had LPR symptoms with no reported history of GERD symptoms.

Differences between Presentation of Gastroesophageal Reflux Disease and Laryngopharyngeal Reflux
It is important to note that some of the features of LPR may be present in those with GERD but through an entirely different pathogenesis. For instance, one may have GERD symptoms and also suffer with a chronic cough or laryngeal disorders by chance. However, LPR cannot occur without measurable gastroesophageal reflux. The diagnosis of LPR is difficult and relies on a combination of ENT assessments and tests as well as pH monitoring, and referrals are made to one or other specialty depending on the type and prominence of the symptoms [64, 65]. Various alternative methods for the diagnosis have been suggested and tested. Previous studies have investigated the role of multiple pH monitoring along the length of the oesophagus and therefore in the proximal as well as the distal oesophagus [66]. Combined pH and impedance monitoring has also been used to increase the diagnostic yield. The role of pepsin detection in the larynx has been investigated as a means for diagnosis. In LPR pepsin can remain in the larynx after reflux, where the pH is around 6.8, but be reactivated when acidic refluxate comes up [66]. Studies investigating pepsin detection in LPR have shown promising results [67].

Management and Treatment of Gastroesophageal Reflux Disease
There are three main methods of management of GERD:
- Lifestyle modifications and non-pharmaceutical therapies
- Medication
- Surgery

Lifestyle modifications and non-pharmaceutical therapies such as increasing the number of pillows, avoiding reflux-provoking foods and meals before bedtime, decreased alcohol consumption, cessation of smoking, reducing weight, dietary restriction, reducing stress and the use of chewing gum are all recognised antireflux strategies.

Chewing gum has been used as a novel method in the management of GERD symptoms. Helm et al. [68] recognised that salivary flow rate and buffering capacity are important in the protection of the oesophagus against gastroesophageal reflux. Chewing gum increases salivary flow rate and buffering capacity, which in turn has the potential for increasing swallowing frequency and improving the clearance rate of reflux within the oesophagus [69].

Smoak and Koufman [70] investigated the effects of chewing gum in a study of 40 consecutive patients with LPR; 20 subjects randomly received regular chewing gum and the other 20 chewed a gum containing bicarbonate. The authors observed an increase in oesophageal and pharyngeal pH. In another study 30 patients acted as their own controls and were given a refluxogenic meal on 2 separated days. On 1 of the days they randomly chewed gum after the consumption of the meal and on the other day they did not chew gum. The pH was measured in the oesophagus on both days. The authors concluded that chewing a piece of sugar-free gum reduced drops in oesophageal pH in the immediate postprandial (after consumption of food) period. Chewing gum can therefore be used as an adjunct to other conservative methods in the management of GERD but further research is needed in this area [71].

Over the last 20 years, medical and surgical treatment of GERD has been revolutionised, firstly by H_2 receptor antagonists and secondly by proton pump inhibitors (PPI). These act by inhibiting the proton pump in the parietal cell, causing powerful and sustained inhibition of gastric secretion of acid [72]. Current guidelines recommend PPIs as a first line of treatment of suspected reflux symptoms. Although very effective in the control of symptoms, there are concerns regarding long-term PPI therapy, including increased susceptibility to gastrointestinal and respiratory infections and risk of hip fracture [73]. The most commonly carried out surgical procedure is a Nissen fundoplication. This procedure in simple terms means wrapping the stomach around the oesophagus to change the anatomical angle and neurogenic reflex mechanisms. The aim is to prevent acid being refluxed from the stomach back into the oesophagus. In recent years a laparoscopic approach to antireflux surgery has become favoured, in particular in specialist centres, with a reduction in risks and side effects. During recent years, there has been some debate as to the relative value of long-term PPI treatment compared with antireflux surgery for the management of chronic GERD. Studies have shown that in the long term both treatments are highly effective, safe and well tolerated [74].

Gastroesophageal Reflux Disease and Dental Erosion

The role of GERD in dental erosion has been widely reported in the dental literature. Regurgitated acid entering the mouth causes dental erosion. The pattern of the erosion is similar to other conditions involving stomach juice such as eating disorders, rumination and chronic alcoholism. Since the acidity in the stomach may be below pH 1, frequent regurgitation or vomiting will erode teeth.

The evidence associating GERD and dental erosion comes from two main areas: patients presenting with symptoms of GERD who are then found to have dental erosion and patients presenting with dental erosion who are then found to have GERD.

Medical Evidence
The relationship between dental erosion and GERD has been investigated in children and adults. One of the first investigations to report the association between dental erosion and GERD was carried out by Jarvinen et al. [9]. They diagnosed GERD by using endoscopy to assess oesophagitis in 20 patients. Typically, in disease the appearance of the mucosa is reddened and inflamed and in chronic disease the lumen begins to close, causing dysphagia. Dental erosion was assessed in the 20 oesophagitis patients by grading each tooth surface numerically using a tooth wear index. In the study group, 4 patients were found to have dental erosion. They concluded that patients diagnosed with GERD had a higher risk of developing dental erosion. Meurman et al. [10] carried out a similar study but included a larger group of 117 Finnish patients referred with symptoms of GERD. Dental erosion was reported to involve 24% of tooth surfaces. The authors concluded that severe reflux disease of long duration was more likely to cause dental erosion than milder forms. Aine et al. [75] reported the case results of 17 children with confirmed GERD and

2 children with dental erosion in whom this condition led to the diagnosis of GERD. They found that almost all children with pathological gastro-esophageal reflux had dental erosion of some type but the severity varied. In a more recent systematic review Pace et al. [76] reported the prevalence of dental erosion in GERD patients as 24% and the presence of GERD in dental erosion patients 32.5%. Moazzez et al. [13], in a study on patients referred to a gastroenterological clinic with symptoms of reflux, assessed tooth wear and compared the results to a control group. Tooth wear involving dentine was more prevalent in patients complaining of symptoms of GERD and those diagnosed as having GERD following 24-hour pH monitoring than a control group. Patients with poorer salivary buffering capacity and those complaining of hoarseness had lower salivary flow rate than controls. Therefore, the subjects were not only more likely to develop dental erosion but also had extra-oesophageal symptoms of reflux. This association is an interesting one and raises the possibility that once reflux passes through the UOS it can affect not only the teeth but also the surrounding structures including the larynx.

Another study by the same authors investigated at 4 sites along the oesophagus with 24-hour ambulatory pH monitoring in patients complaining of extra-oesophageal reflux (including dental erosion, hoarseness and chronic cough). The authors reported that the severity of reflux above the UOS was correlated to the severity of dental erosion, particularly on the palatal surfaces [77]. In another study, patients with GERD complaining of respiratory symptoms had a higher prevalence of dental erosion than those without [78].

Dental Evidence
There is evidence from dental patients who were subsequently assessed for reflux disease. Gudmundsson et al. [11] measured oral pH and distal oesophageal pH in 14 patients with dental erosion. Dental erosion was graded as mild or severe.

Oesophageal pH was measured at 5 cm above the LOS using an antimony pH electrode and 21% of patients were found to have pathological GERD; extended periods of lowered oral pH were also recorded but the two did not coincide. The authors concluded that the erosion was a result of reduced salivary buffering capacity rather than GERD.

In a small study of 12 patients with dental erosion, Schroeder et al. [14] investigated reflux using ambulatory 24-hour oesophageal pH monitoring; 10 of the 12 dental patients were diagnosed with reflux disease but no relationship was reported between saliva and tooth wear. The authors also assessed the presence of dental erosion in a separate group of 30 patients with reflux disease as assessed by 24-hour pH measurement; 12 of 30 patients also had dental erosion. The authors separated the results into distal (near the stomach) and proximal reflux (near the UOS) and found that patients with proximal reflux had 7% of their teeth affected as opposed to those with distal reflux who had 3% of their teeth affected.

In a controlled study, Bartlett et al. [12] investigated 36 patients with palatal dental erosion. The results were compared to 10 subjects without tooth wear or symptoms of GERD. Oral pH was measured simultaneously; 23 (64%) patients were found to have GERD and of these 16 were found to have gastroesophageal reflux symptoms whilst the remaining 7 did not complain of any symptoms. The term 'silent refluxers' was used to describe these patients. The hypothesis in these patients suggested that patients with chronic reflux might have higher than normal pain thresholds or become unresponsive to pain. In addition, in this study a statistically significant relationship was observed between the low pH in the distal oesophagus and the pH in the mouth.

More recently, Gregory-Head et al. [79] reported a study comparing levels of tooth wear in 20 patients with symptoms of GERD compared to a group of controls; 10 of the patient group were diagnosed with GERD. Tooth wear was assessed using a tooth wear index and GERD was diagnosed using 24-hour pH monitoring. GERD patients had significantly higher tooth wear scores compared with control subjects.

These tests assessed the presence of acid with the oesophagus. However, the efficiency of the oesophagus in moving fluids is also important. Manometry measures the efficiency of transporting fluids along the oesophagus and is used indirectly to assess its capacity to prevent reflux. One controlled study measured the motility of patients presenting with dental erosion. The authors reported that whilst the LOS sphincter pressure was normal, the motility of the oesophagus was abnormal compared to the controls. The assumption being that poor oesophageal motility led to the development of reflux and ultimately to dental erosion [80].

Implications of Symptoms of Reflux and Dental Erosion

Although heartburn is the most common symptom of reflux disease, it does not correlate well to the development of dental erosion. There have been a couple of studies investigating the reporting of symptoms from patients and the presence of dental erosion, particularly in Scandinavia [9, 11]. Both of these studies investigated patients presenting with symptoms of reflux and then assessed the prevalence of erosion. A clear correlation between the presence of the reported symptoms and the existence of dental erosion was not observed. Part of the problem is the reliability of symptoms indicating the presence of reflux. Silent reflux is an increasingly recognised phenomenon [26]. In one dental study, up to 25% of subjects presenting with dental erosion were observed to have pathological levels of reflux despite not having any symptoms [8].

Another study investigated patients attending a general hospital after referral for reflux-related symptoms. The severity of tooth wear was assessed using a modified Smith and Knight index and the results were compared to a control group [9]. Although no correlation was observed between heartburn and the presence of tooth wear there were some weak relationships between extra-oesophageal symptoms, particularly hoarseness, and the severity of the dental erosion. Whilst this study could not be considered definitive, it suggests that reflux passing through both lower and upper sphincters has the potential to cause dental erosion. From a dental management perspective, it is useful to record any symptoms of reflux, particularly those associated with the UOS, as it might indicate an underlying disease process and imply that gastric reflux is the cause of the dental erosion. A recent review reported a higher prevalence of dental erosion and halitosis in patients with GERD symptoms [81]. More recently, two prevalence studies conducted in the UK and Europe identified reflux symptoms as risk factors in the development of tooth wear. In both studies the odds ratio illuminating the risk of developing tooth wear was the highest assessed. All these findings match clinical experience that reflux is an important risk in developing severe tooth wear [82, 83].

Implications of Diet and Dental Erosion

Whilst dietary control and avoidance is a recognised management with extrinsic erosion it is less so with conditions related to reflux disease. In symptomatic patients, it is common to find that they avoid any foods likely to provoke reflux. Subjects will readily admit to avoiding spicy or acidic foods because consuming them is painful. Therefore, someone who is under the care of a gastro-enterologist may already be avoiding many of the foods listed above. However, if the patients are not aware of the reflux problems, they may not be avoiding these foods and reflux might be increased.

It is clear that dental erosion and GERD are related. However, the question still remains of why some people with GERD suffer from dental erosion and others not. The most likely explanation is that the reflux in most remains close to the LOS and does not reach the UOS or oral cav-

Table 3. Eating disorders

Anorexia	Bulimia
Mainly females	Mainly females
Low self-image	Low self-image
Western society	Western society
Compulsive	Compulsive
Intelligent	Intelligent
Early adolescence	Late adolescence
Dietary restriction	Binge/purging
Low body weight	Normal body weight
Low metabolic rate	Electrolyte imbalance
Minimal drug use	Drug and alcohol abuse

ity. In some though, the protective mechanism along the oesophagus either fails or is overwhelmed and the gastric contents reach the mouth. Other possible reasons could be insensitive diagnostic methods (inability to measure high reflux), differences in salivary flow rate and buffering capacity. With recent advances such as impedance measurement and wireless prolonged pH measurement, further understanding of the differences between typical GERD symptoms and LPR is possible. However, more research is needed to answer some of the abovementioned questions.

Eating Disorders

An eating disorder can be defined as a persistent avoidance of food or eating behaviour which impairs physical or psychosocial function and is not related to other medical conditions [84]. The two closely linked disorders to dentistry are anorexia and bulimia nervosa (table 3). Eating disorders have been described by the Eating Disorders Association as the 'outward expression of deep psychological and emotional turmoil, with sufferers turning to food and eating as a means of expressing their difficulties'. Anorexia nervosa is the refusal to maintain normal body weight. Bulimia is derived from the Greek, meaning ox hunger, and is characterised by binge eating followed by behavioural responses aimed at avoiding body weight gain.

Anorexia Nervosa

The literal meaning is 'a nervous loss of appetite' and is derived from the Greek word 'orexis' or appetite [84]. The most important feature is a relentless pursuit of thinness [84]. This pursuit continues despite being thin. Sufferers continue to avoid food because of an altered body image driving them to further food restriction. There is an understanding that anorexia has two clinical subtypes: restrictive and binge/purge. The former pursue their goals through dietary restriction whilst the latter aid this through purging and laxatives. The distinction between the subtypes can be blurred as sufferers pass from one form to another.

The annual incidence of anorexia in Britain has been estimated at between 0.6 and 1.6 per 100,000 of the whole population [85]. This is a sociocultural disease affecting white, upper and middle-class women between the ages of 12 and 30 years [86, 87]. It is an overwhelming disease of Westernised industrial societies and is 10 times more common in females than males [88].

Clinically, the condition is diagnosed when the body weight is less than 85% of the ideal or normal value. Initially, anorexics may start a gradual transition with limitations to high-calorie foods, later meat avoidance and finally reliance on 'safe foods' without any calorific gain. The continual weight loss has medical implications with poor concentration, decline of interest and social avoidance. The altered body image distorts their awareness of self despite obvious changes to those around them. These changes in body image occur with depressive symptoms in the acutely underweight individuals [89]. Treatment of anorexia is multilevel and multidisciplinary. Hospital-based treatment includes inpatient and outpatient care.

Bulimia

The term was derived from the Greek words 'bous' and 'limos' literally meaning 'ox hunger'. The condition was first recognised in the late 1970s by Russell [90]. The identifying feature is binge eating with an excessive amount of food with a subjective loss of control [84]. Binge eating is associated with behaviour aimed to avoid weight gain, most often through self-induced vomiting. The diagnosis is made when binge eating and vomiting occur more than twice a week for at least 3 months. The body weight for bulimic is normal but if it drops then anorexia becomes part of the condition. Some characteristics involve subtyping into purging and non-purging variants. Among the purging types metabolic disturbances are more common with electrolyte imbalance and lower body weight.

It is difficult to find reliable data for the prevalence of bulimia in the UK. Patients with bulimia are normally slightly older than anorexics, typically in their early 20s, while late-onset anorexia nervosa affects adolescents. Some estimates are about 1–3% of females [91]. The male to female ratio is 1:10 [84]. Dieting usually precedes disease onset although some report binge eating prior to the onset [84].

Many of the risk factors identified in anorexia are common to bulimia and some merging of the conditions is known to occur. Early critical comments about weight can be identified as precursors of the condition. Unlike anorexia there is more of a tendency for self-abuse such as alcohol, drugs and self-mutilation [92].

Dental Implications

The oral status of patients with eating disorders has been assessed in several studies [93]. It is evident that a common presenting feature is erosion of the palatal (lingual) surfaces of the upper anterior teeth, but also of the posterior teeth as well. The appearance of palatal erosion was first described as perimylolysis [94]. The main differences between eating disorders appears to be that severe palatal and moderate buccal erosion is ap-

parent in many of those who vomit regularly, but is rare in non-vomiting patients. Those sufferers using purging to rid themselves of food have an increased risk of developing erosion. The main support from this observation comes from two early papers from Scandinavia [93, 94]. However, both studies recognised that a contribution from the subject's diet, which included acidic foods and drinks, was possible. Although it might be expected that vomiting and erosion are directly related, one study observed the contrary. The authors reported that the frequency, duration and total number of vomiting episodes was not directly related to erosion [86]. The same authors did not find a relationship between the level of erosion and the frequency of vomiting. Another study reported relationships between erosion and those reporting self-induced vomiting [48]. This apparent dilemma suggests that other factors are involved in the development of erosion. Those with non-vomiting and restrictive diets, particularly those with anorexia, are less likely to develop erosion but the risk still exists later in life. In addition, because of the complex nature of the condition, those who have controlled their eating disorder may still retain a higher risk of continuing dental erosion because of the link between it and gastroesophageal reflux.

The distribution of erosion is typically on the palatal surfaces of the upper anterior teeth [48]. This study also reported more erosion on the occlusal and buccal surfaces of the lower posterior teeth and this difference was independent of whether vomiting occurred or not. This might be explained with the increased consumption of acidic drinks but it is not clear [95, 96]. However, chronic sufferers (for 5 years or more) are more likely to develop more widespread erosion [96]. Milosevic and Slade [86] also recognised that prolonged vomiting over extensive periods of time increased the risk of developing erosion. Rytömaa et al. [97] compared the incidence of dental erosion in a group of 35 bulimics and compared the results to 105 controls and also reported severe erosion in patients compared with a similar group of controls. Another study showed more extensive erosion in anorexic patients with a vomiting habit than those with an absence of purgative episodes and these patients in turn had more erosion than a control group [98].

An increased risk of caries has also been reported but the association is unclear [99]. In the paper by Hellstrom there were no differences between vomiting and non-vomiting subjects whilst another reported less caries in anorexics [93], but neither study compared their results to a control group. Other workers have not found any association [47, 86, 96]. Overall, there seems to be little agreement on whether caries is increased or decreased in eating disorders and this may reflect the changing and merging of signs and symptoms in these subjects [99].

Saliva might be expected to be important, particularly with self-induced vomiting, because of the autonomic nervous system control of the process. Also, changes to electrolyte balance seen in vomiting might be expected to have an impact on saliva. Rytömaa et al. [97] reported decreased salivary flow rate in their study of bulimics. Another study of 35 subjects with eating disorders also reported decreased unstimulated salivary flow rate and suggested that tests of salivary flow may serve as an indicator of the risk of progression of erosion [100]. Normal salivary flow has been reported in non-vomiting anorexics and bulimics [101]. Other workers have reported significantly lower rates of salivary flow in their study of vomiting bulimics with and without dental erosion [102]. These workers also measured bicarbonate ion levels and observed reduced levels irrespective of vomiting but increased viscosity in the subjects with erosion. This may reflect the changes in electrolyte balance found in the vomiting groups. There are difficulties in measuring saliva as the testing methods are not universally accepted nor are they particularly accurate. Finally, an observation that parotid enlargement occurs in bulimia has been reported by a number of authors [103–104].

Chronic Alcoholism

Chronic alcoholism is a serious condition with potentially life-threatening complications. Some alcoholics present with dental erosion. The pattern of wear suggests that the source of the acid is regurgitated or refluxed stomach juice. Attrition due to bruxism has also been reported in alcoholics [105]. Chronic alcoholism is thought to affect 10% of the population, although this figure overestimates the probable prevalence [106]. Alcohol can result in gastritis and provoke gastroesophageal reflux [107]. Alcoholics also have poor diet control and tend to eat more acidic foods and drinks. Tooth wear has been found to be more prevalent in studies comparing alcoholics to controls [47, 108]. Extensive palatal and incisal wear was observed in case reports of 6 subjects with a history of long term alcohol abuse [47].

Rumination

Rumination is a rare but interesting condition that can cause severe dental erosion. The pattern of erosion in these patients is similar to other conditions where the acid is regurgitated from the stomach, such as eating disorders. Subjects regurgitate their food (which can be solid or liquid), sometimes re-chew the food, and then swallow again. They repeatedly raise their intra-abdominal pressure after meals and regurgitation occurs when one of these compressions coincides with swallowing and the associated relaxation of the LOS [109]. Rumination occurs commonly in people with learning difficulties but it can affect other members of the population.

It has been reported that rumination may be more common than was previously thought. It has also been suggested that it affects highly intelligent, professional people [110]. The pathophysiology of rumination is poorly understood and has been incompletely studied. It is generally considered to be a psychological disorder although it has also been suggested that patients might suffer from GERD. Patients often find it embarrassing to admit to the condition and the prevalence might be higher than was first thought.

The pattern of dental erosion is similar to other intrinsic causes with the first signs developing on the palatal surfaces of the upper incisors and if the condition continues to involve other tooth surfaces. Because the gastric juice is forced into the mouth just after feeding it is generally quite acidic and the resulting erosion is normally severe.

Pregnancy and Other Causes

The hormonal changes in pregnancy are known to affect eating habits during the term. Unusual eating habits can develop during pregnancy [46] but these tend to be temporary and return to normal after the birth. Unexpectedly, anorexics or bulimics may actually improve whilst being pregnant [111]. Vomiting during pregnancy can occur especially during the first trimester and may cause further erosion. There is also increased reflux in pregnancy.

Conclusion

Intrinsic causes of dental erosion involve stomach acids entering the mouth. These strong acids erode the enamel and dentine, normally starting on the palatal surfaces of the upper anterior teeth. The strength of the acid often results in severe erosion, resulting in significant loss of enamel and dentine. As the condition progresses the damage to teeth becomes more widespread.

The relationship between gastroesophageal reflux and dental erosion has been well documented. The association has been investigated in patients presenting with gastroesophageal reflux and in those presenting with dental erosion. An association between gastroesophageal reflux and dental erosion has been found in both groups.

The association of eating disorders and dental erosion has also been well reported. Persistent vomiting has been observed to cause dental erosion and is commonly found in patients with eating disorders.

Gastric causes of dental erosion are probably relatively uncommon, but when they do occur the damage to teeth is often severe and time consuming to treat. At present there are no specific guidelines for the prevention, diagnosis and treatment of GERD and therefore more research and RCTs are needed for a clearer approach on the management of the condition, including dental erosion as one of its manifestations.

References

1 Dent J, El-Serag HB, Wallander MA, Johansson S: Epidemiology of gastro-oesophageal reflux disease: a systematic review. Gut 2005;54:710–717.

2 Bartlett DW, Coward PY: Comparison of erosive potential of gastric juice and a carbonated drink in vitro. J Oral Rehabil 2001;28:1045–1047.

3 Bartlett DW, Ricketts DNJ, Fisher NL: Management of the short clinical crown by indirect restorations. Dent Update 1997;24:431–436.

4 Bartlett DW: Adapting crown preparations to adhesive materials. Dent Update 2000;27:460–463.

5 Kidd EAM, Smith BGN: Toothwear histories: a sensitive issue. Dent Update 1993;20:174–178.

6 Smith BGN, Knight JK: A comparison of patterns of tooth wear with aetiological factors. Br Dent J 1984;157:16–19.

7 Lussi A, Schaffner M, Holtz P, Suter P: Dental erosion in a population of Swiss adults. Community Dent Oral Epidemiol 1991;19:286–290.

8 Yoshikava H, Furuta K, Ueno M, Egawa M, Yoshino A, Kondo S, Nariai Y, Ishibashi H, Kinoshita Y, Sekine J: Oral symptoms including dental erosion in gastroesophageal reflux disease are associated with decreased salivary flow volume and swallowing function. J Gastroenterol 2012;47:412–420.

9 Jarvinen V, Meurman JH, Hyvarinen H, Rytomaa I, Murtomaa H: Dental erosion and upper gastrointestinal disorders. Oral Surg Oral Med Oral Pathol 1988;65: 298–303.

10 Meurman JH, Toskala J, Nuutinen P, Klemetti E: Oral and dental manifestations in gastroesophageal reflux disease. Oral Surg Oral Med Oral Pathol 1994;78: 583–589.

11 Gudmundsson K, Kristleifsson G, Theodors A, Holbrook WP: Tooth erosion, gastroesophageal reflux, and salivary buffer capacity. Oral Surg Oral Med Oral Pathol 1995;79:185–189.

12 Bartlett DW, Evans DF, Anggiansah A, Smith BGN: A study of the association between gastro-oesophageal reflux and palatal dental erosion. Br Dent J 1996; 181:125–131.

13 Moazzez R, Anggiansah A, Bartlett DW: Dental erosion, gastro-oesophageal reflux disease and saliva: how are they related? J Dent 2004;32:489–494.

14 Schroeder PL, Filler SJ, Ramirez B, Lazarchik DA, Vaezi MF, Richter JE: Dental erosion and acid reflux disease. Ann Intern Med 1995;122:809–815.

15 O'Sullivan EA, Curzon ME, Roberts GJ, Milla PJ, Stringer MD: Gastroesophageal reflux in children and its relationship to erosion of primary and permanent teeth. Eur J Oral Sci 1998;106:765–769.

16 Gregory-Head BL, Curtis DA: Erosion caused by gastroesophageal reflux: diagnostic considerations. J Prosthodont 1997;6:278–285.

17 Meyer GW, Austin RM, Brady CE 3rd, Castell DO: Muscle anatomy of the human esophagus. J Clin Gastroenterol 1986;8:131–134.

18 Peters FT, Kleibeuker JH: Barrett's oesophagus and carcinoma: recent insights into its development and possible prevention. Scand J Gastroenterol Suppl 1993;200:59–64.

19 Buthpitiya AG, Stroud D, Russell CO: Pharyngeal pump and esophageal transit. Dig Dis Sci 1987;32:1244–1248.

20 Richter JE, Wu WC, Johns DN, Blackwell JN, Nelson JL, Castell JA, et al: Esophageal manometry in 95 healthy adult volunteers: variability of pressures with age and frequency of 'abnormal' contractions. Dig Dis Sci 1987;32:583–592.

21 Johnson LF, DeMeester TR: Twenty-four-hour pH monitoring of the distal esophagus. Am J Gastroenterol 1974;62: 325–332.

22 Vantrappen G, Janssens J: Pathophysiology and treatment of gastro-oesophageal reflux disease. Scand J Gastroenterol Suppl 1989;24(suppl):7–12.

23 Benjamin SB, Richter JE, Cordova CM, Knuff TE, Castell DO: Prospective manometric evaluation with pharmacologic provocation of patients with suspected esophageal motility dysfunction. Gastroenterol Int 1983;84:893–901.

24 Janssens J, Vantrappen G, Ghillebert G: 24-hour recording of esophageal pressure and pH in patients with noncardiac chest pain. Gastroenterology 1986;90: 1978–1984.

25 Diamant NE: Pathophysiology of gastroesophageal reflux disease. Part 1. Oral cavity, pharynx and oesophagus. GI Motility online 2006, DOI: 10.1038/gimo21.

26 Orr WC: Therapeutic options in the treatment of nighttime gastroesophageal reflux. Digestion 2005;72:229–238.

27 Koufmann JA, Aviv JE, Casiano RR, Shaw GY: Laryngopharyngeal reflux: position statement of the committee on speech, voice, and swallowing disorders of the American Academy of Otolaryngology – Head and Neck Surgery. Otolaryngol Head Neck Surg 2002;127:32–35.

28 Vakill N, Van Zanten SV, Kahrilas P, Dent J, Jones R: The Montreal definition and classification of gastroesophageal reflux disease: a global evidence-based consensus. Am J Gastroenterol 2006; 101:1900–1920.

29 Anggiansah A, Bright N, Mccullagh M, Owen W: Transition from nutcracker esophagus to achalasia. Dig Dis Sci 1990; 35:1162–1166.

30 Chandra A, Moazzez R, Bartlett DW, Anggiansah A, Owen WJ: A review of the atypical manifestations of gastroesophageal reflux disease. Int J Clin Pract 2004;58:41–48.

31 Kitchen LI, Castell DO: Rationale and efficacy of conservative therapy for gastroesophageal reflux disease. Arch Intern Med 1991;151:448–454.

32 Castell DO, Holtz A: Gastroesophageal reflux. Postgrad Med 1989;86:141–148.

33 Nebel OT, Fornes MF, Castell DO: Symptomatic gastroesophageal reflux: incidence and precipitating factors. Dig Dis 1976;21:953–956.

34 Bennett JR: Heartburn and gastro-oesophageal reflux. Br J Clin Pract 1991; 45:273–277.

35 Gunasekaran T, Dahlberg M, Ramesh P, Namachivayam G: Prevalence and associated features of gastroesophageal reflux symptoms in a Caucasian-predominant adolescent school population. Dig Dis Sci 2008;53:2373–2379.

36 Gunasekaran T, Dahlberg M: Prevalence of gastroesophageal reflux symptoms in adolescents: is there a difference in different racial and ethnic groups? Dis Esophagus 2011;24: 18–24.

37 Bartlett DW, Evans DF, Smith BGN: The relationship between gastro-oesophageal reflux disease and dental erosion. J Oral Rehabil 1996;23:289–297.

38 Irwin RS, French CL, Curley FJ, Zawacki JK, Bennett FM: Chronic cough due to gastroesophageal reflux. Chest 1993;104: 1511–1517.

39 Hennesey TPJ, Cuschieri A, Bennett JR: Reflux Oesophagitis, ed 1. London, Butterworth, 1989.

40 Chernow B, Johnson LF, Janowitz WR, Castell DO: Pulmonary aspiration as a consequence of gastroesophageal reflux: a diagnostic approach. Dig Dis Sci 1979; 24:839–844.

41 Irwin RS, Madison JM: Anatomical diagnostic protocol in evaluating chronic cough with specific reference to gastroesophageal reflux disease. Am J Med 2000;108(suppl 4a):126S–130S.

42 Irwin RS, Richter JE: Gastroesophageal reflux and chronic cough. Am J Gastroenterol 2000;95(suppl):S9–S14.

43 Field SK: Gastroesophageal reflux and respiratory symptoms. Chest 1999;116: 843.

44 Field SK, Underwood M, Brant R, Cowie RL: Prevalence of gastroesophageal reflux symptoms in asthma. Chest 1996; 109:316–322.

45 Field SK: Underlying mechanisms of respiratory symptoms with esophageal acid when there is no evidence of airway response. Am J Med 2001;111(suppl 8A): 37S–40S.

46 McLoughlin IJ, Hassanyeh F: Pica in a patient with anorexia nervosa. Br J Psychiatry 1990;156:568–570.

47 Robb ND: Dental erosion in patients with chronic alcoholism. J Dent 1989;17: 219–221.

48 Robb ND, Smith BG, Geidrys-Leeper E: The distribution of erosion in the dentitions of patients with eating disorders. Br Dent J 1995;178:171–175.

49 Smit CF, van Leeuwen JA, Mathus-Vliegen LM, Devriese PP, Semin A, Tan J, et al: Gastropharyngeal and gastroesophageal reflux in globus and hoarseness. Arch Otolaryngol Head Neck Surg 2000;126:827–830.

50 Helm JF: Esophageal acid clearance. J Clin Gastroenterol 1986;8(suppl 1):5–11.

51 Dent J, Dodds WJ, Hogan WJ, Toouli J: Factors that influence induction of gastroesophageal reflux in normal human subjects. Dig Dis Sci 1988;33:270–275.

52 DeMeester TR, Johnson LF, Joseph GJ, Toscano MS, Hall AW, Skinner DB: Patterns of gastroesophageal reflux in health and disease. Ann Surg 1976;184:459–469.

53 Kraus BB, Jane W, Sinclair PA, Castell DO: Gastroesophageal reflux in runners. Ann Intern Med 1990;112:429–433.

54 Hirsch DP, Mathus-54Vliegen EM, Dagli U, Tytgat GN, Boeckxstaens GE: Effect of prolonged gastric distention on lower esophageal sphincter function and gastroesophageal reflux. Am J Gastroenterol 2003;98:1696–1704.

55 Vitale GC, Cheadle WG, Patel B, Sadek SA: The effect of alcohol on nocturnal gastroesophageal reflux. JAMA 1987;258:2077–2079.

56 Choi JY, Jung HK, Song EM, Shim KN, Jung SA: Determinants of symptoms in gastroesophageal reflux disease: nonerosive reflux disease, symptomatic, and silent erosive reflux disease. Eur J Gastroenterol Hepatol 2013;25:764–771.

57 Blondeau K, Tack J: Pro: impedence testing is useful in the management of GERD. Am J Gastroenterol 2009;104:2664–2666.

58 Klauser AG, Heinrich C, Schindlbeck NE, Muller-Lissner SA: Is long-term esophageal monitoring of clinical value? Am J Gastroenterol 1989;84:362–366.

59 Sweiss R, Fox M, Anggiansah A, Wong T: Prolonged, wireless pH studies have a high diagnostic yield in patients with reflux symptoms and negative 24-hour catheter pH studies. Neurogastroenterol Motil 2011;23:419–426.

60 Shay S: A balancing view: impedence-pH testing in GERD – limited role for now, perhaps more helpful in the future. Am J Gastroenterol 2009;104:2669–2670.

61 Dent J, Vakil N, Jones R, Bytzer P, Schoning U, Halling K, Junghard O, Lind T: Accuracy of the diagnosis of GORD by questionnaire, physicians and a trial of proton pump inhibitor treatment: the Diamond Study. Gut 2010;59:714–721.

62 Printza A, Kyrgidis A, Oikonomidou E, Triaridis S: Assessing laryngopharyngeal reflux symptoms with the reflux symptom index. Otolaryngol Head Neck Surg 2011;145:974–980.

63 Bardhan KD, Strugala V, Dettmar PW: Reflux revisited: advancing the role of pepsin. Int J Otolaryngol 2012;2012:646901.

64 Koufman J, Dettmar P, Johnston N: Laryngopharyngeal reflux (LPR). ENT News 2005;14:42–45.

65 Reulbach TR, Belafsky PC, Blalock PD, Koufman JA, Postma GN: Occult laryngeal pathology in a community-based cohort. Otolaryngol Head Neck Surg 2001;124:448.

66 Marshall R, Anggiansah A, Owen WA, Manifold DK, Owen WJ: The extent of duodenogastric reflux in gastro-oesophageal reflux disease. Eur J Gastroenterol Hepatol 2001;13:5–10.

67 Knight J, Lively MO, Johnston N, Dettmar PW, Koufman JA: Sensitive pepsin immunoassay for detection of laryngopharyngeal reflux. Laryngoscope 2005;115:1473–1478.

68 Helm JF, Dodds WJ, Pelc LR, Palmer DW, Hogan WJ, Teeter BC: Effect of esophageal emptying and saliva on clearance of acid from the esophagus. N Engl J Med 1984;310:284–288.

69 Edgar WM, O'Mullane DM (eds): Saliva and Dental Health. London, British Dental Association Publications, 1990.

70 Smoak BR, Koufman JA: Effects of gum chewing on pharyngeal and esophageal pH. Ann Otol Rhinol Laryngol 2001;110:1117–1119.

71 Moazzez R, Bartlett D, Anggiansah A: The effect of chewing sugar-free gum on gastro-esophageal reflux. J Dent Res 2005;84:1062–1065.

72 NICE: Dyspepsia: Managing Dyspepsia in Adults in Primary Care. Newcastle on Tyne: North of England Dyspepsia Guideline Development Group. London, National Institute of Clinical Excellence, 2004.

73 Yang YX, Lewis JD, Epstein S, Metz DC: Long-term proton pump inhibitor therapy and risk of hip fracture. JAMA 2006;296:2947–2953.

74 Lundell L, Attwood S, Ell C, Fiocca R, Galmiche JP, Hatlebakk J, Lind T, Junghard O: Comparing laparoscopic antireflux surgery with esomeprazole in the management of patients with chronic gastro-oesophageal reflux disease: a 3-year interim analysis of the LOTUS trial. Gut 2008;57:1207–1213.

75 Aine L, Baer M, Maki M: Dental erosions caused by gastroesophageal reflux disease in children. J Dent Child 1993;60:210–214.

76 Pace F, Pallotta S, Tonini M, Vakil N, Bianchi Porro G: Systematic review: gastro-oesophageal reflux disease and dental lesions. Aliment Pharmacol Ther 2008;27:1179–1186.

77 Moazzez R, Anggiansah A, Bartlett D: The association of acidic reflux above the upper oesophageal sphincter with palatal tooth wear. Caries Res 2005;39:475–478.

78 Wang GR, Zhang H, Wang ZG, Jiang GS, Guo CH: Relationship between dental erosion and respiratory symptoms in patients with gastro-oesophageal reflux disease. J Dentistry 2010;38:892–898.

79 Gregory-Head BL, Curtis DA, Kim L, Cello J: Evaluation of dental erosion in patients with gastroesophageal reflux disease. J Prosthet Dent 2000;83:675–680.

80 Bartlett DW, Evans DF, Anggiansah A, Smith BGN: The role of the esophagus in dental erosion. Oral Surg Oral Med Oral Pathol Oral Radiol Endod 1999;89:312–315.

81 Marsicano JA, de Moura-Grec PG, Bonato RC, Sales-Peres Mde C, Sales-Peres A, Sales-Peres S: Gastroesophageal reflux, dental erosion, and halitosis in epidemiological surveys: a systematic review. Eur J Gastroenterol Hepatol 2013;25:135–141.

82 Bartlett DW, Lussi A, West NX, Bouchard P, Sanz M, Bourgeois D: Prevalence of tooth wear on buccal and lingual surfaces and possible risk factors in young European adults. J Dent 2013;41:1007–1013.

83 Bartlett D, Fares J, Shirodaria S, Chiu K, Ahmad N: The association of tooth wear, diet and dietary habits in adults aged 18–30 years old. J Dent 2011;39:811–816.

84 Klein DA, Walsh BT: Eating disorders: clinical features and pathophysiology. Physiol Behav 2004;81:359–374.

85 Kendal RE, Hall DJ, Babigan HM: The epidemiology of anorexia nervosa. Psychol Med 1973;3:200–203.

86 Milosevic A, Slade PD: The orodental status of anorexics and bulimics. Br Dent J 1989;167:66–70.

87 Jensen OE, Featherstone JDB, Stege P: Chemical and physical oral findings in a case of anorexia nervosa and bulimia. J Oral Pathol Med 1987;16:399–402.

88 Williamson DA, Martin CK, Stewart T: Psychological aspects of eating disorders. Best Pract Res Clin Gastroenterol 2004;18:1073–1088.

89 Kaye WH: Anorexia nervosa, obsessional behavior, and serotonin. Psychopharmacol Bull 1997;33:335–344.

90 Russell G: Bulimia nervosa: an ominous variant of anorexia nervosa. Psychol Med 1979;9:429–448.

91 Kendler KS, MacLean C, Neale M, Kessler R, Heath A, Eaves L: The genetic epidemiology of bulimia nervosa. Am J Psychiatry 1991;148:1627–1637.

92 Lilenfeld LR, Stein D, Bulik CM, Strober M, Plotnicov K, Pollice C, et al: Personality traits among currently eating disordered, recovered and never ill first-degree female relatives of bulimic and control women. Psychol Med 2000;30:1399–1410.

93 Hellstrom I: Oral complications in anorexia nervosa. Scand J Dent Res 1977;85:71–86.

94 Holst JJ, Lange F: A contribution towards the genesis of tooth wasting from non-mechanical causes. Acta Odontol Scand 1939;26:396.

95 Hurst PS, Lacey LH, Crisp AH: Teeth, vomiting and diet: a study of the dental characteristics of seventeen anorexia nervosa patients. Postgrad Med J 1977;53:298–305.

96 Scheutzel P: Etiology of dental erosion – intrinsic factors. Eur J Oral Sci 1996;104:178–190.

97 Rytömaa I, Järvinen V, Kanerva R, Heinonen OP: Bulimia and tooth erosion. Acta Odontol Scand 1998;56:36–40.

98 Aranha ACC, Eduardo CP, Cordás TA: Eating disorders. Part I. Psychiatric diagnosis and dental implications. J Contemp Dent Pract 2008;9:73–81.

99 Milosevic A: Eating disorders and the dentist. Br Dent J 1999;186:109–113.

100 Ohrn R, Angmar-Mansson B: Oral status of 35 subjects with eating disorders: a 1-year study. Eur J Oral Sci 2000;108:275–280.

101 Touyz SW, Liew VP, Tseng P, Frisken K, Williams H, Beumont PJ: Oral and dental complications in dieting disorders. Int J Eat Disord 1993;14:341–347.

102 Milosevic A, Dawson LJ: Salivary factors in vomiting bulimics with and without pathological tooth wear. Caries Res 1996;30:361–366.

103 Levin PA, Falko JM, Dixon K: Benign parotid enlargement in bulimia. Ann Intern Med 1980;93:827–829.

104 Hasler JF: Parotid enlargement: a presenting sign in anorexia nervosa. Oral Surg Oral Med Oral Pathol 1982;53:567–573.

105 King WH, Tucker KM: Dental problems of alcoholic and nonalcoholic psychiatric patients. Q J Stud Alcohol 1973;34:1208–1211.

106 Christen AG: Dentistry and the alcoholic patient. Dent Clin N Am 1983;27:341–361.

107 Gottfried EB, Korsten MA, Lieber CS: Alcohol-induced gastric and duodenal lesions in man. Am J Gastroenterol 1978;70:587–592.

108 Robb ND, Smith BGN: Prevalence of pathological tooth wear in patients with chronic alcoholism. Br Dent J 1990;169:367–369.

109 Levine DF, Wingate DL, Pfeffer JM, Butcher P: Habitual rumination: a benign disorder. Br Med J 1983;287:255–256.

110 Gilmour AG, Beckett HA: The voluntary reflux phenomenon. Br Dent J 1994;175:368–372.

111 Fairburn CG, Stein A, Jones R: Eating habits and eating disorders during pregnancy. Psychosom Med 1992;54:665–672.

Dr. R. Moazzez
Department of Prosthodontics
King's College London Dental Institute, Floor 25, Guy's Tower
St. Thomas' Street, London Bridge
London SE1 9RT (UK)
E-Mail rebecca.v.moazzez@kcl.ac.uk

Lussi A, Ganss C (eds): Erosive Tooth Wear. Monogr Oral Sci. Basel, Karger, 2014, vol 25, pp 197–205
DOI: 10.1159/000360372

The Potential of Saliva in Protecting against Dental Erosion

Anderson T. Hara · Domenick T. Zero

Department of Preventive and Community Dentistry, Oral Health Research Institute, Indiana University
School of Dentistry, Indianapolis, Ind., USA

Abstract

Saliva is the most relevant biological factor for the prevention of dental erosion. It starts acting even before the acid attack, with an increase of the salivary flow rate as a response to the acidic stimuli. This creates a more favorable scenario, improving the buffering system of saliva and effectively diluting and clearing acids that come in contact with dental surfaces during the erosive challenge. Saliva plays a role in the formation of the acquired dental pellicle, a perm-selective membrane that prevents the contact of the acid with the tooth surfaces. Due to its mineral content, saliva can prevent demineralization as well as enhance remineralization. These protective properties may become more evident in hyposalivatory patients. Finally, saliva may also represent the biological expression of an individual's risk for developing erosive lesions; therefore, some of the saliva components as well as of the acquired dental pellicle can serve as potential biomarkers for dental erosion.   © 2014 S. Karger AG, Basel

The biological factors related to dental erosion involve properties and characteristics of saliva, acquired dental pellicle, tooth structure and surrounding soft tissues [1, 2]. The interaction of these factors with both erosive agent and behavioral aspects, over time, influences the development as well as the prevention, arrestment and possibly recovery of erosive lesions [3]. Substantial interest exists in saliva, as it is one of the most relevant biological modulators for dental erosion. A critical review based on clinical and laboratorial findings is presented, clarifying the impact of saliva on the dental erosion process.

Protective Mechanisms of Saliva

Saliva has been considered as the most important biological factor in dental erosion prevention due to its ability to: (1) act directly on the erosive agent itself by diluting, clearing, neutralizing and buffering acids, (2) play a role in forming a protective membrane covering the tooth surface (acquired pellicle) and (3) reduce the demineralization rate and enhance remineralization by providing calcium, phosphate and fluoride to eroded enamel and dentine. Perhaps the best clinical indicator of the protective properties of saliva would be the flow rate, since practically all the above salivary parameters depend on it [4]. The average unstimulated salivary flow rate is reported to be >0.3 ml/min with normal daily production between 0.5 and 1.5 liters [5]. The relevance of saliva on the erosion process was experimentally illustrated by a study comparing laboratorial and clinical – with salivary protection – erosion models, where it was shown that enamel erosion was dramatically reduced by the order of 10 times in the clinical model [6].

Action before Erosion

Saliva starts its protective effect against erosion even before the acid challenge, by the increase of the flow rate as a response to the extra-oral stimuli such as odor [7, 8] or sight [9]. Sour foodstuff has a strong influence on the anticipatory salivary flow [7, 9], which can be significantly increased compared to the normal unstimulated flow rate [8]. Hypersalivation also occurs in advance of vomiting as a response from the 'vomiting center' of the brain [10], as frequently seen in individuals suffering from anorexia and bulimia nervosa, rumination or chronic alcoholism. It is suggested that this could minimize the erosion caused by acids of gastric origin. On the other hand, patients with symptoms of gastroesophageal reflux disease should not expect the salivary output to increase before the gastric juice regurgitation, because this is an involuntary response not co-coordinated by the autonomic nervous system [11]. Therefore, there may be insufficient time for saliva to act before erosion occurs.

Higher salivary flow rate creates a favorable scenario for the prevention or minimization of initial erosive attack due to the increase of the organic and inorganic constituents of saliva. The constituents of primary interest in the erosion process are carbonic acid (H_2CO_3)/hydrogen carbonate (HCO_3^-), dihydrogen phosphate ($H_2PO_4^-$)/hydrogen phosphate (HPO_4^{2-}), calcium (Ca^{2+}) and fluoride (F^-) [12, 13]. These ions are associated with enhancing the buffer capacity of saliva and maintenance of the integrity of teeth [14]. Hydrogen carbonate is the principal buffer of saliva and its concentration increases from about 5 mmol/l in unstimulated up to 60 mmol/l in stimulated whole saliva. The concentration of dihydrogen phosphate is regulated in the opposite direction, from 5 mmol/l unstimulated saliva down to 3 mmol/l in stimulated saliva [15]. The protein buffer system may also be of some importance in lower pH levels (below 4.5). In a clinical study, the saliva from patients with gastroesophageal reflux disease symptoms presented lower buffering capacity than healthy controls, which may have contributed to their larger number of erosive lesions [16–18].

Action during Erosion

Once the acid reaches the mouth several salivary mechanisms come into play to protect the teeth. Intra-oral stimuli of the salivary flow are mainly due to chemical and mechanical stimulation. Potentially erosive foodstuff and beverages [19] elicit a strong response. Three droplets of 4% citric acid applied to the tongue every 30 s for 5 min caused the mean flow rate to rise up to about 1.87 ml/min, which was significantly higher than the unstimulated flow of about 0.38 ml/min [8]. Mastication can also stimulate the saliva output [20]. It has been suggested that the stimulation of the mechanoreceptive neurons in the gingival tissues may result in a reflex secretion of saliva [21]. Depending on the oral stimuli, different salivary glands may be affected, leading to variation in salivary flow and composition [8] and thus influencing the level of salivary protection. Chewing gum increases salivary flow and should be beneficial for dental erosion prevention, with the possible exception of acidic gums repeatedly replaced in a relatively short period of time. Under these circumstances, the salivary protective factors may not be enough to prevent erosive tooth wear in dentine surfaces [22].

A lower flow rate decreases the capacity of saliva in neutralizing and buffering acids increasing the chances for erosion development, as shown in previous studies [23, 24]. Even though acid clearance has been reported as an individual property [25], it can be suggested that factors such as food consistency and sites of the mouth affect the acid clearance pattern. Sites poorly bathed by saliva or mainly bathed with mucous saliva are more likely

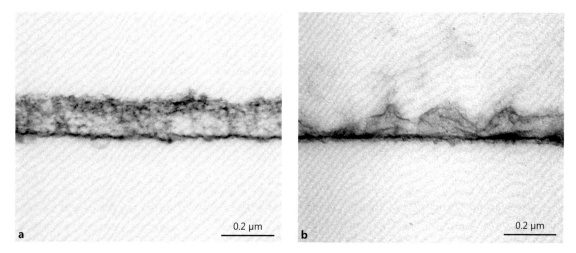

Fig. 1. a Transmission electron microscopy image of the 2-hour pellicle formed on enamel surface in situ. **b** The 2-hour pellicle after 10 min of erosive challenge in situ by orange juice; even after partial dissolution, the pellicle was still able to provide some protection to enamel.

to show erosion compared to sites protected by serous saliva [26]. Lussi et al. [27] have shown significantly faster pH recovery after ingestion of orange juice on the second mandibular premolar compared to the maxillary central incisor, due to the closeness of the former to the parotid salivary gland. The time required for saliva to neutralize and/or clear the acid from the tooth surface has been measured in vivo with pH electrodes and has been shown to range between 2 and 5 min [28]. Bartlett et al. [29] reported similar ranges of between 3 and 7 min, but also reported a wide variance, suggesting that the buffering and clearance capacities are strongly related to individual variations. It was observed that after orange juice ingestion, patients with dental erosion presented both lower pH levels at the tooth surface and lower clearance capacity [27], which explains why they are at higher risk compared to healthy individuals. Recovery of the pH, however, was faster than that reported in other studies. Interestingly, drinking water was an effective measure to increase the pH values close to the initial levels [27].

Saliva also allows the deposition of the acquired pellicle, a protein-based layer dynamically

formed on dental surfaces after its removal by toothbrushing with dentifrice, chemical dissolution or prophylaxis. The acquired pellicle protects against erosion by preventing direct contact between the acids and the tooth surface [30; see chapter by Hannig and Hannig, this vol., pp. 206–214]. This protective effect is dictated by the composition, thickness and maturation time of the pellicle and limited by the aggressiveness of the erosive challenge. Hara et al. [31] showed that a 2-hour acquired pellicle formed on enamel surfaces in situ was able to reduce the demineralization provided by orange juice of up to 10 min of acid exposure using an in situ erosion model (fig. 1a, b). However, no measurable protection was detected after 20 and 30 min of acid exposure. It was speculated that the 10-min acid exposure, which consisted of sipping 10 ml of the juice, holding it for 15 s in the mouth, spitting and resting for 15 s to repeat the procedure 39 more times, could simulate the ingestion of a regular cup of beverage (400 ml) over a 20-min period. This level of acid exposure is considered a high risk of erosion behavior. Interestingly, no protection could be found in this study for the dentine substrate covered by the 2-hour pellicle. It is unclear whether that relates to differences in the pellicle composition, but it has been suggested that differences in the nature and composition of the substrates may affect the pellicle composition and properties [32]. It could also be suggested that no protection was found for dentine because of the higher susceptibility of dentine to demineralization, which could have resulted in the pellicle being quickly lost together with the etched dentine [31].

Some morphological aspects may interfere with saliva action and erosion development. Different sites of the mouth may render teeth more susceptible to erosion, not only because of different salivary protection but also because of their exposure to mechanical forces resulting from the contact with surrounding soft tissues [33] and tongue [34].

Action after Erosion

Once the erosive agent is neutralized or cleared from the tooth surface, the salivary calcium and phosphate can remineralize eroded enamel [35, 36]. Substantial enhancement of remineralization occurs in the presence of fluoride ions [37–39]. The effect of the length of the remineralization time has been investigated [40]. Enamel specimens eroded by citric acid for 2 h and immersed in artificial saliva showed partial rehardening after 1–4 h, while specimens remineralized for 6–24 h showed a complete rehardening. An in situ study analyzing the surface microhardness recovery of enamel and dentine eroded by acidic beverage showed up to 37.8% of remineralization of enamel specimens after 24 h of exposure to the oral environment [41]. When treated with fluoride gel after the erosive attack, the remineralization rate of enamel specimens significantly increased to 57.2%. Similarly, it was shown that eroded dentine had a surface microhardness recovery of about 55.4%; however, no additional protection was observed for fluoride gel treatment in this substrate [41]. Some limited remineralization benefit of saliva has also been demonstrated in other in situ

studies, where exposure of dietary acid-eroded dental surfaces to saliva reduced the subsequent toothbrushing abrasive wear [42–44]. However, this protection could not be observed in a recent epidemiological study with over 3,000 persons [45; see chapters by Lussi and Carvalho, this vol., pp. 1–15 and Wiegand and Schlueter, this vol., pp. 215–219]. The many differences in the experimental methods between them may explain the contrasting results. Nevertheless, it is also important to question the magnitude of the protection by saliva remineralization on the overall erosion prevention. The histopathology of enamel erosion lesions suggests that there are only limited areas for remineralization to take place, as part of the lesion is etched away during the acid attack [46].

Although important, the saliva protection (before, during and after acid exposure) may not be enough to prevent dental erosion. These abovementioned biological protective factors are best understood if considered as a physiological host response to occasional or mild episodes of acid challenge in the mouth. No pathological consequences occur unless the acid challenge (strength and/or frequency) exceeds a certain threshold or the host response is not adequate to counteract the erosive challenge. As emphasized by Meurman et al. [24], if the erosive challenge is strong enough even normal salivary flow and function cannot protect the teeth. As a consequence, dental erosion could be dramatically enhanced by highly erosive challenges and/or by salivary dysfunction.

Hyposalivation and Dental Erosion

Detrimental Effects

Hyposalivation can be defined as the decrease of unstimulated and stimulated salivary flow rates to less than 0.1 and 0.7 ml/min, respectively [5]. This salivary gland hypofunction is mainly caused by the side effect of drugs, Sjögren's syndrome, radiation treatment for head and neck cancer and specific dietary and exercise patterns [47]. Its prevalence has been reported to be around 30% in patients aged between 20 and 69 years [48]. Hyposalivation has negative implications not only on the individual's oral health but also on quality of life [49]. Its frequent symptoms include the sensation of dry mouth, difficulty in swallowing, speaking, eating and wearing dentures, a burning feeling in the tongue, pain and irritation in the mucosa, and frequent thirst. Associated with the common clinical signs is the presence of rapid and severe caries [50] and dental erosion [23, 51, 52]. Tests of the stimulated and unstimulated flow rate as well as of the buffer capacity of saliva may provide useful information about the individual risk to dental erosion. Sialometric evaluations should be carried out at a fixed time point or in a limited time interval in the morning, avoiding intra-individual variations due to the circadian cycle [53].

Despite the above facts, only limited knowledge exists on the clinical efficacy of existing preventive and therapeutic measures for erosion in the hyposalivatory population. Gedalia et al. [54] showed an additive dental erosion protection of a fluoride mouth rinse (0.025% of fluoride as amine fluoride and SnF_2) and a source of calcium (hard cheese masticated for 5 min) in the remineralization of eroded enamel clinically.

Compensating for the Lack of Saliva with Preventive Measures

Salivary mechanical and chemical stimulation as well as the use of saliva substitutes have been suggested to compensate for the lack of saliva. Highly fluoridated and calcium-containing oral care products have also been considered. While no definite clinical evidence exists, some laboratory studies have investigated their potential on dental erosion prevention.

An in vitro study simulating hyposalivatory conditions (flow rate of 0.05 ml/min) showed a significant increase of dental erosion [55]. In those circumstances, fluoridated toothpastes helped in reducing the development of erosive lesions. However, there was no additional benefit by using highly concentrated fluoridated toothpastes (5,000 ppm F, as NaF) compared to the regular formulations (1,100 ppm F, as NaF). It is speculated that under clinical conditions better retention of fluoride may happen in the mouth due to the presence of other potential reservoirs. In addition, it should be borne in mind that hyposalivatory patients would keep a higher concentration of the dentifrice in the mouth for a longer time, as there is less dilution in saliva and salivary clearance is reduced [56]. Therefore, clinical studies are still needed to further verify the potential of highly fluoridated toothpastes to prevent erosion in hyposalivatory patients.

Another approach to increase the fluoride retention (and benefits) in the mouth is the use of a calcium rinse before the fluoride rinse. The theory behind it, as suggested by Vogel et al. [57], states that the presence of calcium will increase the number of sites for the retention of fluoride, making it more available and for longer. To verify whether this combination could provide enhanced protection in hyposalivatory conditions, a laboratory study using a similar hyposalivatory model was used [58]. It was observed that the calcium prerinse provided additional protection against erosion, but only on root dentine. Interestingly, a substantial increase in the fluoride concentration was observed on the enamel and root dentine surfaces when treated with the calcium prerinse. Similar results were observed when using calcium-containing toothpastes [unpubl. data], which shows that calcium-containing mouth rinses and dentifrices may potentially provide protection against erosion in particularly higher risk conditions, including those represented by reduced salivary flow.

Saliva Expression of the Individual's Response to Dental Erosion

Saliva represents the biological expression of an individual's susceptibility to dental erosion, as observed in studies using well-controlled experimental conditions. Wetton et al. [59] reported that saliva from different donors offered differing protection levels against enamel and dentine erosion. In this study, dental specimens were repeatedly exposed for 2 h to the collected saliva, followed by citric acid for 10 min. Some saliva samples reduced dental erosion in enamel and dentine, while the sample of 1 subject led to increased enamel loss. In previous studies using well-standardized intra-oral demineralization [38] and remineralization [60] models, it was also possible to observe great variation of susceptibility to dental erosion among participants, with some showing extensive demineralization and/or remineralization and others not. These models provided a high level of control for chemical (acid challenge, fluoride exposure), behavioral (acid intake mode, frequency, subject's compliance) and biological (salivary flow rate) factors, thus allowing dental erosion to express according to the subject's individual salivary properties and composition. Interestingly, no clear correlation was found between saliva properties (pH, buffer capacity) and inorganic composition (Ca, P and F) and the susceptibility of enamel to demineralization [unpubl. data], suggesting that the individual organic (protein) composition of saliva, either alone or in association with salivary chemical properties, may play an important role in the erosion demineralization and remineralization processes. Jager et al. [61] further investigated the influence of salivary factors on the erosion of pellicle-covered hydroxyapatite discs and observed that sodium, urea, total protein, albumin, pH and flow of unstimulated saliva, as well as sodium, potassium, urea and phosphorus of stimulated saliva, had significant roles.

Publications have suggested that salivary proteins may be key biomarkers for several systemic diseases [62, 63]. Specific salivary proteins may also be relevant biomarkers for dental erosion, since it has been reported that they can potentially influence dental demineralization and remineralization [64]. Statherins [65–67], proline-

rich proteins [65, 68], histatins [69] and cystatins [70] have shown a high affinity to enamel surface. Thus, it is postulated that those salivary proteins can provide protection against acid attack. Acquired enamel pellicle proteins such as albumin, mucin, acidic proline-rich proteins and cystatins have been shown to be important contributors to the protection of enamel from acid-induced demineralization [71–74].

Recent studies have contrasted some of the saliva properties and characteristics between populations with and without clinical signs of erosion. Hellwig et al. [75] collected saliva from 10 volunteers with and without severe clinical signs of dental erosion and individually mixed it with sour drops or citric acid. Enamel specimens were soaked in the mixture for 5 min and were subsequently incubated in saliva for 2 min. This cycle was repeated 3 times, and then the specimens were kept in saliva for 8 h in order to verify remineralization effects. Erosion was measured by surface microhardness, and decreased significantly in all groups except for the saliva (control) group. For sour drops and citric acid mixed with saliva from patients without erosion, the final microhardness was higher compared to the mixture of the two erosive compounds with saliva from patients with erosion. Subsequent storage in saliva resulted in some minor remineralization, especially in the group that was least demineralized (sour drops plus saliva from patients without erosion). It was concluded that salivary components play a crucial role in the development of dental erosion.

Recently, Wang et al. [76] observed no difference in the flow rate, pH level, buffering capacity, bicarbonate, buffer base, calcium, phosphorus and urea concentrations of whole saliva between a dental erosion population and its age-matched (12–13 years old) and sex-matched controls. Piangprach et al. [77] studied different properties of saliva between erosion and nonerosion patients, stratified by age, and observed greater unstimulated salivary buffering capacity and urea concentration when no erosion was present in participants aged 16–20 years. In the group aged 46–50 years, stimulated salivary total protein was significantly higher in the group with enamel erosion. Zwier et al. [78] tested the saliva collected from 88 adolescents with erosion and 49 controls (aged 16 ± 1 years) for flow rate, pH and buffer capacity, as well as for total protein content, carbonic anhydrase VI, amylase, albumin, calcium, phosphate, urea, sodium, chloride and potassium. Interestingly, only unstimulated flow rate and chloride concentration in unstimulated saliva were found to be significantly different between the studied populations. However, the authors pointed out that due to the multifactorial nature of dental erosion a larger sample size and possibly more evident differences between the erosion and matched-control populations would be necessary to better establish the role of saliva in dental erosion. Due to these limitations and some conflicting results, finding a strong predictor for dental erosion among the several existing salivary parameters may be a very difficult task to accomplish.

Perhaps a better approach would be to focus on the search for biological markers in the dental-acquired pellicle, as it has a more intimate relationship with the dental surfaces. The characteristics, properties and composition of the dental pellicle in relation to dental erosion are thoroughly reviewed in the chapter by Hannig and Hannig [this vol., pp. 206–214].

Despite the evidence suggesting the beneficial role of saliva and acquired pellicle on dental erosion, there is still need for further understanding of their importance on the clinical expression of dental erosion. Recent developments of sensitive proteomic methodologies have opened new avenues for the characterization of very low-abundance biological samples. Using this proteomic technology, more than 130 different proteins have been identified in the dental pellicle [64, 79]; however, there is no clear understanding of their roles in dental erosion development. Nonetheless, it is known that those proteins can modulate the mineral homeostasis of tooth surfaces and the development of the acquired dental pellicle. Moazzez et al. [80] have observed differences in the erosion protection of the pellicle formed by dietary dental erosion patients compared to healthy age-matched controls. It seems that the complex balance between the remineralization induction by saliva mineral supersaturation, the inhibition of apatite mineral formation and the inhibition of dental dissolution by acquired enamel pellicle proteins are important factors modulating dental demineralization and remineralization [81]. Provided that these proteins can significantly affect the mineral gain or loss from the dental structures in clinical conditions, their presence could be used as potential biomarkers to identify individual risk status for dental erosion development.

References

1 Zero DT: Etiology of dental erosion – extrinsic factors. Eur J Oral Sci 1996; 104:162–177.
2 Lussi A, Jaeggi T, Zero D: The role of diet in the aetiology of dental erosion. Caries Res 2004;38:34–44.
3 Zero DT, Lussi A: Etiology of enamel erosion – intrinsic and extrinsic factors; in Tooth Wear and Sensitivity. London, Martin Dunitz, 2000, pp 121–139.
4 Tenovuo J: Salivary parameters of relevance for assessing caries activity in individuals and populations. Community Dent Oral Epidemiol 1997;25:82–86.
5 Navazesh M, Kumar SK: Measuring salivary flow: challenges and opportunities. J Am Dent Assoc 2008;139:35S–40S.
6 West NX, Maxwell A, Hughes JA, Parker DM, Newcombe RG, Addy M: A method to measure clinical erosion: the effect of orange juice consumption on erosion of enamel. J Dent 1998;26:329–335.
7 Lee VM, Linden RW: An olfactory-submandibular salivary reflex in humans. Exp Physiol 1992;77:221–224.
8 Engelen L, de Wijk RA, Prinz JF, van der Bilt A, Bosman F: The relation between saliva flow after different stimulations and the perception of flavor and texture attributes in custard desserts. Physiol Behav 2003;78:165–169.

9 Christensen CM, Navazesh M: Anticipatory salivary flow to the sight of different foods. Appetite 1984;5:307–315.

10 Lee M, Feldman M: Nausea and vomiting; in Feldman M, Scharschmidt B, Sleisenger M (eds): Sleisenger and Fordtran's Gastrointestinal and Liver Disease: Pathophysiology, Diagnosis, Management, ed. 6. Philadelphia, Saunders, 1998, pp 117–127.

11 Saksena R, Bartlett DW, Smith BG: The role of saliva in regurgitation erosion. Eur J Prosthodont Restor Dent 1999;7:121–124.

12 Larsen MJ, Pearce EI: Saturation of human saliva with respect to calcium salts. Arch Oral Biol 2003;48:317–322.

13 Dodds MW, Johnson DA, Yeh CK: Health benefits of saliva: a review. J Dent 2005;33:223–233.

14 Dawes C, Kubieniec K: The effects of prolonged gum chewing on salivary flow rate and composition. Arch Oral Biol 2004;49:665–669.

15 Ferguson DB: Salivary glands and saliva; in Applied Physiology of the Mouth. Bristol, Wright, 1975, pp 145–179.

16 Corrêa MC, Lerco MM, Cunha Mde L, Henry MA: Salivary parameters and teeth erosions in patients with gastroesophageal reflux disease. Arq Gastroenterol 2012;49:214–218.

17 Gudmundsson K, Kristleifsson G, Theodors A, Holbrook WP: Tooth erosion, gastroesophageal reflux, and salivary buffer capacity. Oral Surg Oral Med Oral Pathol Oral Radiol Endod 1995;79:185–189.

18 Moazzez R, Bartlett D, Anggiansah A: Dental erosion, gastro-oesophageal reflux disease and saliva: how are they related? J Dent 2004;32:489–494.

19 Lussi A, Megert B, Shellis RP, Wang X: Analysis of the erosive effect of different dietary substances and medications. Br J Nutr 2012;107:252–262.

20 Yeh CK, Johnson DA, Dodds MW, Sakai S, Rugh JD, Hatch JP: Association of salivary flow rates with maximal bite force. J Dent Res 2000;79:1560–1565.

21 Scott BJ, Bajaj J, Linden RW: The contribution of mechanoreceptive neurones in the gingival tissues to the masticatory-parotid salivary reflex in man. J Oral Rehabil 1999;26:791–797.

22 Paice EM, Vowles RW, West NX, Hooper SM: The erosive effects of saliva following chewing gum on enamel and dentine: an ex vivo study. Br Dent J 2011;210:E3.

23 Jarvinen VK, Rytomaa II, Heinonen OP: Risk factors in dental erosion. J Dent Res 1991;70:942–947.

24 Meurman JH, Toskala J, Nuutinen P, Klemetti E: Oral and dental manifestations in gastroesophageal reflux disease. Oral Surg Oral Med Oral Pathol 1994;78:583–589.

25 Bashir E, Ekberg O, Lagerlof F: Salivary clearance of citric acid after an oral rinse. J Dent 1995;23:209–212.

26 Young WG, Khan F: Sites of dental erosion are saliva-dependent. J Oral Rehabil 2002;29:35–43.

27 Lussi A, von Salis-Marincek M, Ganss C, Hellwig E, Cheaib Z, Jaeggi T: Clinical study monitoring the pH on tooth surfaces in patients with and without erosion. Caries Res 2012;46:507–512.

28 Millward A, Shaw L, Harrington E, Smith AJ: Continuous monitoring of salivary flow rate and pH at the surface of the dentition following consumption of acidic beverages. Caries Res 1997;31:44–49.

29 Bartlett DW, Bureau GP, Anggiansah A: Evaluation of the pH of a new carbonated soft drink beverage: an in vivo investigation. J Prosthodont 2003;12:21–25.

30 Hannig M: Ultrastructural investigation of pellicle morphogenesis at two different intraoral sites during a 24-hour period. Clin Oral Investig 1999;3:88–95.

31 Hara AT, Ando M, González-Cabezas C, Cury JA, Serra MC, Zero DT: Protective effect of the dental pellicle against erosive challenges in situ. J Dent Res 2006;85:612–616.

32 Glantz PO, Baier RE, Christersson CE: Biochemical and physiological considerations for modeling biofilms in the oral cavity: a review. Dent Mater 1996;12:208–214.

33 Amaechi BT, Higham SM, Edgar WM: Influence of abrasion in clinical manifestation of human dental erosion. J Oral Rehabil 2003;30:407–413.

34 Gregg T, Mace S, West NX, Addy M: A study in vitro of the abrasive effect of the tongue on enamel and dentine softened by acid erosion. Caries Res 2004;38:557–560.

35 Gedalia I, Dakuar A, Shapira L, Lewinstein I, Goultschin J, Rahamim E: Enamel softening with Coca-Cola and rehardening with milk or saliva. Am J Dent 1991;4:120–122.

36 Zero DT, Fu J, Scott-Anne K, Proskin H: Evaluation of fluoride dentifrices using a short-term intraoral remineralization model. J Dent Res 1994;73:272.

37 Hooper SM, Newcombe RG, Faller R, Eversole S, Addy M, West NX: The protective effects of toothpaste against erosion by orange juice: studies in situ and in vitro. J Dent 2007;35:476–481.

38 Hara AT, Kelly SA, González-Cabezas C, Eckert GJ, Barlow AP, Mason SC, Zero DT: Influence of fluoride availability of dentifrices on eroded enamel remineralization in situ. Caries Res 2009;43:57–63.

39 Ren YF, Liu X, Fadel N, Malmstrom H, Barnes V, Xu T: Preventive effects of dentifrice containing 5,000 ppm fluoride against dental erosion in situ. J Dent 2011;39:672–678.

40 Eisenburger M, Addy M, Hughes JA, Shellis RP: Effect of time on the remineralisation of enamel by synthetic saliva after citric acid erosion. Caries Res 2001;35:211–215.

41 Fushida CE, Cury JA: Evaluation of enamel-dentine erosion by beverage and recovery by saliva and fluoride. J Dent Res 1999;78:410.

42 Jaeggi T, Lussi A: Toothbrush abrasion of erosively altered enamel after intraoral exposure to saliva: an in situ study. Caries Res 1999;33:455–461.

43 Hara AT, Turssi CP, Teixeira EC, Serra MC, Cury JA: Abrasive wear on eroded root dentine after different periods of exposure to saliva in situ. Eur J Oral Sci 2003;111:423–427.

44 Attin T, Siegel S, Buchalla W, Lennon AM, Hannig C, Becker K: Brushing abrasion of softened and remineralised dentin: an in situ study. Caries Res 2004;38:62–66.

45 Bartlett DW, Lussi A, West NX, Bouchard P, Sanz M, Bourgeois D: Prevalence of tooth wear on buccal and lingual surfaces and possible risk factors in young European adults. J Dent 2013;41:1007–1013.

46 Lussi A, Schlueter N, Rakhmatullina E, Ganss C: Dental erosion – an overview with emphasis on chemical and histopathological aspects. Caries Res 2011;45(suppl 1):2–12.

47 Tschoppe P, Wolgin M, Pischon N, Kielbassa AM: Etiologic factors of hyposalivation and consequences for oral health. Quintessence Int 2010;41:321–333.

48 Flink H, Bergdahl M, Tegelberg A, Rosenblad A, Lagerlof F: Prevalence of hyposalivation in relation to general health, body mass index and remaining teeth in different age groups of adults. Community Dent Oral Epidemiol 2008;36:523–531.

49 Cassolato SF, Turnbull RS: Xerostomia: clinical aspects and treatment. Gerodontology 2003;20:64–77.
50 Sreebny L, Baum B, Edgar W, Epstein J, Fox P, Larmas M: Saliva: its role in health and diseases. Int Dent J 1992;42: 291–304.
51 Rytomaa I, Jarvinen V, Kanerva R, Heinonen OP: Bulimia and tooth erosion. Acta Odontol Scand 1998;56:36–40.
52 Jensdottir T, Buchwald C, Nauntofte B, Hansen HS, Bardow A: Saliva in relation to dental erosion before and after radiotherapy. Acta Odontol Scand 2013;71: 1008–1013.
53 Flink H, Tegelberg A, Lagerlof F: Influence of the time of measurement of unstimulated human whole saliva on the diagnosis of hyposalivation. Arch Oral Biol 2005;50:553–559.
54 Gedalia I, Braustein E, Lewinstein I, Shapira L, Ever-Hadani P, Sela M: Fluoride and hard cheese exposure on etched enamel in neck-irradiated patients in situ. J Dent 1996;24:365–368.
55 Scaramucci T, Borges AB, Lippert F, Frank NE, Hara AT: Sodium fluoride effect on erosion-abrasion under hyposalivatory simulating conditions. Arch Oral Biol 2013;58:1457–1463.
56 Billings RJ, Adair SM, Shields CP, Moss ME: Clinical evaluation of new designs for intraoral fluoride-releasing systems. Pediatr Dent 1998;20:17–24.
57 Vogel GL, Chow LC, Carey CM: Calcium pre-rinse greatly increases overnight salivary fluoride after a 228-ppm fluoride rinse. Caries Res 2008;42:401–404.
58 Borges AB, Scaramucci T, Lippert F, Zero DT, Hara AT: Erosion protection by calcium lactate/sodium fluoride rinses under different salivary flows in vitro. Caries Res 2014;48:193–199.
59 Wetton S, Hughes J, Newcombe RG, Addy M: The effect of saliva derived from different individuals on the erosion of enamel and dentine. A study in vitro. Caries Res 2007;41:423–426.
60 Zero DT, Hara AT, Kelly SA, González-Cabezas C, Eckert GJ, Barlow AP, Mason SC: Evaluation of a desensitizing test dentifrice using an in situ erosion remineralization model. J Clin Dent 2006; 17:112–116.

61 Jager DH, Vieira AM, Ligtenberg AJ, Bronkhorst E, Huysmans MC, Vissink A: Effect of salivary factors on the susceptibility of hydroxyapatite to early erosion. Caries Res 2011;45:532–537.
62 Van Nieuw Amerongen A, Bolscher JG, Veerman EC: Salivary proteins: protective and diagnostic value in cariology? Caries Res 2004;38:247–253.
63 Wong DT: Salivary diagnostics powered by nanotechnologies, proteomics and genomics. J Am Dent Assoc 2006;137: 313–321.
64 Siqueira WL, Zhang W, Helmerhorst EJ, Gygi SP, Oppenheim FG: Identification of protein components in in vivo human acquired enamel pellicle using LC-ESI-MS/MS. J Proteome Res 2007;6:2152–2160.
65 Moreno EC, Varughese K, Hay DI: Effect of human salivary proteins on the precipitation kinetics of calcium phosphate. Calcif Tissue Int 1979;28:7–16.
66 Hay DI, Schluckebier SK, Moreno EC: Equilibrium dialysis and ultrafiltration studies of calcium and phosphate binding by human salivary proteins. Implications for salivary supersaturation with respect to calcium phosphate salts. Calcif Tissue Int 1982;34:531–538.
67 Hay DI, Smith DJ, Schluckebier SK, Moreno EC: Relationship between concentration of human salivary statherin and inhibition of calcium phosphate precipitation in stimulated human parotid saliva. J Dent Res 1984;63:857–863.
68 Aoba T, Moreno EC, Hay DI: Inhibition of apatite crystal growth by the amino-terminal segment of human salivary acidic proline-rich proteins. Calcif Tissue Int 1984;36:651–658.
69 Richardson CF, Johnsson M, Raj PA, Levine MJ, Nancollas GH: The influence of histatin-5 fragments on the mineralization of hydroxyapatite. Arch Oral Biol 1993;38:997–1002.
70 Johnsson M, Richardson CF, Bergey EJ, Levine MJ, Nancollas GH: The effects of human salivary cystatins and statherin on hydroxyapatite crystallization. Arch Oral Biol 1991;36:631–636.

71 Arends J, Schuthof J, Christoffersen J: Inhibition of enamel demineralization by albumin in vitro. Caries Res 1986;20: 337–340.
72 Nieuw Amerongen AV, Oderkerk CH, Driessen AA: Role of mucins from human whole saliva in the protection of tooth enamel against demineralization in vitro. Caries Res 1987;21:297–309.
73 Bruvo M, Moe D, Kirkeby S, Vorum H, Bardow A: Individual variations in protective effects of experimentally formed salivary pellicles. Caries Res 2009;43: 163–170.
74 Hara AT, Lippert F, Zero DT: Interplay between experimental dental pellicles and stannous-containing toothpaste on dental erosion-abrasion. Caries Res 2013;47:325–329.
75 Hellwig E, Lussi A, Goetz F: Influence of human saliva on the development of artificial erosions. Caries Res 2013;47: 553–558.
76 Wang P, Zhou Y, Zhu YH, Lin HC: Unstimulated and stimulated salivary characteristics of 12- to 13-year-old school-children with and without dental erosion. Arch Oral Biol 2011;56:1328–1332.
77 Piangprach T, Hengtrakool C, Kukiat-trakoon B, Kedjarune-Leggat U: The effect of salivary factors on dental erosion in various age groups and tooth surfaces. J Am Dent Assoc 2009;140: 1137–1143.
78 Zwier N, Huysmans MC, Jager DH, Ruben J, Bronkhorst EM, Truin GJ: Saliva parameters and erosive wear in adolescents. Caries Res 2013;47:548–552.
79 Siqueira WL, Oppenheim FG: Small molecular weight proteins/peptides present in the in vivo formed human acquired enamel pellicle. Arch Oral Biol 2009;54: 437–444.
80 Moazzez RV, Austin RS, Rojas-Serrano M, Carpenter G, Cotroneo E, Proctor G, Zaidel L, Bartlett DW: Comparison of the possible protective effect of the salivary pellicle of individuals with and without erosion. Caries Res 2013;48:57–62.
81 Fujikawa H, Matsuyama K, Uchiyama A, Nakashima S, Ujiie T: Influence of salivary macromolecules and fluoride on enamel lesion remineralization in vitro. Caries Res 2008;42:37–45.

Prof. A.T. Hara
Department of Preventive and Community Dentistry, Oral Health Research Institute
Indiana University School of Dentistry, 415 North Lansing Street
Indianapolis, IN 46202-2876 (USA)
E-Mail ahara@iu.edu

Lussi A, Ganss C (eds): Erosive Tooth Wear. Monogr Oral Sci. Basel, Karger, 2014, vol 25, pp 206–214
DOI: 10.1159/000360376

The Pellicle and Erosion

Matthias Hannig[a] · Christian Hannig[b]

[a]Clinic of Operative Dentistry, Periodontology and Preventive Dentistry, Saarland University, Homburg, and
[b]Clinic of Operative Dentistry, Medical Faculty Carl Gustav Carus, TU Dresden, Dresden, Germany

Abstract

All tooth surfaces exposed to the oral environment are naturally coated by the acquired salivary pellicle. The pellicle is composed of adsorbed macromolecular components from saliva, gingival crevicular fluid, blood, bacteria, mucosa and diet. The pellicle (formed in situ/in vivo) functions as a semipermeable network of adsorbed salivary macromolecules and provides partial protection against acidic challenges; however, it cannot completely prevent demineralization of the tooth surface. The physiological pellicle reduces calcium and phosphate release from the enamel, and much less from the dentinal surface. With high probability, calcium- and phosphate-binding peptides and proteins adsorbed in the basal pellicle layer are of main relevance for the erosion-reducing effects of the natural salivary pellicle. Improvement of the pellicle's protective properties by dietary components (e.g. polyphenolic agents) might be a promising erosion-preventive approach that, however, needs validation by in situ experiments.   © 2014 S. Karger AG, Basel

Dental erosion is described as the loss of dental hard substance due to the chemical action of extrinsic or intrinsic acids without bacterial involvement. The acquired salivary pellicle has been regarded as one key factor in the physiological prevention of dental erosion [1, 2]. The pellicle constitutes an interfacial mediator between the tooth surface and the oral environment [1–3]. Due to its mesh-like ultrastructure [1], the pellicle provides a surface coating through which ions are delivered during de- and remineralization [1, 2, 4].

The present review focuses on the potential of the physiologically formed salivary pellicle to reduce and modulate tooth surface erosion. After a brief overview on pellicle formation and composition, results of recent in vitro, in situ and in vivo studies are presented to elucidate the protective potential of the naturally formed salivary pellicle with regard to tooth erosion.

Pellicle Formation and Composition

The acquired pellicle is formed by the adsorption of proteins, peptides, lipids and other macromolecules present in saliva [1, 2]. Salivary pellicle formation is a dynamic process which starts immediately with the adsorption of single peptides and proteins onto the cleansed tooth surface [1–3]. Within 1 min, an electron-dense pellicle layer (10–20 nm thick) is detectable on the enamel surface [1, 5] (fig. 1). This initial pellicle is formed by an almost instantaneous adsorption of salivary

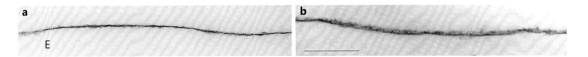

Fig. 1. TEM micrographs of salivary pellicles formed in situ on enamel surfaces within 30 s (**a**) and 60 s (**b**). The pellicle layer reveals an electron-dense, homogeneous ultrastructural appearance and a thickness between 10 and 20 nm. The enamel has been removed during processing of the specimens for the TEM analysis. Original magnification ×30,000. Bar represents 200 nm.

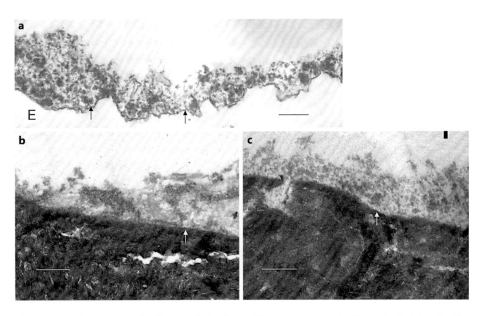

Fig. 2. TEM micrographs of salivary pellicles formed in situ on enamel within 60 min (**a**) and within 2 h on dentine (**b, c**). E = Enamel. The pellicles are characterized by a heterogeneous (mostly globular) outer layer on top of an electron-dense basal layer (arrows). The enamel has been removed during processing of the specimens for the TEM analysis. Original magnification ×30,000. Bars represent 200 nm.

proteins on the enamel surface [1, 2, 5, 6] due to electrostatic interactions between charged groups of the macromolecules on the one hand, and phosphate and calcium ions of the apatite surface on the other hand [1, 2, 7]. In addition to ionic interactions, van der Waals forces and hydrophobic interactions will contribute to the adsorption of salivary proteins to the tooth surface [3]. Subsequent pellicle formation is characterized by protein-protein interactions and the adsorption of single proteins, protein agglomerates and other biomacromolecules, mainly from saliva but also from gingival crevicular fluid, blood, bacteria, mucosa and diet [1, 5, 6, 8].

From previously published transmission electron microscope (TEM) micrographs [5], it has been supposed that the in vivo-formed salivary pellicle consists of two layers: a densely packed basal layer of initially adsorbed proteins onto which a more complex and heterogeneous globular layer, composed of heterotypic protein aggregates, is deposited in a time- and site-dependent manner (fig. 2). This model for in situ pellicle formation has been confirmed recently by surface force spectroscopy and friction force spectroscopy data from in vitro investigations [9–12]. Also, complementary surface characterization methods (surface plasmon resonance and quartz crystal microbalance with dissipation monitoring) for the analysis of the in vitro adsorbed salivary films clearly support this two-layer model [13].

In general, formation of the salivary pellicle has been considered to be a selective process, since only a limited number of the proteins which are detected in saliva are found in the pellicle [14]. Recent investigations using state-of-the-art proteomics have demonstrated that the in vivo-formed enamel pellicle contains more than 130 proteins [15, 16]. When categorizing the pellicle proteins based on their possible role and function, three main groups, together contributing to more than 60% of all pellicle proteins, could be identified [16, 17]. The first group includes proteins which possess the capability to bind calcium ions (e.g. acidic proline-rich proteins, histatins or statherin). The second group consists of proteins revealing a high tendency to bind phosphate ions. The third group is characterized by proteins that are relevant for interactions with other proteins (protein-protein interactions) [16, 17]. Using proteomic approaches, it could be demonstrated very recently that there is a tendency for salivary proteins with high affinity to calcium or phosphate to be more abundant in the early stages (5–10 min) of pellicle formation, while proteins revealing protein-protein interaction properties are more abundant in the later stage (2 h) of in vivo pellicle formation [17]. These data confirm the two-layer model of in vivo pellicle formation from a biochemical point of view.

Over the last years, the peptidome of the in situ pellicle has also been studied intensively [7, 18]. Based on LC-MS (liquid chromatography coupled with mass spectrometry) data, 6 phosphorylated peptides were identified in an intact form in the 2-hour in situ-formed salivary pellicle [7]. By additionally performed tandem MS analysis, 30 fragments of peptides not covalently bound to the enamel could be detected in the 2-hour in situ pellicle [7]. LC-ESI (electrospray ionization)-MS/MS analysis of the 2-hour in vivo-formed salivary pellicle revealed 78 natural peptides with molecular weights ranging from 766.9 to 3,981.4 Da originating from 29 different proteins [18]; 50% of the peptides identified in the 2-hour in vivo-formed pellicle carry a net negative charge at neutral pH [18], exhibiting a high affinity to hydroxyapatite based on charge interactions. These findings support again that electrostatic interactions are important for the initial phase of pellicle formation.

Even though the pellicle's proteome could be characterized in some detail over the last years, information on other macromolecular pellicle components is quite sparse. In current research, gas chromatography coupled with ESI-MS was used for the first time to analyse the fatty acid profile of the in situ pellicle [19, 20]. A total of 11 fatty acids were identified in pellicle samples of 10 subjects [20]. Palmitic, stearic, oleic and erucic acid represent the major ones and account for more than 80% of the pellicle fatty acids [20]. These data provide some very valuable insights with regard to the lipid composition of the salivary pellicle. However, extensive future investigations will be necessary to identify the pellicle's complete lipidome.

Acid-Protective Properties of the Physiological Pellicle

Several in situ and in vivo studies indicate that the salivary pellicle layer has the potential to protect the enamel surface against erosive demineralization [21–29]. In good accordance, all these investigations reveal that the naturally formed pellicle provides an evident inhibitory effect regarding acid-related alterations (e.g. mineral loss, decrease in microhardness and increase in surface roughness) on the enamel surface during erosion [21–29]. However, the effectiveness of the salivary pellicle to reduce demineralization and to protect the enamel surface against erosive acids differs strongly, being dependent on the study designs, and thus it is difficult to assess the exact level of enamel surface protection by the physiologically formed pellicle. The pellicle has been described as a semipermeable membrane that regulates and modifies the demineralization processes at the tooth surface [1, 30]. The physiological pellicle reduces and retards enamel demineralization during acid exposure; however, it does not completely inhibit acid-related changes to the enamel surface [1, 21–29]. It might be assumed that the reduction of calcium loss caused by the in situ-formed enamel pellicle amounts to around 60% [25, 29]. However, the pellicle cannot protect the tooth surface against severe erosive challenges (sipping 10 ml of orange juice for 15 s each time, 40 times, within 10 min) [26]. These in situ findings have been confirmed recently by in vitro data indicating that an in vitro-formed 15-hour salivary pellicle layer provides erosion inhibition in short-term citric acid exposures ($\leq$4 min) [31].

Salivary pellicles formed in situ for 30 min, 1 h and 2 h or for 2, 6, 12 and 24 h do not differ significantly in their ability to reduce enamel demineralization during 60-second citric acid exposure [22–25]. Even short-term enamel pellicles formed in situ within 3 min offer protection against erosive demineralization by citric acid [25]. However, acid resistance of the in situ-formed pellicle layer itself is dependent on formation time, since the 2-hour pellicle dissolves from the enamel surface more quickly than 6-, 12- and 24-hour pellicles [22].

Notwithstanding its clinical relevance, the protective effect of pellicle formation on dentinal surfaces has attracted only little attention to date [26, 29, 32]. The in situ-formed 2-hour pellicle causes reduction of calcium release from dentinal surfaces due to exposure to hydrochloric acid (pH 2.3 or 2.6) of about 30% compared to dentinal specimens without pellicle [29, 32]. TEM investigations on the behaviour of the 2-hour in situ dentine pellicle during acid exposure reveal that the pellicle layer is not completely dissolved from the dentinal surface

due to the 5-min exposure to hydrochloric acid, whereas the underlying dentine is demineralized [32]. This finding clearly indicates that the pellicle is highly permeable for the dissolved calcium and phosphate, as well as for the acid itself [32].

How Does the Pellicle Protect the Tooth Surface against Erosion?

It has been supposed that the pellicle layer is an insoluble network of adsorbed salivary biopolymers [1, 2]. Demineralization of the tooth surface can occur only after diffusion of the acid (H^+ ions) through the pellicle or after (partial) dissolution and removal of the acquired pellicle induced by the interacting acid. Due to its mesh-like structure the pellicle cannot prevent direct contact between the erosive agent and the tooth surface (fig. 3); however, it can reduce and retard immediate interaction between acids and the tooth surface. Furthermore, proteins adsorbed in the pellicle layer might act as a buffer by binding H^+ ions or acids attacking the tooth surface [1, 2].

Up to now, the specific components of the salivary pellicle, which are mainly responsible for the reduction of erosive damage at the enamel surface, have been identified only in part. Proteins that contain calcium-binding domains (such as acidic proline-rich proteins, histatins or statherin) play an important role as pellicle precursor proteins [1, 7, 16, 18, 33] and have been considered to be of relevance for the protective properties of the pellicle against acids [33]. After adsorption to the tooth surface, these calcium-binding proteins might maintain high concentrations of calcium within the pellicle layer and close to the apatite surface, thereby stabilizing the enamel surface and reducing the erosive demineralization. However, further studies are needed to understand in detail how binding of proteins to the enamel crystallites influences acid-mediated surface erosion.

Evidence has been provided that the pellicle layer formed in situ on porcelain discs contains

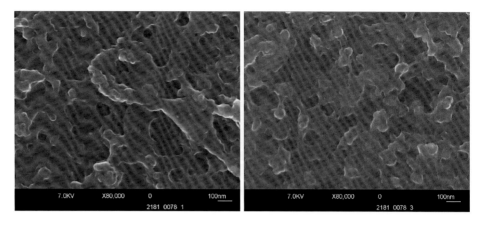

Fig. 3. Field emission in-lens SEM micrographs of salivary pellicle layers formed in situ within 30 min. These SEM micrographs have been obtained after critical point drying of the samples and demonstrate very heterogeneous reticular (left), meshwork-like micromorphology (right) and surface topography of the in situ pellicle.

calcium that can be dissolved by exposure to citric acid [27]. This observation supports the potential function of the pellicle as a depot for calcium ions. In addition, it has been shown recently by in vitro experiments that undialyzed whole saliva is significantly more effective in protecting the enamel surface against erosive demineralization than dialyzed (ion-depleted) saliva [34]. These results indicate that the ionic composition of saliva amplifies the demineralization protective effects of the salivary pellicles [34], probably by maintaining a state of saturation of calcium and phosphate ions within the pellicle for counteracting enamel demineralization. Recent data from in vitro investigations also suggest that calcium ions can easily diffuse in and out of the pellicle layer, thereby permitting a 'free' calcium exchange between saliva and the adsorbed pellicle proteins under physiological conditions, which will be important for remineralization processes [4]. Altogether, these findings underline that the pellicle layer plays an important role in maintaining the integrity and mineral homeostasis of the tooth surface.

The in vivo-formed pellicle layer by itself reveals a certain acid resistance [22–24, 32]. Thus,

during acidic attack, the pellicle layer is not immediately and totally removed from the enamel surface, but rather gradually dissolved from its external to basal components [22–24, 32]. Whereas the outer globular pellicle layer reveals a comparatively high solubility in acids, the densely arranged basal pellicle layer provides a high stability against dissolution by acids [22–24, 32]. Nevertheless, this innermost pellicle layer is permeable for ions [32].

In most studies regarding the erosion-protective properties of the in situ-formed salivary pellicle layer, enamel specimens coated by in situ pellicles were incubated ex vivo with different acids under in vitro conditions to study the protective potential of the pellicle. Only few studies analysed the protective function of the pellicle during in vivo consumption of acidic agents [26, 35]. In order to investigate the protective properties of the physiological pellicle layer during the consumption of acidic beverages, volunteers carried enamel specimens for 2 h intra-orally [35]. In the following, they drank 200 ml of orange juice (pH 3.8), Coke Light (pH 2.8) or Sprite Light (pH 2.8), respectively, over a period of 20 s under in vivo conditions (i.e. with the specimens kept inserted in the oral cavity) [35]. Measurement of Knoop microhardness revealed only little reduction of the relative hardness values of the enamel surface immediately after in vivo consumption of Sprite Light (5.3%) and Coke Light (7.5%) [35]; with orange juice, almost no change of the microhardness was recorded. TEM investigation showed that the outer globular layer of the in situ-formed 2-hour pellicles had been removed during the 20-second drinking period of the acidic beverages, whereas the electron-dense basal layer of the pellicle was not affected by the acidic beverages [35]. Interestingly, on specimens that had been carried in situ for a further 2 h after drinking the beverages, it could be detected by TEM that eroded nanolacunae underneath the basal pellicle at the enamel surface were filled with proteinaceous structures [35]. These pellicle structures in the eroded enamel depict a repair process of superficial erosive defects due to infiltration and adsorption of salivary proteins. On the one hand, this proteinaceous filling of superficial enamel defects might act as guard rail for subsequent remineralization; on the other hand, it may function as a 'subsurface' pellicle layer, reducing the solubility of the enamel surface and increasing tooth protection against erosive challenges. This subsurface pellicle formation (fig. 4) represents a hitherto widely underestimated protective function of the physiologically formed salivary pellicle under in vivo conditions, although already in 1965 Meckel [36] described the subsurface pellicle layer based on electron microscopic analyses. Further investigations are needed to elucidate this important aspect of pellicle formation and the relevance of the protein-enriched enamel surface layer concerning its susceptibility to acidic challenges and prevention of erosive demineralization.

Contradicting results have been reported with regard to the relation between the thickness of the pellicle and its acid-protective potential [21, 23, 24]. On the one hand, a correlation between the thickness of the in situ pellicle and its protecting effect against acid has been shown [21]. On the

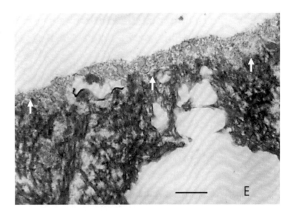

Fig. 4. TEM micrograph of an in situ pellicle formed within 24 h in palatal position on an enamel surface that was etched with phosphoric acid for 60 s before intra-oral exposure of the specimen. E = Enamel. The etched enamel surface has been filled by adsorbed salivary proteins, forming an electron-dense subsurface pellicle on top of which the granular surface pellicle has formed. Arrows indicate the borderline between subsurface and surface pellicle. The enamel has been removed during processing of the specimens for the TEM analysis. Original magnification ×30,000. Bar represents 200 nm.

other hand, no clear influence of the thickness of the in situ pellicle and its protective properties could be observed [23, 24]. Thus, further investigations are necessary to clarify the relevance of the pellicle's thickness for its erosion-inhibiting effects.

Differences in the level of protection against enamel erosion have been reported between individual saliva sources [37, 38]. In vitro as well as ex vivo investigations indicate that saliva from different donors or in situ pellicle layers formed by different volunteers yield different levels of protection against erosion [27, 37, 38]. Very recently, it could be demonstrated by surface microhardness measurements that 1-hour pellicle layers formed in situ in healthy subjects reveal a higher potential to protect the enamel surface than salivary pellicle formed over 1 h in individuals with clinically manifested erosion [28], clearly underlining the relevance of subject-related factors concerning the extent of individual erosion.

Is It Possible to Enhance the Protective Properties of the Salivary Pellicle against Erosion?

A promising approach for the prevention of erosive demineralization of the tooth surface would be reinforcement of the pellicle's protective properties by modifying its composition [39–47]. Dietary components (such as casein, polyphenols or lipids) which have the ability to become adsorbed and incorporated into the salivary pellicle layer have been supposed to increase the pellicle's erosion-inhibiting potential [39–47].

Casein has been thought to be an important component of the salivary pellicle concerning its acid-protective properties [39–41]. Casein reveals an erosion-decreasing effect after adsorption on the enamel [39, 40]. Based on in vitro data it has been concluded that casein will be firmly adsorbed to the hydroxyapatite surface, thereby stabilizing the crystallite surface and inhibiting ion detachment during acid attack [39]. Interestingly, the efficacy of casein as a barrier to acids is enhanced in the presence of a salivary pellicle layer [41]. In contrast, Cheaib and Lussi [42] reported that the addition of casein alone has no effect on the erosion-inhibiting properties of an experimental pellicle under in vitro conditions. However, the combination of casein and (pig) mucin increases the efficacy of the in vitro pellicle against acid-induced enamel softening [42].

As shown by previous in vitro experiments, treatment with polyphenolic agents causes an increase in pellicle thickness [43, 44]. Polyphenols will induce precipitation and aggregation of salivary proteins [43, 44]. These protein/polyphenol aggregates will be readily adsorbed at the pellicle surface, thereby increasing the pellicle's thickness [43, 44]. Furthermore, polyphenolic agents will become incorporated in the pellicle layer, causing a dramatic reduction of the elutability of the adsorbed proteins due to a cross-linking reaction with the polyphenols [43, 44]. An increase in pellicle thickness might enhance the protective properties of the pellicle layer against erosion under in situ conditions [45]. However, the influence of polyphenolic agents on salivary pellicle formation and function has not yet been investigated by in situ studies in detail.

Lipophilic agents (lipids) can modify the composition and ultrastructure of the salivary pellicle [46, 47] and thus it has been assumed that a lipid-enriched pellicle layer would be more resistant to erosive acid exposure [46]. However, the few data available on in situ pellicle modification by oil treatment do not support this hypothesis. TEM analyses have demonstrated scattered adsorption of micelle-like structures/lipid nanovesicles (200–400 nm in diameter) to the pellicle surface after 10 min of in vivo rinsing with safflower oil-containing solutions [46, 47]. The lipid vesicles become – at least in part – integrated into the pellicle layer, causing a less dense, looser ultrastructural appearance of the 2-hour in situ pellicle compared to controls [46, 47]. Furthermore, TEM investigations indicate that exposing the oil-modified pellicle layer to hydrochloric acid at low pH values results in faster and stronger degradation than observed for the control pellicle [47]. Thus, treatment by safflower oil will neither retard disintegration of the in situ pellicle nor enhance its preventive effect against erosion [47]. On the contrary, in situ pellicle modification by safflower oil results in an increased calcium loss from the enamel surface at pH values between 2 and 3 [47].

Conclusion

Up to now, only limited scientific data have been available concerning the protective potential of the salivary pellicle against tooth erosion under in situ and in vivo conditions. During short-term exposure to acidic agents, the physiological pellicle provides partial protection against erosive mineral loss in a pH-dependent manner. Thereby, the pellicle functions as a diffusion-limiting, semipermeable network, which is continuously dissolved during acid exposure, rather than as a barrier.

References

1 Hannig M, Joiner A: The structure, function and properties of the acquired pellicle; in Druckworth RM (ed): The Teeth and Their Environment. Monogr Oral Sci 2006;19:29–64.

2 Siqueira WL, Custodio W, Mc Donald EE: New insights into the composition and functions of the acquired enamel pellicle. J Dent Res 2012;91:1110–1118.

3 Hannig C, Hannig M: The oral cavity – a key system to understand substratum-dependent bioadhesion on solid surfaces in man. Clin Oral Invest 2009;13:123–139.

4 Ash A, Ridout MJ, Parker R, Machie AR, Burnett GR, Wilde PJ: Effect of calcium ions on in vitro pellicle formation from parotid and whole saliva. Colloids Surf B Biointerfaces 2013;102:546–553.

5 Hannig M: Ultrastructural investigation of pellicle morphogenesis at two different intraoral sites during a 24-hour period. Clin Oral Investig 1999;3:88–95.

6 Zhang YF, Zheng J, Zheng L, Shi XY, Qian LM, Zhou ZR: Effect of adsorption time on the lubricating properties of the salivary pellicle on human tooth enamel. Wear 2013;301:300–307.

7 Vitorino R, Calheiros-Lobo MJ, Williams J, Ferrer-Correia AJF, Tomer KB, Duarte JA, Domingues PM, Amado FML: Peptidomic analysis of human acquired enamel pellicle. Biomed Chromatogr 2007;21:1107–1117.

8 Vitkov L, Hannig M, Nekrashevych Y, Krautgartner W D: Supramolecular pellicle precursors. Eur J Oral Sci 2004;112:320–325.

9 Cárdenas M, Arnebrant T, Rennie A, Fragneto G, Thomas RK, Lindh L: Human saliva forms a complex film structure on alumina surfaces. Biomacromolecules 2007;8:65–69.

10 Cárdenas M, Valle-Delgado JJ, Hamit J, Rutland MW, Anrebrant T: Interactions of hydroxyapatite surfaces: conditioning films of human whole saliva. Langmuir 2008;24:7262–7268.

11 Harvey NM, Yakubov GE, Stokes JR, Klein J: Lubrication and load-bearing properties of human salivary pellicles adsorbed ex vivo on molecularly smooth substrata. Biofouling 2012;8:843–856.

12 Sotres J, Lindh L, Arnebrant T: Friction force spectroscopy as a tool to study the strength and structure of salivary films. Langmuir 2011;27:13692–13700.

13 Macakova L, Yakubov GE, Plunkett MA, Stokes JR: Influence of ionic strength changes on the structure of pre-adsorbed salivary films. A response of a natural multi-component layer. Colloids Surf B Biointerfaces 2010;77:31–39.

14 Yao Y, Berg EA, Costello CE, Troxler RF, Oppenheim FG: Identification of protein components in human acquired enamel pellicle and whole saliva using novel proteomics approaches. J Biol Chem 2003;14:5300–5308.

15 Siqueira WL, Zhang W, Helmerhorst EJ, Gygi SP, Oppenheim FG: Identification of protein components in in vivo human acquired enamel pellicle using LC-ESI-MS/MS. J Proteome Res 2007;6:2152–2160.

16 Vitorino R, Calheiros-Lobo MJ, Duarte JA, Domingues PM, Amado FML: Peptide profile of human acquired enamel pellicle using MALDI tandem MS. J Sep Sci 2008;31:523–537.

17 Lee YH, Zimmermann JN, Custodio W, Xiao Y, Basiri T, Hatibovic-Kofmann S, Siqueira WL: Proteomic evaluation of acquired enamel pellicle during in vivo formation. PLoS One 2013;8:1–10.

18 Siqueira WL, Oppenheim FG: Small molecular weight proteins/peptides present in the in vivo formed human acquired enamel pellicle. Arch Oral Biol 2009;54:437–444.

19 Reich M, Hannig C, Al-Ahmad A, Bolek R, Kümmerer K: A comprehensive method for determination of fatty acids in the initial oral biofilm (pellicle). J Lipid Res 2012;53:2226–2230.

20 Reich M, Kümmerer K, Al-Ahmad A, Hannig C: Fatty acid profile of the initial oral biofilm (pellicle): an in-situ study. Lipids 2013;48:929–937.

21 Amaechi BT, Higham SM, Edgar WM, Milosevic A: Thickness of acquired salivary pellicle as a determinant of the sites of dental erosion. J Dent Res 1999;78:1821–1828.

22 Hannig M, Hess NJ, Hoth-Hannig W, de Vrese M: Influence of salivary pellicle formation time on enamel demineralization – an in situ pilot study. Clin Oral Invest 2003;7:158–161.

23 Hannig M, Balz B: Influence of in vivo formed salivary pellicle on enamel erosion. Caries Res 1999;33:372–379.

24 Hannig M, Balz M: Protective properties of salivary pellicles from two different intraoral sites on enamel erosion. Caries Res 2001;35:142–148.

25 Hannig M, Fiebiger M, Güntzer M, Döbert A, Zimehl R, Nekrashevych Y: Protective effect of the in situ formed short-term salivary pellicle. Arch Oral Biol 2004;49:903–910.

26 Hara AT, Ando M, González-Caezas C, Cury JA, Serra MC, Zero DT: Protective effect of the dental pellicle against erosive challenges in situ. J Dent Res 2006;85:612–616.

27 Jager DHJ, Vieira AM, Ligtenberg AJM, Bronkhorst E, Huysmans MC, Vissink A: Effect of salivary factors on the susceptibility of hydroxyapatite to early erosion. Caries Res 2011;45:532–537.

28 Moazzez RV, Austin RS, Rojas-Serrano M, Carpenter G, Cotroneo E, Proctor G, Zaidel L, Bartlett DW: Comparison of the possible protective effect of the salivary pellicle of individuals with and without erosion. Caries Res 2014;48:57–62.

29 Wiegand A, Bliggenstorfer S, Magalhães AC, Sener B, Attin T: Impact of the in situ formed salivary pellicle on enamel and dentine erosion induced by different acids. Acta Odontol Scand 2008;66:225–230.

30 Zahradnik RT, Moreno EC, Burke EJ: Effect of salivary pellicle on enamel subsurface demineralization in vitro. J Dent Res 1976;55:664–670.

31 Brevik SC, Lussi A, Rakhmatullina E: A new optical detection method to assess the erosion inhibition by in vitro salivary pellicle layer. J Dent 2013;41:428–435.

32 Hannig C, Becker K, Häusler N, Hoth-Hannig W, Attin T, Hannig M: Protective effect of the in situ pellicle on dentin erosion – an ex vivo pilot study. Arch Oral Biol 2007;52:444–449.

33 Siqueira WL, Margolis HC, Helmerhorst EJ, Mendes FM, Oppenheim FG: Evidence of intact histatins in the in vivo acquired enamel pellicle. J Dent Res 2010;89:626–630.

34 Martins C, Castro GF, Siqueira MF, Xiao Y, Yamaguti PM, Siqueira WL: Effect of dialyzed saliva on human enamel demineralization. Caries Res 2013;47:56–62.

35 Hannig C, Berndt D, Hoth-Hannig W, Hannig M: The effect of acidic beverages on the ultrastructure of the acquired pellicle – an in situ study. Arch Oral Biol 2009;54:518–526.

36 Meckel AD: The formation and properties of organic films on teeth. Arch Oral Biol 1965;10:585–597.

37 Bruvo M, Moe D, Kirkeby S, Vorum H, Bardow A: Individual variations on protective effects of experimentally formed salivary pellicles. Caries Res 2009;43: 163–170.

38 Wetton S, Hughes J, Newcombe RG, Addy M: The effect of saliva derived from different individuals on the erosion of enamel and dentine. Caries Res 2007;41:423–426.

39 Barbour ME; Shellis RP, Parker DM, Allen GC, Addy M: Inhibition of hydroxyapatite dissolution by whole casein: the effects of pH protein concentration, calcium, and ionic strength. Eur J Oral Sci 2008;116:473–478.

40 White AJ, Gracia LG, Barbour ME: Inhibition of dental erosion by casein and casein-derived proteins. Caries Res 2010;45:13–20.

41 Hemingway CA, White AJ, Shellis RP, Addy M, Parker DM, Barbour ME: Enamel erosion in dietary acids: inhibition by food proteins in vitro. Caries Res 2010;44:525–530.

42 Cheaib Z, Lussi A: Impact of acquired enamel pellicle modification on initial dental erosion. Caries Res 2011;45:107–112.

43 Joiner A, Muller D, Elofsson UM, Malmsten M, Arnebrant T: Adsorption from black tea and red wine onto in vitro salivary pellicles studied by ellipsometry. Eur J Oral Sci 2003;111:417–422.

44 Joiner A, Elofsson UM, Arnebrant T: Adsorption of chlorhexidine and black tea onto in vitro salivary pellicles as studied by ellipsometry. Eur J Oral Sci 2006;114:337–342.

45 Dickinson ME, Mann AB: Nanoscale characterization of salivary pellicle. Mater Res Soc Symp Proc 2005, vol 841, pp 63–68.

46 Kensche A, Reich M, Kümmerer K, Hannig M, Hannig C: Lipids in preventive dentistry. Clin Oral Investig 2013; 17:669–685.

47 Hannig C, Wagenschwanz C, Pötschke S, Kümmerer K, Kensche A, Hoth-Hannig W, Hannig M: Effect of safflower oil on the protective properties of the in situ formed salivary pellicle. Caries Res 2012;46:496–506.

Prof. M. Hannig
Clinic of Operative Dentistry, Periodontology and Preventive Dentistry
Saarland University, Building 73
DE–66421 Homburg (Germany)
E-Mail matthias.hannig@uks.eu

Lussi A, Ganss C (eds): Erosive Tooth Wear. Monogr Oral Sci. Basel, Karger, 2014, vol 25, pp 215–219
DOI: 10.1159/000360379

The Role of Oral Hygiene: Does Toothbrushing Harm?

Annette Wiegand[a] · Nadine Schlueter[b]

[a]Department of Preventive Dentistry, Periodontology and Cariology, Georg August University, Göttingen, and [b]Department of Conservative and Preventive Dentistry, Dental Clinic, Justus Liebig University, Giessen, Germany

Abstract

Although toothbrushing is considered a prerequisite for maintaining good oral health, it also has the potential to have an impact on tooth wear, particularly with regard to dental erosion. Experimental studies have demonstrated that tooth abrasion can be influenced by a number of factors, including not only the physical properties of the toothpaste and toothbrush used but also patient-related factors such as toothbrushing frequency and force of brushing. While abrasion resulting from routine oral hygiene can be considered as physiological wear over time, intensive brushing might further harm eroded surfaces by removing the demineralised enamel surface layer. The effects of brushing on eroded dentine are not fully elucidated, particular under in vivo conditions. However, there are indications that brushing after an acid impact causes less additional hard tissue loss in dentine than in enamel. Toothbrushing frequency and force as well as toothbrush hardness were shown to act as co-factors in the multifactorial aetiology of non-cervical carious lesions. In vitro studies showed that toothbrushing abrasion is primarily related to the abrasivity of the toothpaste, while the toothbrush acts as a carrier, only modifying the effects of the toothpaste. The benefits of normal oral hygiene procedure exceed possible side effects by far, but excessive toothbrushing – especially of eroded teeth – might cause some harmful effects.   © 2014 S. Karger AG, Basel

Toothbrushing is generally considered to be a safe and effective means for maintaining oral health [1]. In situ studies have reported clinically irrelevant levels of enamel loss (0–0.5 μm enamel loss after 28 days [2] and 0.5–0.7 μm after 6 months of simulated normal hygiene [3]). In contrast, dentine is less resistant to abrasion and 35–45 μm of dentine loss after 6 months of normal oral hygiene were reported [3]. Extrapolation to 10 years of normal toothbrushing reveals enamel and dentine losses of around 20 μm and 1 mm, respectively.

Although anecdotal reports about the severe misuse of oral hygiene products are rare [4, 5], clinical studies have shown some correlation between toothbrushing frequency [5, 6], brushing force or toothbrush bristle hardness [7] and the development of non-carious cervical defects. Only very few clinical or in vivo studies on the effect of combined chemo-mechanical impacts on dental hard tissue exist. However, a number of in vitro and in situ studies have shown that toothbrushing might further harm the surface of eroded enamel and dentine. In vitro, short-term erosive challenges (1–3 min) leave a partially demineralised and softened enamel surface layer of up to several hundred nanometres behind, which is partially removed by brushing of clinically relevant duration [8, 9]. In dentine, the dissolution of mineral leads to the exposure of the organic matrix, which is exceptionally resistant to mechanical forces and is compressed rather than removed by brushing [10], even after notably aggressive impacts such as combined chemical, enzymatic and mechanical alterations [11].

This chapter provides an overview of toothbrush and toothpaste features relevant for the abrasion process and focuses on the complex interaction between toothbrushing abrasion and dental erosion.

Toothpaste

Toothpastes facilitate tooth cleaning by abrasives and other ingredients, and also act as carriers of active ingredients to deliver protection against caries, plaque, gingivitis, periodontitis, hypersensitive dentine and/or dental erosion.

Toothbrushing abrasion of dental hard tissues – and especially on eroded enamel and dentine – is mainly determined by the abrasivity and dilution rate of the toothpaste [12, 13] rather than by the toothbrush itself [14].

The abrasivity of toothpastes is usually determined by the REA (relative enamel abrasion) or RDA (relative dentine abrasion) value, comparing the abrasivity to that of a standard toothpaste given a score of 10 or 100, respectively. As sound dentine is considerably more susceptible to abrasion than enamel, the RDA value has become the main parameter to characterize the abrasivity of toothpastes. However, the RDA and REA values are not necessarily correlated, meaning that a high abrasivity on enamel does not always imply a high abrasivity on dentine [2, 15]. Moreover, the relationship between toothpaste abrasivity and stain removal ability of a particular product is not necessarily direct [16].

In vitro studies clearly showed that abrasion of sound dental hard tissue increased with increasing abrasivity of the toothpaste [17]. As less abrasion can be observed in situ compared to in vitro conditions, it is quite likely that under clinical conditions the toothpaste abrasivity is altered by the presence of saliva and pellicle [18], so that even toothpastes of distinctly different abrasivity can cause similar abrasion [3, 18]. While it is difficult to determine a precise level of abrasivity that causes irreversible damage of dental hard tissues, the use of highly abrasive toothpastes in the range of the ISO (International Organization for Standardization) limit (RDA 250) should be avoided.

The abrasion resistance of dental hard tissues is significantly reduced when the surface is demineralised [19–21]. Loss of eroded dental hard tissues also increases with increasing abrasivity of the toothpaste [14, 22–25], but it is not known yet whether the abrasivity of the toothpaste has a greater impact on acid-altered than on sound dental hard tissue.

On eroded enamel, the toothpaste abrasivity is partly counteracted by the presence of fluoride. An in vitro study demonstrated that fluoride-containing toothpastes of different abrasivity resulted in less abrasion potential than fluoride-free toothpastes of the same abrasivity [23]. As the demineralised surface layer of eroded enamel is considerably thinner than the bulk enamel loss, conventional fluoride toothpastes rather remineralise but protect the surface by the formation of calcium fluoride-like precipitates [26]. In contrast, dentine is more susceptible to abrasion and less receptive to fluoride, so that fluoride-free and fluoride-containing toothpastes caused the same amount of erosive-abrasive wear, except for low-abrasive toothpastes [23]. Recent studies also indicate that abrasive forces might hamper the formation of mineral precipitation or partly remove surface precipitates essential for the anti-erosive effect [27, 28]. A detailed presentation of erosion-protective agents present also in toothpastes is given elsewhere [see chapters by Huysmans et al., this vol., pp. 230–243 and Buzalaf et al., this vol., pp. 244–252].

Toothbrush

In contrast to the toothpaste, the toothbrush is probably of minor importance in terms of hard tissue abrasion, but modifies the effects of the toothpaste [29]. In this context, the toothbrushing force, but also the kind of toothbrush and the filament stiffness, were considered relevant [14, 22, 30, 31].

Under controlled in vitro conditions, the amount of abrasion to both enamel and dentine rises as the brushing force is increased [32], and this is especially true for eroded enamel. However, it is unlikely that with clinically relevant brushing forces sound dental hard tissue can be damaged and that the demineralised zone of eroded enamel [33] or the exposed collagenous matrix of eroded dentine [10] can be removed completely. In this context, in vitro studies have demonstrated power and sonic toothbrushes to be less abrasive than manual toothbrushes; most likely as they are applied with lower brushing force. While differences between power or sonic toothbrushes and manual toothbrushes were not significant on sound dental hard tissues, sonic and power toothbrushes caused significantly less wear than manual toothbrushes on eroded enamel and dentine [30, 34, 35]. On the other hand, electric toothbrushing was shown to be a significant risk factor for erosive tooth wear in European adults [36].

A recent study indicated that the development of cervical non-carious lesions among other factors is also related to the toothbrush hardness [7]. In vitro data suggested that the filament stiffness seems irrelevant for the abrasion of eroded enamel [22, 29] but showed a tendency for higher loss of eroded dentine with decreasing filament diameter [14]. Earlier, it was proposed that the greater flexion of the soft bristles leads to an increased duration and area of bristle contact with the brushed surface and, thus, to an increased quantity of abrasives moving over the surface [37]. Besides these factors, the filament configuration and tip geometry as well as the bristle arrangement were also thought to be relevant, but were only tested on acrylic resin specimens rather than on dental substrate [31, 38].

Interaction between Erosion and Abrasion

Sound dental hard tissues are quite resistant against mechanical forces, while eroded enamel and dentine are more prone to abrasion, especially when erosion and abrasion act simultaneously [39]. Short-time contact with acids or erosive drinks leads to a surface softening of several hundred nanometres in depth. Under laboratory conditions, exaggerated brushing [8, 33] is able to remove this layer almost completely. Using clinically relevant brushing times, almost no differences between different brushing forces [33] or hard and soft toothbrushes [29] can be detected, indicating that the outermost region of the softened layer is mechanically very unstable and easily removed irrespective of the mechanical force. At the same time, it is unlikely that with clinically relevant brushing time and force the demineralised zone of eroded enamel is completely removed [33].

On eroded dentine surfaces, the erosion process exposes the collagen matrix. It becomes only somewhat compressed with increasing brushing forces; however, it is not removed by clinically relevant brushing forces and might even act as a barrier against further mechanical impacts [10, 40]. Thus, there are indications that the effects of brushing on eroded dentine are less pronounced than those on eroded enamel. The organic matrix can be enzymatically altered by host enzymes. Interestingly, a partial enzymatic degradation of the collagen does not lead to a reduced stability against brushing even with higher brushing forces. However, the enzymatic reduction of matrix thickness can lead to an increased tissue loss due to reduction of the barrier function of the matrix [11].

It is often discussed whether erosive lesions can remineralise in the oral cavity by prolonged exposure to saliva [see chapters by Lussi and Carvalho, this vol., pp. 1–15, and by Shellis et al., this vol., pp. 163–179]. Hence, the effectiveness of waiting periods between an erosive attack and toothbrushing is an ongoing debate, as brushing is able to increase the wear of enamel and dentine softened by demineralisation. No clinical studies dealing with this issue exist. However, in situ studies showed that waiting periods are of limited efficacy for eroded enamel as waiting periods of up to 2 h decreased enamel abrasion only slightly or not at all [21, 41, 42], indicating that only a limited rehardening by human saliva takes place. On eroded dentine, waiting periods of 30 or 60 min significantly decreased dentine wear to the level of eroded, but unbrushed, surfaces [20]. However, a large survey on over 3,000 European adults with in part advanced erosive tooth wear could not demonstrate a beneficial effect of waiting periods concerning its prevention. [36]. Avoidance of demineralisation with a concomitant decrease of surface hardness, for example by application of adequate symptomatic therapeutic approaches [see chapters by Huysmans et al., this vol., pp. 230–243 and Buzalaf et al., this vol., pp. 244–252], might be more meaningful. As an alternative approach, patients at high risk for erosive wear might also benefit from toothbrushing before rather than immediately after an erosive impact as enamel and dentine wear is significantly higher in the latter case [43].

Conclusion

Teeth are chemically and mechanically challenged during life, so that abrasion by toothbrushing to a certain extent can be considered as a physiological wear mechanism. Abnormal oral hygiene and the interaction between erosion and abrasion might cause increased wear. Overall, the toothbrush alone does not appear to be a significant factor with regard to abrasive activity; it is the combination of toothbrushing with toothpaste that is relevant to the issue of abrasion and dental erosion. To date, most of our knowledge in the area of abrasion, particularly with regard to dental erosion, has been derived from well-intentioned in vitro and in situ studies of somewhat limited extrapolative power, so that further clinical studies are necessary to elucidate the impact of certain factors associated with the overall process of toothbrushing abrasion.

References

1 Addy M, Hunter ML: Can tooth brushing damage your health? Effects on oral and dental tissues. Int Dent J 2003; 53(suppl 3):177–186.

2 Joiner A, Pickles MJ, Tanner C, Weader E, Doyle P: An in situ model to study the toothpaste abrasion of enamel. J Clin Periodontol 2004;31:434–438.

3 Pickles MJ, Joiner A, Weader E, Cooper YL, Cox Bebington TF: Abrasion of human enamel and dentine caused by toothpastes of differing abrasivity determined using an in situ wear model. Int Dent J 2005;55:188–193.

4 Gow AM, Kelleher MG: Tooth surface floss loss: unusual interproximal and lingual cervical lesions as a result of bizarre dental flossing. Dent Update 2003; 30:331–336.

5 Charon J, Sandele P, Joachim F: Iatrogenic interdental brushing. Apropos of a case (in French). J Parodontol 1990;9: 51–55.

6 Lussi A, Schaffner M: Progression of and risk factors for dental erosion and wedge-shaped defects over a 6-year period. Caries Res 2000;34:182–187.

7 Brandini DA, de Sousa ALB, Trevisan CL, Pinelli LAP, Santos SCD, Pedrini D, Panzarini SR: Noncarious cervical lesions and their association with toothbrushing practices: in vivo evaluation. Oper Dent 2011;36:581–589.

8 Wiegand A, Wegehaupt F, Werner C, Attin T: Susceptibility of acid-softened enamel to mechanical wear – ultrasonication versus toothbrushing abrasion. Caries Res 2007;41:56–60.

9 Voronets J, Lussi A: Thickness of softened human enamel removed by toothbrush abrasion: an in vitro study. Clin Oral Investig 2010;14:251–256.

10 Ganss C, Hardt M, Blazek D, Klimek J, Schlueter N: Effects of toothbrushing force on the mineral content and demineralized organic matrix of eroded dentine. Eur J Oral Sci 2009;117:255–260.

11 Schlueter N, Glatzki J, Klimek J, Ganss C: Erosive-abrasive tissue loss in dentine under simulated bulimic conditions. Arch Oral Biol 2012;57:1176–1182.

12 Franzo D, Philpotts CJ, Cox TF, Joiner A: The effect of toothpaste concentration on enamel and dentine wear in vitro. J Dent 2010;38:974–979.

13 Turssi CP, Messias DC, Hara AT, Hughes N, Garcia-Godoy F: Brushing abrasion of dentin: effect of diluent and dilution rate of toothpaste. Am J Dent 2010;23:247–250.

14 Wiegand A, Kuhn M, Sener B, Roos M, Attin T: Abrasion of eroded dentin caused by toothpaste slurries of different abrasivity and toothbrushes of different filament diameter. J Dent 2009; 37:480–484.

15 Barbakow F, Imfeld T, Lutz F, Stookey G, Schemehorn B: Dentin abrasion (RDA), enamel abrasion (REA) and polishing scores of dentifrices sold in Switzerland. Schweiz Monatsschr Zahnmed 1989;99:408–413.

16 Schemehorn BR, Moore MH, Putt MS: Abrasion, polishing, and stain removal characteristics of various commercial dentifrices in vitro. J Clin Dent 2011;22: 11–18.

17 Philpotts CJ, Weader E, Joiner A: The measurement in vitro of enamel and dentine wear by toothpastes of different abrasivity. Int Dent J 2005;55:183–187.

18 Joiner A, Schwarz A, Philpotts CJ, Cox TF, Huber K, Hannig M: The protective nature of pellicle towards toothpaste abrasion on enamel and dentine. J Dent 2008;36:360–368.

19 Kielbassa AM, Gillmann L, Zanner C, Meyer-Lueckel H, Hellwig E, Schulte-Mönting J: Profilometric and microradiographic studies on the effects of toothpaste and acidic gel abrasivity on sound and demineralized bovine dental enamel. Caries Res 2005;39:380–386.

20 Attin T, Siegel S, Buchalla W, Lennon AM, Hannig C, Becker K: Brushing abrasion of softened and remineralised dentin: an in situ study. Caries Res 2004;38:62–66.

21 Jaeggi T, Lussi A: Toothbrush abrasion of erosively altered enamel after intraoral exposure to saliva: an in situ study. Caries Res 1999;33:455–461.

22 Wiegand A, Schwerzmann M, Sener B, Magalhaes AC, Roos M, Ziebolz D, Imfeld T, Attin T: Impact of toothpaste slurry abrasivity and toothbrush filament stiffness on abrasion of eroded enamel – an in vitro study. Acta Odontol Scand 2008;66:231–235.

23 Hara AT, Gonzalez-Cabezas C, Creeth J, Parmar M, Eckert GJ, Zero DT: Interplay between fluoride and abrasivity of dentifrices on dental erosion-abrasion. J Dent 2009;37:781–785.

24 Hooper S, West NX, Pickles MJ, Joiner A, Newcombe RG, Addy M: Investigation of erosion and abrasion on enamel and dentine: a model in situ using toothpastes of different abrasivity. J Clin Periodontol 2003;30:802–808.

25 West NX, Hooper SM: In situ randomised trial investigating abrasive effects of two desensitising toothpastes on dentine with acidic challenge prior to brushing. J Dent 2012;40:77–85.

26 Magalhaes AC, Wiegand A, Rios D, Buzalaf MAR, Lussi A: Fluoride in dental erosion. Monogr Oral Sci 2011;22:158–170.

27 Ganss C, Lussi A, Grunau O, Klimek J, Schlueter N: Conventional and anti-erosion fluoride toothpastes: effect on enamel erosion and erosion-abrasion. Caries Res 2011;45:581–589.

28 Wiegand A, Schneider S, Sener B, Roos M, Attin T: Stability against brushing abrasion and the erosion-protective effect of different fluoride compounds. Caries Res 2014;48:154–162.

29 Voronets J, Jaeggi T, Buergin W, Lussi A: Controlled toothbrush abrasion of softened human enamel. Caries Res 2008;42:286–290.

30 Wiegand A, Burkhard JP, Eggmann F, Attin T: Brushing force of manual and sonic toothbrushes affects dental hard tissue abrasion. Clin Oral Investig 2013; 17:815–822.

31 McLey L, Boyd RL, Sargod S: Clinical and laboratory evaluation of powered electric toothbrushes: laboratory determination of relative abrasion of three powered toothbrushes. J Clin Dent 1997; 8:76–80.

32 Parry J, Harrington E, Rees GD, McNab R, Smith AJ: Control of brushing variables for the in vitro assessment of toothpaste abrasivity using a novel laboratory model. J Dent 2008;36:117–124.

33 Wiegand A, Kowing L, Attin T: Impact of brushing force on abrasion of acid-softened and sound enamel. Arch Oral Biol 2007;52:1043–1047.

34 Knezevic A, Nyamaa I, Tarle Z, Kunzelmann KH: In vitro assessment of human dentin wear resulting from toothbrushing. J Calif Dent Assoc 2010;38:109–113.

35 Sorensen JA, Nguyen HK: Evaluation of toothbrush-induced dentin substrate wear using an in vitro ridged-configuration model. Am J Dent 2002;15:26B–32B.

36 Bartlett D, Lussi A, West NX, Bouchard P, Sanz M, Bourgeois D: Prevalence of erosive tooth wear and important risk factors: a European population-based cross-sectional study. J Dent 2013;41: 1007–1013.

37 Dyer D, Addy M, Newcombe RG: Studies in vitro of abrasion by different manual toothbrush heads and a standard toothpaste. J Clin Periodontol 2000;27: 99–103.

38 Dyer D, Macdonald E, Newcombe RG, Scratcher C, Ley F, Addy M: Abrasion and stain removal by different manual toothbrushes and brush actions: studies in vitro. J Clin Periodontol 2001;28:121–127.

39 Eisenburger M, Shellis RP, Addy M: Comparative study of wear of enamel induced by alternating and simultaneous combinations of abrasion and erosion in vitro. Caries Res 2003;37:450–455.

40 Ganss C, Schlueter N, Hardt M, von Hinckeldey J, Klimek J: Effects of toothbrushing on eroded dentine. Eur J Oral Sci 2007;115:390–396.

41 Ganss C, Schlueter N, Friedrich D, Klimek J: Efficacy of waiting periods and topical fluoride treatment on toothbrush abrasion of eroded enamel in situ. Caries Res 2007;41:146–151.

42 Attin T, Knofel S, Buchalla W, Tutuncu R: In situ evaluation of different remineralization periods to decrease brushing abrasion of demineralized enamel. Caries Res 2001;35:216–222.

43 Wiegand A, Egert S, Attin T: Toothbrushing before or after an acidic challenge to minimize tooth wear? An in situ/ex vivo study. Am J Dent 2008;21:13–16.

Prof. A. Wiegand
Department of Preventive Dentistry, Periodontology and Cariology
Georg August University Göttingen, Robert-Koch-Strasse 40
DE–35075 Göttingen (Germany)
E-Mail annette.wiegand@med.uni-goettingen.de

Lussi A, Ganss C (eds): Erosive Tooth Wear. Monogr Oral Sci. Basel, Karger, 2014, vol 25, pp 220–229
DOI: 10.1159/000360612

Risk Assessment and Causal Preventive Measures

Adrian Lussi[a] · Elmar Hellwig[b]

[a]Department of Preventive, Restorative and Pediatric Dentistry, School of Dental Medicine,
University of Bern, Bern, Switzerland; [b]Department of Operative Dentistry and Periodontology,
Center of Dental Medicine, University of Freiburg, Freiburg, Germany

Abstract

A prerequisite for preventive measures is to diagnose erosive tooth wear and to evaluate the different etiological factors in order to identify persons at risk. No diagnostic device is available for the assessment of erosive defects. Thus, they can only be detected clinically. Consequently, erosion not diagnosed at an early stage may render timely preventive measures difficult. In order to assess the risk factors, patients should record their dietary intake for a distinct period of time. Then a dentist can determine the erosive potential of the diet. A table with common beverages and foodstuffs is presented for judging the erosive potential. Particularly, patients with more than 4 dietary acid intakes have a higher risk for erosion when other risk factors are present. Regurgitation of gastric acids is a further important risk factor for the development of erosion which has to be taken into account. Based on these analyses, an individually tailored preventive program may be suggested to the patients. It may comprise dietary advice, use of calcium-enriched beverages, optimization of prophylactic regimes, stimulation of salivary flow rate, use of buffering medicaments and particular motivation for nondestructive toothbrushing habits with an erosive-protecting toothpaste as well as rinsing solutions. Since erosion and abrasion often occur simultaneously, all of the causative components must be taken into consideration when planning preventive strategies but only those important and feasible for an individual should be communicated to the patient.

The early clinical differentiation of the various defects found under the umbrella of tooth wear (abrasion, attrition, erosion) is important to adequately prevent each of these dental hard tissue defects [1]. The prevention of predominantly abrasion lesions such as wedge-shaped defects has to be different from prevention of defects that have mainly chemical destruction from, for example, frequent vomiting. A prerequisite for the prevention of all of the above is the identification of those patients who are at risk of erosive tooth wear in order to initiate primary preventive measures. It is important to evaluate the different etiological factors that may lead to erosive tooth wear in order to identify persons at risk. Several predictors have been suggested, such as vomiting and regurgitation, misuse of acidic dietary products, use of acidic energy drinks, acidic medicaments and drugs, occupation, lactovegetarian diet, and excessive toothbrushing [2]. Sports drinks are often erosive and when consumed during strenuous activity (when the person is in a state of some dehydration) the possible destructive effects may be further enhanced. A calcium-enriched experimental sports drink consumed during controlled sporting activities showed only minimal erosion compared with a commercially available sports drink [3]. Phosphopeptide-stabilized amorphous calcium phosphate added to a sports drink showed a significant reduction in its erosive potential [4]. Calcium-enriched orange juice is available on the market [see also chapter by Barbour and Lussi, this vol., pp. 143–154]. Further, strenuous sports activity may lead to reflux due to decreased tone of the esophageal sphincter. These causes and risk factors have been discussed in other chapters and are only covered here when they are of special interest concerning the preventive approach.

Clinical detection of erosive tooth wear is important once dissolution has started. However, there is still no diagnostic device available for early clinical detection and quantification of dental erosion. Therefore, the clinical appearance is the most important sign for dental professionals to diagnose erosion. This is of particular importance in the early stages of erosive tooth wear. The appearance of smooth silky-glazed, sometimes dull enamel, intact enamel along the gingival margin and grooving on occlusal surfaces are some typical signs of enamel erosive tooth wear. It is a difficult task to diagnose erosion at an early stage and it seems to be difficult to assess whether dentine is exposed or not [5]. Therefore, a modern preventive strategy needs training of dentists in early detection and monitoring of the process [see chapter by Ganss and Lussi, this vol., pp. 22–31]. Only with these capabilities can dentists comply with their responsibilities for providing adequate care for patients. Often patients themselves do not seek treatment until the condition is at an advanced stage, when the teeth become hypersensi-

tive or when the aesthetics are affected. This is particularly true for patients who suffer from anorexia nervosa or bulimia.

When erosive tooth wear is detected or when there are indications for an increased risk, detailed patient assessment should be undertaken. All of the causes discussed in the other chapters have to be taken into account. A very important part of patient assessment is case history taking. However, chair-side interviews are generally not sufficient to determine dietary habits that may lead to erosion because the patients may be unaware of their acid ingestion. It is therefore advisable to have such patients record their complete dietary intake for, for example, 4 consecutive days (table 1). The time of day and quantity of all ingested foods and beverages, including dietary supplements, should be recorded. Both weekdays and weekends should be included, as dietary habits during weekends may be considerably different from those during weekdays. This dietary and behavior record should be sent to the dentist prior to the next appointment. The dentist should evaluate the erosive potential of the different acidic food items and drinks and the frequency of ingestion during main meals and snacks, and then be able to estimate the daily acid challenge.

The progression of erosion seems to be greater in older (52–56 years) compared to younger (32–36 years) persons and has a skewed distribution [1]. This study revealed that one third of the persons account for more than two thirds of the total progression. The group with high erosion progression was found to have 4 or more dietary acid intakes per day and a low buffering capacity of their stimulated saliva and used a hard bristle toothbrush. Intake frequency of the same magnitude was also associated with an increased risk of erosion in children [6]. In this study, the group with erosion ate fruit significantly more frequently and had different drinking habits such as swishing, sucking or holding drinks in their mouths. The drinking method (holding, sipping, gulping, nipping, sucking) strongly affected the tooth sur-

Table 1. Example of a patient's dietary history (to be recorded over 4 consecutive days including a weekend) and evaluation by the dentist

a Patient's dietary history

Time	Foods/beverages, method of drinking	Oral hygiene
Day 1, Date: 12.12.2015 (Saturday)		
6.30	yoghurt, honey, coffee with milk	toothbrushing
9.30	300 ml orange juice, sipping	
12.30	cooked whole potatoes, cheese, salad with French dressing, black tea and 1 apricot	rinsing solution
16.15	300 ml orange juice, sipping	toothbrushing
19.00	mixed salad with French dressing, bread and rose hip tea	
20.00–21.00	2 glasses of white wine, sipping, cheese	
22.00		1 acidic candy
23.00	toothbrushing	

Days 2–4 as above.

b Evaluation: frequency intake of erosive products

	Day 1	Day 2	Day 3	Day 4	Mean
Meals	4	3	3	2	3
Between meals	4	5	3	4	4

face pH. It follows that holding or sipping of erosive beverages over time should be avoided, as it causes low pH values for a long period of time [7]. Knowing that, in the presence of other risk factors, 4 or more nutritional acidic intakes per day are associated with higher risk for the development and progression of erosion assists the dentist in the assessment of the patient's risk [1, 6]. Every patient should be questioned and examined using the information provided in table 2. Possible intrinsic acid exposure should also be taken into account. Every person has a preferred sleeping side that will lead stomach juice to one side of the mouth and hence to an asymmetric distribution of erosive lesions (fig. 1).

The erosive potential of certain drinks or foods can be estimated using the information in table 3. The pH, the titratable acidity to pH 7.0, calcium and phosphorus concentration, fluoride content, and the degree of saturation with re-spect to hydroxyapatite (HAp) as well as to fluorapatite (FAp) are given. The methods used were as follows [10]: caries-free human premolars with no cracks on the buccal sites were ground flat under water cooling on a rotating polishing machine. The procedure was such that 200 µm of enamel was polished away in the center of the window. Before the erosive challenge, enamel specimens were immersed in 20 ml of freshly collected human saliva for 3 h to form salivary pellicle. Then, baseline surface nanohardness was determined with a Vickers diamond under a pressure of 50 mN for 15 s. Six baseline indentations were made at intervals of 70 µm. Afterwards, the enamel specimens were individually placed in the appropriate solution under constant agitation at 30°C. Carbonated drinks were degassed by stirring at room temperature to avoid the bubbles adhering to the enamel surface, which would affect the chemical analyses and

Table 2. Parameters to be covered in order to unveil etiological factors for erosions (in part from Lussi et al. [8] and Lussi and Jaeggi [9])

- Case history (medical and dental)
- Detection of the main noncarious hard tissue lesions: site-specific distribution, BEWE
- Record of dietary intake over 4 days : estimation of the erosive potential
- Diet: Herbal teas, acidic candies, alcohol, sports drinks, soft drinks, flavored mineral water, effervescent vitamin C tablets (see table 3).
- Reflux, vomiting: acid or bitter taste in the mouth and gastric pain (especially when awakening), stomach ache (particularly after certain foods and beverages (e.g. wine, citric juices, vinegar, fatty foods, tomatoes, peppermint), coughing, hiccup, heartburn, discomfort behind the breastbone (dysphagia), chronic respiratory symptoms
- Bulimia/anorexia: enlargement of the parotid gland, redness in palate and pharynx, formation of rhagades on lips, changes in skin and nail of index and middle fingers, tooth marks on the back of the hand (sign of forced vomiting)
- Drugs: alcohol, tranquillizer, anti-emetics, anti-histamines, vitamin C fizzy tablets (change of acidic or saliva-reducing drugs is possible)
- Determination of flow rate and buffering capacity of saliva
- Oral hygiene habits: Technique, abrasivity of toothpaste
- Occupational exposure to acidic environments
- Strenuous exercise (erosive sports drinks, reflux)
- X-ray therapy of the head area
- Silicone impressions, study models, and/or photographs to assess further progression

BEWE = Basic Erosive Wear Examination.

hardness measurements. After immersion for 2 min, the enamel samples were taken out of the solution and the hardness measurement was performed once again.

All substances were analyzed in duplicate for calcium, phosphorus and fluoride using standard procedures. The pH and the amount of base added to raise the pH to 7.0 were measured using a pH electrode. To do so, 10 g of each substance was titrated with 0.5 mol/l NaOH in steps of 0.02 ml and the amount of base added (mmol/l) was calculated. The degree of saturation (pK-pI) with respect to HAp and FAp was calculated from the pH and the concentrations of calcium, phosphate and fluoride using a computer program [11]. This program assumes a solubility product of $10^{-58.5}$ for HAp and $10^{-59.6}$ for FAp [12, 13].

Apple juice, for example, is undersaturated with respect to both HAp and FAp (as expressed by pK-pI) and caused surface softening in the experiment. Table 3 also shows that soft drinks, en-

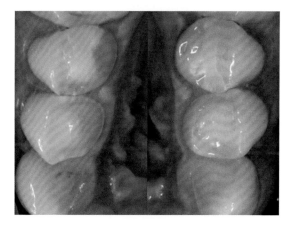

Fig. 1. Asymmetric (right-left) distribution of erosive lesions caused by nightly reflux.

ergy drinks, some sports drinks, juices, fruits, some medications and alcoholic drinks caused, in this short immersion time of 2 min, a statistically significant decrease in surface hardness of enamel samples. Yoghurts, teas, coffee and mineral wa-

Table 3. pH, titratable acid, calcium, inorganic phosphorus, fluoride content, degree of saturation with respect to hydroxy-and fluorapatite as well as change of surface hardness (Vickers 50 mN) after 2 min incubation in different beverages and foodstuffs (in part from Lussi et al. [10] and unpubl. data)

Tested agents	Important erosion-related ingredients	pH	mmol OH$^-$/l to pH 7.0	Ca (mmol/l)	Pi (mmol/l)	F (mg/l)	pK-pl HAp	pK-pl FAp	ΔSH2-0
Soft drinks									
Carpe Diem									
Kombucha fresh	herbal tea extract	3.0	39.0	3.3	0.1	0.39	−19	−12	−190
Coca-Cola	phosphoric acid, flavors	2.5	17.5	1.1	5.0	0.22	−20	−13	−157
Coca-Cola light	phosphoric acid, citric acid	2.6	19.0	0.8	4.9	0.22	−19	−13	−277
Fanta regular	orange fruit, citric acid	2.7	52.5	0.5	0.1	0.04	−25	−19	−245
Ice tea classic	citric acid	2.9	26.5	0.5	0.1	0.76	−24	−17	−84
Ice tea lemon	citric acid	3.0	24.0	0.2	0.1	0.58	−24	−17	−86
Ice tea peach	citric acid	2.9	21.5	0.1	0.2	0.53	−25	−18	−82
Pepsi Cola	phosphoric acid, citric acid	2.4	19.0	0.3	4.9	0.04	−23	−17	−191
Pepsi Cola light	phosphoric acid, citric acid	2.8	15.0	0.3	4.7	0.04	−20	−14	−180
Rivella blue	citric acid	3.3	38.0	4.0	2.2	0.08	−12	−6	−254
Rivella green	citric acid	3.2	44.0	3.3	2.4	0.09	−13	−7	−145
Rivella red	citric acid	3.3	41.5	3.1	2.3	0.08	−13	−7	−211
Schweppes	citric acid	2.5	88.6	0.2	0	0.03	−33	−27	−219
Sinalco	citric, ascorbic acid	3.1	36.0	1.1	0.1	0.06	−20	−14	−167
Sprite	citric acid	2.5	39.0	0.3	0	0.02	−29	−23	−193
Sprite zero	citric acid	3.0	62.0	0.3	0	0.06	−31	−24	−172
Sports and energy drinks									
Gatorade	citric acid	3.2	46.0	0.1	3.0	0.05	−20	−14	−125
Isostar	citric acid, ascorbic acid	3.9	56.5	8.2	4.5	0.11	−6	0	−35
Isostar orange	citric acid	3.6	31.4	5.8	3.4	0.18	−9	−3	−46
Powerade	malic, citric acid	3.7	43.0	0.3	0	0.21	−23	−16	−63
Red Bull	citric acid, taurine,	3.3	98.0	1.9	0	0.11	−26	−20	−89
Fruit juice and fruits									
Apple juice	malic, oxalic acid	3.4	72.0	2.0	1.7	0.06	−13	−7	−145
Carrot juice	some fruit acids	4.2	70.5	4.4	1.2	0.04	−7	−1	−13
Grapefruit juice	citric acid	3.2	168.5	2.3	2.2	0.03	−14	−8	−153
Multivitamin juice	citric, malic acid	3.6	131.4	4.8	6.5	0.12	−9	−3	−4
Orange juice 1	citric, malic acid	3.7	108.0	2.4	2.4	0.03	−10	−5	−35
Orange juice 2	citric, malic acid	3.6	121.0	2.0	2.6	0.03	−11	−6	−60
Pineapple juice	citric, malic acid	3.4	60.0	1.7	1.9	0.04	−13	−7	−86
Apricot	malic, citric acid	3.3	317.0	1.2	6.0	0.02	−14	−8	−120
Kiwi	citric, quinic acid	3.3	206.5	3.4	4.5	0.02	−12	−6	−117
Orange	n/a	3.6	113.0	2.2	1.3	0.03	−12	−6	−97
Alcoholic drinks									
Bacardi Breezer	orange juice	3.2	60.0	0.2	0.1	0.03	−23	−17	−225
Carlsberg beer	−	4.2	17.5	0.7	5.7	0.74	−8	−2	−2
Eichhof beer	−	4.1	18.0	1.9	9.3	0.06	−6	−1	+1
Champagne	tartaric, lactic acid	3.0	78.0	1.9	2.0	0.26	−16	−9	−127
Red wine 1	salicylic, malic acid	3.4	76.0	1.3	4.7	0.07	−13	−6	−31
Red wine 2	lactic, tartaric acid	3.7	63.0	1.7	2.8	0.11	−11	−5	−21
Smirnoff vodka	lemon juice	3.1	50.0	0.2	6.5	0.12	−19	−12	−174
White wine	malic, salicylic acid	3.6	53.0	1.3	4.4	0.27	−11	−5	−25

Table 3. Continued

Tested agents	Important erosion-related ingredients	pH	mmol OH⁻/l to pH 7.0	Ca (mmol/l)	Pi (mmol/l)	F (mg/l)	pK-pl HAp	pK-pl FAp	ΔSH2-0
Medication									
Alca-C fizzy tablet	acetylsalicylic, ascorbic acid	4.2	53.0	9.0	0	0.07	−10	−5	−13
Alcacyl 500	acetylsalicylic acid	6.9	0.5	1.9	0	0.07	0	3	−2
Alka-Seltzer fizzy tablet	acetylsalicylic, citric acid	6.2	14.0	2.1	0	0.08	2	5	−4
Aspirine-C fizzy tablet	acetylsalicylic acid, vitamin C	5.5	27.5	2.0	0	0.08	−6	−2	−17
Fluimucil 200 fizzy tablet	tartaric acid, citric acid monohydrate	4.7	19.5	2.0	0	0.06	−13	−8	−9
Neocitran	vitamin C	2.9	73.5	4.6	1.6	0.09	−16	−1	−250
Siccoral	n.a.	5.4	2.5	0.2	0.1	0.03	−7	−4	−7
Vit. C fizzy tablet 1	citric acid, vitamin C	3.9	93.0	1.9	0	0.06	−15	−9	−88
Vit. C fizzy tablet 2	citric acid, vitamin C	3.6	85.0	1.8	2.0	0.06	−11	−6	−139
Yoghurt, Milk									
Forest berries	forest berries	3.8	159.0	45.5	36.8	0.05	−1	4	−6
Kiwi Tropicana	–	4.0	124.5	45.8	33.8	0.04	0	5	+7
Lemon	–	4.1	110.4	32.0	39.9	0.04	0	6	−1
Nature	–	3.9	120.0	43.3	34.3	0.04	−1	5	+3
Slimline	–	4.0	133.5	56.3	38.7	0.03	1	6	−3
Milk	–	7.0	4.0	29.5	18.9	0.01	16	18	+6
Sour milk	–	4.2	56.0	69.0	39.2	0.03	2	7	+9
Mineral water									
Henniez	–	7.7	n.a.	2.5	0	0.10	2	5	+4
Henniez sparkling	–	6.1	4.0	2.4	0	0.09	−6	−3	−1
Valser	–	5.6	12.5	9.9	0	0.60	−3	2	−2
Valser Viva lemon	citric acid, herbs	3.3	40.0	9.8	0.1	0.63	−15	−8	−81
Tea and Coffee									
Black tea	–	6.6	1.5	1.1	0.3	1.63	6	10	−1
Peppermint	–	7.5	n.a.	1.9	0.4	0.05	12	14	+1
Rose hip	malic, tartaric acid	3.2	19.5	2.7	0.4	0.05	−16	−10	−181
Wild berries	–	6.8	1.0	1.1	0.2	0.78	7	11	+2
Espresso	–	5.8	3.0	0.7	0.6	0.07	1	5	+4
Salad dressing									
Thomy French classic	acetic, citric acid	4.0	141.0	20.5	0.5	0.11	−6	−1	−21
Thomy French light	acetic, citric acid	3.9	145.0	40.0	1.1	0.11	−5	1	−33
Vinegar	acetic acid	3.2	740.8	3.4	2.2	1.20	−13	−6	−319

mmol OH⁻/l to pH 7.0: titratable acidity; Ca: calcium concentration; Pi: phosphate concentration; F: fluoride concentration; pK-pl HAp: degree of saturation with respect to hydroxyapatite; pK-pl FAp: degree of saturation with respect to fluorapatite. A positive value of ΔSH2-0 denotes a hardening of the surface while a negative value represents softening. n.a. = Not available.

ters, except for those with acidic additives, did not have a detrimental effect on enamel hardness. Flavored mineral water (i.e. Valser Viva lemon) has in contrast to plain mineral water a high erosive potential that may not be recognized by consumers. This has some implication concerning tooth health because the public is not aware of the erosive potential of these acidic drinks labeled as mineral water. Rose hip tea showed a distinct erosive potential, some herbal teas were found to be

Table 4. Recommended preventive measures for managing acid intake and reducing acid exposure [8, 9, 20]

– Management of acid intake and exposure
– Reduce acid exposure by reducing the frequency and contact time of acids (main meals only)
– Avoid acidic foods and drinks last thing at night
– Do not hold or swish acidic drinks in your mouth, avoid sipping these drinks
– Use a straw, ensuring the flow is not aimed directly at any individual tooth surface
– Avoid sipping, drink beverages swiftly, no sucking between teeth
– Chose calcium-enriched or modified (sports) drinks and foods with no or reduced erosive potential, finish meals with dairy products
– Be aware of acidic medicaments
– Eating several small meals during the day, no large meal before sleeping
– Avoid reflux-inducing foods and beverages, such as wine, citric, acid, vinegar, fatty foods (fried, etc.), tomatoes, peppermint, coffee, black tea, carbonated drinks, chocolate
– Chew tooth-friendly gum to stimulate saliva production and to reduce postprandial reflux
– Suspected gastroesophageal reflux: referral to gastroenterologist; the doctor decides concerning proton pump inhibitors such as esomeprazole
– Anorexia/bulimia: initiate psychological or psychiatric treatment
– After vomiting: rinse mouth with water or milk, or use (stannous) fluoride oral rinse and clean tongue from acid remnants
– Avoid toothbrushing immediately after vomiting; instead, use a (stannous) fluoride containing mouth rinse, a sodium bicarbonate (baking soda) solution or water

Established and potential preventive therapy [see chapters by Huysmans et al., this vol., pp. 230–243 and Buzalaf et al., this vol., pp. 244–252].

even more erosive than orange juice and acidic lozenges may aggravate erosive lesions [14–18].

In the context of judging the hardness numbers in table 3 it has to be mentioned that decrease of hardness of some units will most probably not cause softening in vivo because saliva may clear the substance very fast [18]. When the liquid surrounding the tooth surface is only slightly undersaturated with respect to the mineral, initial surface demineralization occurs followed by a local pH rise and increased content of ions in the liquid surface layer adjacent to the tooth mineral. As a result this layer becomes saturated with respect to enamel and will not demineralize further [19]. A substance slightly undersaturated with respect to HAp and supersaturated with respect to FAp (e.g. natural yoghurt) will not cause erosion. Table 3 also shows clearly that there is no fixed critical pH value concerning erosion as it is with caries. The solution ad-

jacent to tooth mineral may have higher concentrations of Ca and P compared to the plaque fluid and will therefore not be able to dissolve tooth mineral even at lower pH values such as the 'critical' pH for caries (which is around 5.5) (see chapter by Lussi and Carvalho, this vol., pp. 1–15). Yoghurt and other foodstuff or beverages have a pH of around 4 and showed an increase of hardness after 2 min of immersion. The data of table 3 do not reproduce the clinical conditions, and should only be interpreted as a help for judging the erosive potential of a dietary substance or a medication.

Based on these analyses, an appropriate preventive program may be suggested to patients (table 4). However, the advice has to be made on an individual basis, so not all points listed in table 4 are of interest to every patient. The aim of the program is to reduce acid exposure by decreasing the frequency of ingestion of potentially harmful drinks and foodstuffs as well as minimizing contact time with the teeth, and by rapid consumption of them rather than sipping or swishing. In addition, reflux/vomiting should be controlled and the patient's hygienic regime should be optimized. As discussed previously, various processes cause the degradation of tooth substance. Erosion and abrasion often occur simultaneously, though usually one of these factors may be predominant. When giving preventive instructions, all of the causative components must be taken into consideration. Other behavioral habits that either stimulate salivary flow such as nonacidic chewing gums or lozenges, or that directly help to neutralize acids such as rinsing with sodium bicarbonate or using stannous/fluoride containing oral care products may counter the destructive effects of dietary acids [21–25]. Patients suffering from intrinsic erosion, depending on the cause, need further care such as antacids, psychological therapy or even surgical intervention [see chapter by Moazzez and Bartlett, this vol., pp. 180–196]. There is the possibility that chewing gum may have an abrasive effect on softened tooth structure. However, chewing gum after a meal helps to reduce postprandial esophageal acid exposure [26]. It has also been suggested that chewing nonerosive gum might be a treatment option for some patients with reflux when used immediately after a meal [27, 28].

Adequate preventive measures will often slow down progression of the erosion and reduce the need for immediate restorations. However, assessment of erosion change is important – photographs are simple means of monitoring progression.

Acid-eroded enamel is more susceptible to abrasion and attrition than intact enamel. The thickness of the softened enamel that is removed following different abrasive procedures varies in different investigations depending on the experimental conditions. It has been reported to be between 0.2 and 3 µm [8, 29–39]. As remineralization in vivo is a slow process, repair of this vulnerable layer needs a lot of time (weeks to months). Hence the impact of toothbrushing cannot be avoided and some abrasion of dental hard tissue during the years may be called physiological.

As early as in the 1970s, Graubart et al. [40] showed a protective effect of a 2% sodium fluoride solution in the in vitro erosive process. Less wear of softened teeth was produced in vitro in the presence of fluoride toothpaste than in the presence of nonfluoride toothpaste with an otherwise identical formulation [41]. In recent years, more studies using different fluoride formulations (e.g. sodium fluoride, acidulated phosphate fluoride, stannous fluoride, amine fluoride or titanium tetrafluoride) showed a protective effect in vitro and in situ [42–45]. It appears that modern measures containing (titanium tetra)-fluoride and/or stannous demonstrate the best protection against further erosive tooth wear but there is still need for improvement in terms of better protection [21–25]. The chapters by Huysmans et al. [this vol., pp. 230–243] and Buzalaf et al. [this vol., pp. 244–252] give more insight of established and potential measures for preventive therapy.

Saliva is an important biological factor in the prevention of erosion. It has been speculated that saliva stimulation will enhance the formation of the acquired salivary pellicle. It is known that the pellicle forms rapidly and has some protective effect against erosion [46–49]. Any procedure that removes or reduces the thickness of the salivary pellicle may compromise its protective properties and therefore accelerate the erosion process. Procedures such as toothbrushing with abrasive dentifrice products and professional cleaning with prophylaxis paste will weaken the pellicle and may render teeth more susceptible to erosion [20]. Beverages may interfere with the pellicle formation and thus further modify the protective barrier [50]. For example, black tea and red wine have been shown to have a profound effect on in vitro pellicle maturation, causing thickened layers of stained material to build up which were not readily removed. The mechanism behind this effect was ascribed to the polyphenols contained [51]. Salivary proline-rich proteins (particularly basic proline-rich proteins), via the proline rings [52], have a particularly high affinity for dietary polyphenols [53, 54], as do histatins [55, 56].

In conclusion, as previously discussed, various processes may cause degradation of the tooth substance. When giving preventive instructions, all of the causative components must be taken into consideration but only those important and feasible for an individual should be communicated to the patient.

References

1　Lussi A, Schaffner M: Progression of and risk factors for dental erosion and wedge-shaped defects over a 6-year period. Caries Res 2000;34:182–187.

2　Amaechi BT, Higham SM: Dental erosion: possible approaches to prevention and control. J Dent 2005;33:243–252.

3　Venables MC, Shaw L, Jeukendrup AE, Roedig-Penman A, Finke M, Newcombe RG, Parry J, Smith AJ: Erosive effect of a new sports drink on dental enamel during exercise. Med Sci Sports Exerc 2005; 37:39–44.

4　Ramalingam L, Messer LB, Reynolds EC: Adding case in phosphopeptide-amorphous calcium phosphate to sports drinks to eliminate in vitro erosion. Pediatr Dent 2005;27:61–67.

5　Ganss C, Klimek J, Lussi A: Accuracy and consistency of the visual diagnosis of exposed dentine on worn occlusal/incisal surfaces. Caries Res 2006;40: 208–212.

6　O'Sullivan EA, Curzon MEJ: A comparison of acidic dietary factors in children with and without dental erosion. J Dent Child 2000;67:186–192.

7　Johansson AK, Lingström P, Imfeld T, Birkhed D: Influence of drinking method on tooth-surface pH in relation to dental erosion. Eur J Oral Sci 2004;112: 484–489.

8　Lussi A, Jaeggi T, Zero D: The role of diet in the aetiology of dental erosion. Caries Res 2004;38:34–44.

9　Lussi A, Jaeggi T: Dental Erosion: Diagnosis, Risk Assessment, Prevention, Treatment. London, Quintessence, 2011, pp 55–60.

10　Lussi A, Megert B, Shellis RP, Wang X: Analysis of the erosive effect of different dietary substances and medications. Br J Nutr 2012;107:252–262.

11　Larsen MJ: An investigation of the theoretical background for the stability of the calcium-phosphate salts and their mutual conversion in aqueous solutions. Arch Oral Biol 1986;31:757–761.

12　McDowell H, Gregory TM, Brown E: Solubility of $Ca_5(PO_4)_3OH$ in the system $Ca(OH)_2$-H_3PO_4-H_2O at 5, 15, 25 and 37°C. J Res Natl Bur Stand 1977;81: 273–281.

13　McCann HG: The solubility of fluorapatite and its relationship to that of calcium fluoride. Arch Oral Biol 1968;13: 987–1001.

14　Lussi A, Portmann P, Burhop B: Erosion on abraded dental hard tissues by acid lozenges: an in situ study. Clin Oral Investig 1997;1:191–194.

15　Behrendt A, Oberste V, Wetzel EK: Fluoride concentration and pH of iced tea products. Caries Res 2002;36:405–410.

16　Phelan J, Rees J: The erosive potential of some herbal teas. J Dent 2003;31:241–246.

17　Jensdottir T, Nauntofte B, Buchwald C, Bardow A: Effects of sucking acidic candy on whole-mouth saliva composition. Caries Res 2005;39:468–474.

18　Lussi A, von Salis-Marincek M, Ganss C, Hellwig E, Cheaib Z, Jaeggi T: Clinical study monitoring the pH on tooth surfaces in patients with and without erosion. Caries Res 2012;46:507–512.

19　Lussi A, Schlueter N, Rakhmatullina E, Ganss C: Dental erosion – an overview with emphasis on chemical and histo-pathological aspects. Caries Res 2011; 45(suppl 1):2–12.

20　Zero T, Lussi A: Erosion – chemical and biological factors of importance to the dental practitioner. Int Dent J 2005;55: 285–290.

21　Amaechi BT, Higham SM: Eroded lesions remineralisation by saliva as a possible factor in the site specificity of human dental erosion. Arch Oral Biol 2001;46:697–703.

22　Amaechi BT, Higham SM, Edgar WM: Influence of abrasion in clinical manifestation of human dental erosion. J Oral Rehabil 2003;30:407–413.

23　Ganss C, Schulze K, Schlueter N: Toothpaste and erosion. Monogr Oral Sci 2013;23:88–99.

24　Schlueter N, Klimek J, Ganss C: Effect of a chitosan additive to an Sn^{2+}-containing toothpaste on its anti-erosive/anti-abrasive efficacy – a controlled randomised in situ trial. Clin Oral Investig 2014;18:107–115.

25　Stenhagen KR, Hove LH, Holme B, Tveit AB: The effect of daily fluoride mouth rinsing on enamel erosive/abrasive wear in situ. Caries Res 2013;47:2–8.

26　Avidan B, Sonnenberg A, Schnell TG, Sontag SJ: Walking and chewing reduce postprandial acid reflux. Aliment Pharmacol Ther 2001;15:151–155.

27　Von Schonfeld J, Hector M, Evans DF, Wingate DL: Oesophageal acid and salivary secretion: is chewing gum a treatment option for gastro-oesophageal reflux? Digestion 1997;58:111–114.

28　Smoak BR, Koufman JA: Effects of gum chewing on pharyngeal and esophageal pH. Ann Otol Rhinol Laryngol 2001;110: 1117–1119.

29　Davis WB, Winter PJ: The effect of abrasion on enamel and dentine after exposure to dietary acid. Br Dent J 1980;148: 253–256.

30　Kelly MP, Smith BGN: The effect of remineralizing solutions on tooth wear in vitro. J Dent Res 1988;16:147–149.

31 Jaeggi T, Lussi A: Toothbrush abrasion of erosively altered enamel after intra-oral exposure to saliva: an in situ study. Caries Res 1999;33:455–461.

32 Attin T, Buchalla W, Gollner M, Hellwig E: Use of variable remineralization periods to improve the abrasion resistance of previously eroded enamel. Caries Res 2000;34:48–52.

33 Attin T, Knofel S, Buchalla W, Tutuncu R: In situ evaluation of different remineralization periods to decrease brushing abrasion of demineralized enamel. Caries Res 2001;35:216–222.

34 Amaechi BT, Higham SM: In vitro remineralisation of eroded enamel lesions by saliva. J Dent 2001;29:371–376.

35 Eisenburger M, Addy M, Hughes JA, Shellis RP: Effect of time on the remineralisation of enamel by synthetic saliva after citric acid erosion. Caries Res 2001;35:211–215.

36 Lippert F, Parker DM, Jandt KD: In situ remineralisation of surface softened human enamel studied with AFM nanoindentation. Surf Sci 2004;553:105–114.

37 Wiegand A, Köwing L, Attin T: Impact of brushing force on abrasion of acid-softened and sound enamel. Arch Oral Biol 2007;52:1043–1047.

38 Cheng ZJ, Wang XM, Cui FZ, Ge J, Yan JX: The enamel softening and loss during early erosion studied by AFM, SEM and nanoindentation. Biomed Mater 2009;4:1–7.

39 Voronets J, Lussi A: Thickness of softened human enamel removed by toothbrush abrasion: an in vitro study. Clin Oral Investig 2010;14:251–256.

40 Graubart J, Gedalia I, Pisanti S: Effects of fluoride pretreatment in vitro on human teeth exposed to citrus juice. J Dent Res 1972;51:1677.

41 Bartlett DW, Smith BG, Wilson RF: Comparison of the effect of fluoride and non-fluoride toothpaste on tooth wear in vitro and the influence of enamel fluoride concentration and hardness of enamel. Br Dent J 1994;176:346–348.

42 Ganss C, Klimek J, Schäfer U, Spall T: Effectiveness of two fluoridation measures on erosion progression in human enamel and dentine in vitro. Caries Res 2001;35:325–330.

43 Van Rijkom H, Ruben J, Vieira A, Huysmans MC, Truin GJ, Mulder J: Erosion-inhibiting effect of sodium fluoride and titanium tetrafluoride in vitro. Eur J Oral Sci 2003;111:253–257.

44 Hughes JA, West NX, Addy M: The protective effect of fluoride treatments against enamel erosion in vitro. J Oral Rehabil 2004;31:357–363.

45 Willumsen T, Øgaard B, Hansen BF, Rølla G: Effects from pretreatment of stannous fluoride versus sodium fluoride on enamel exposed to 0.1 or 0.01 M hydrochloric acid. Acta Odontol Scand 2004;62:278–281.

46 Nieuw Amerongen AV, Oderkerk CH, Driessen AA: Role of mucins from human whole saliva in the protection of tooth enamel against demineralization in vitro. Caries Res 1987;21:297–309.

47 Meurman JH, Frank RM: Scanning electron microscopic study of the effect of salivary pellicle on enamel erosion. Caries Res 1991;25:1–6.

48 Hannig M, Balz M: Influence of in vivo formed salivary pellicle on enamel erosion. Caries Res 1999;33:372–379.

49 Hannig M, Fiefiger M, Guntzer M, Dobert A, Zimehl F, Nekrashevych Y: Protective effect of the in situ formed short-term salivary pellicle. Arch Oral Biol 2004;49:903–910.

50 Finke M, Parker DM, Jandt KD: Influence of soft drinks on the thickness and morphology of in situ acquired pellicle layer on enamel. J Colloid Interface Sci 2002;251:263–270.

51 Joiner A, Muller D, Elofsson UM, Malmsten M, Arnebrant T: Adsorption from black tea and red wine onto in vitro salivary pellicles studied by ellipsometry. Eur J Oral Sci 2003;111:417–422.

52 Williamson MP: The structure and function of proline-rich regions in proteins. Biochem J 1994;297:249–260.

53 Hagerman AE, Butler LG: The specificity of proanthocyanidin-protein interactions. J Biol Chem 1981;256:4494–4497.

54 Lu Y, Bennick A: Interaction of tannin with human salivary proline-rich proteins. Arch Oral Biol 1998;43:717–728.

55 Yan Q, Bennick A: Identification of histatins as tannin-binding proteins in human saliva. Biochem J 1995;311:341–347.

56 Wroblewski K, Muhandiram R, Chakrabartty A, Bennick A: The molecular interaction of human salivary histatins with polyphenolic compounds. Eur J Biochem 2001;268:4384–4397.

Prof. A. Lussi
Department of Preventive, Restorative and Pediatric Dentistry
School of Dental Medicine, University of Bern
Freiburgstrasse 7
CH–3010 Bern (Switzerland)
E-Mail adrian.lussi@zmk.unibe.ch

Lussi A, Ganss C (eds): Erosive Tooth Wear. Monogr Oral Sci. Basel, Karger, 2014, vol 25, pp 230–243
DOI: 10.1159/000360555

The Role of Fluoride in Erosion Therapy

Marie-Charlotte Huysmans[a] · Alix Young[b] · Carolina Ganss[c]

[a]College of Dental Sciences, Radboud University Medical Center, Radboud University Nijmegen, Nijmegen, The Netherlands; [b]Department of Cariology and Gerodontology, Faculty of Dentistry, University of Oslo, Oslo, Norway; [c]Department of Conservative and Preventive Dentistry, Dental Clinic, Justus Liebig University Giessen, Giessen, Germany

Abstract

The role of fluoride in erosion therapy has long been questioned. However, recent research has yielded positive results. In this chapter, an overview of the literature is provided regarding the application of fluorides in the prevention and treatment of erosion and erosive wear. The results are presented and discussed for different fluoride sources such as monovalent and polyvalent fluorides, and for different vehicles such as toothpastes, solutions and rinses, as well as varnishes and gels. It is concluded that fluoride applications are very likely to be of use in the preventive treatment of erosive wear. Most promising are high-concentration, acidic formulations and the polyvalent fluoride sources, with the best evidence available for stannous fluoride. However, the evidence base for clinical effectiveness is still small.

© 2014 S. Karger AG, Basel

The role of fluoride in the prevention and treatment of erosion and erosive wear has long been questioned. In caries, in addition to the effect of fluoride ions diffusing into the enamel (sub)surface and adhering to the hydroxyapatite crystal surfaces, fluoride present in the plaque fluid will greatly increase supersaturation and speed up remineralization at pH levels over 4.5 [1]. As the pH level of the acidic substances causing erosion lies in the range of 2–5, it was thought that the fluoride erosion preventive effect could be marginal at best. This hypothesis was coupled with the knowledge that erosion, unlike caries, occurs on clean surfaces, thereby eliminating a possible diffusion barrier effect of the plaque biofilm.

When some fluoride applications were shown to be effective, at least in an in vitro environment, the mechanism with which fluoride could prevent erosive wear was reconsidered. In erosion, the demineralization is largely limited to the surface layer, unlike caries where the demineralization will result in subsurface lesions with an initially relatively intact surface. When the erosive challenge continues, the increasingly softened tooth surface is easily lost – a wear process promoted by mechanical factors such as abrasion. This leaves little time and opportunity for fluoride to act through remineralization, and the predominant effect of preventive treatments should be surface protection instead of remineralization [2]. There are some observations to support this – in situ studies evaluating fluoride toothpaste and/or rinses showed either no significant rehardening after 4 h [3] or limited extra rehardening compared to a non-fluoride control but considerable subsequent protection against repeated erosive challenge [4]. As in caries research, the rehardening detected in other studies may actually have been due to wear of the eroded surface [5]. Traditional fluoride applications, using monovalent fluorides in low-to-moderate concentrations such as in toothpastes and mouth rinses, were observed to have limited preventive effect [6, 7], but specific formulations proved to be effective.

Two mechanisms have been proposed for a fluoride effect in erosion prevention. Firstly, the formation of a CaF_2-like layer as seen especially when using high-concentration, acidic formulations, which by its dissolution under erosive conditions temporarily protects the underlying enamel [8, 9]. Secondly, when using polyvalent metal fluorides, an acid-resistant coating of metal-rich surface precipitates has been observed [10–13] or a metal-rich surface enamel layer which is more acid resistant (fig. 1). In both cases, the protection offered is short-lived in a high-challenge environment, resulting in a need for frequent application of the preventive agent.

Fluoride has been traditionally used in different vehicles. For home use by the patient toothpaste and rinses are the most common, and are subject to legal limitations of the fluoride concentration, usually 1,500 ppm or less for toothpaste and rinsing solutions. For professional applications liquids, gels and varnishes are currently being used, usually at higher concentrations of up to 1.25%. An exception is a 1.25% gel available for home use, although in most countries these products are only available by prescription. The need for frequent application of the preventive agent implies a preference for home care products, which will be discussed in more detail below.

Toothpastes

Toothpastes are ideal vehicles for applying active agents and it is well documented that fluoride toothpastes have significant caries preventive ef-

fects [14]. It is therefore reasonable to consider the role of toothpastes also in the field of dental erosion.

In principle, conventional fluoride toothpastes may provide some protection against erosive wear, but there are also many new products marketed claiming special effects either due to special formulation or new active ingredients. Requirements for such toothpastes are that they are effective not only when applied as slurries, but also when physical effects from the brushing process come into play, and they should exhibit protective effects in enamel as well as in dentine. For the pathohistology of enamel and dentine see chapter by Ganss et al. [this vol., pp. 99–107] and for effects of brushing on eroded enamel and dentine see chapter by Wiegand and Schlueter [this vol., pp. 215–219]. The latter is of particular importance because dentine can be exposed even in small erosive lesions, for example at the cervical area or at the bottom of cupped molar cusps or grooved incisal edges [15], and is therefore an important target tissue for preventive as well as for therapeutic strategies. All these effects should occur without side effects, and the toothpaste should be convenient to use, which is a prerequisite for compliance under everyday conditions.

These requirements are complex as are toothpaste formulations as such. Besides the active ingredient, these products contain many excipients (e.g. for stabilization, thickening, moisturization, aromatization, coloration and control for microorganisms). Further, toothpastes contain abrasives (e.g. silica particles of different sizes or nonsilica particles like polyethylene; fig. 2), and the role of these components is so far not clear. However, all of these ingredients may have an impact on the effects of a toothpaste, which makes it difficult to draw conclusions for classes of formulations (e.g. NaF-toothpastes) based on testing of single or only few products from this class. The findings of studies mentioned in the following must therefore be interpreted with care.

Another source of uncertainty about what can be expected from toothpastes is that the experi-

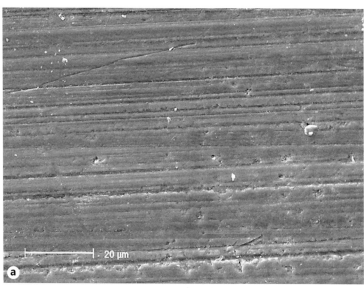

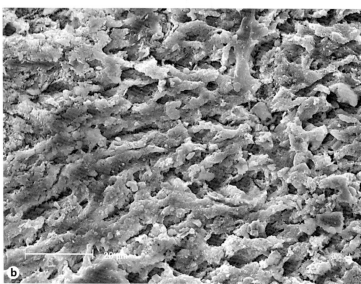

Fig. 1. a Ground flat and polished sound enamel surface from an in vitro study [62]. **b** Enamel sample from the same study after intervention. Erosion was performed with 1% citric acid (6 × 5 min/day for 10 days). After the first and the last erosion each day, the sample was immersed in an Sn/F solution for 2 min each (1,400 ppm Sn, 750 ppm F – as NaF, 750 ppm F – as AMF; pH 4.5). The rough and irregular surface structure indicates erosive demineralisation. Energy-dispersive X-ray spectroscopy revealed 11 wt% Sn on the sample surface.

mental designs used for testing are highly variable with respect to all relevant parameters (e.g. the inclusion and type of salivary pellicle on the tooth surface), not only between different working groups but also within the work of each research group. This is regrettably a common feature in erosion research, which affects all the studies discussed in this chapter.

Toothpastes with Monovalent Fluoride Compounds

Common monovalent fluoride compounds in toothpastes are amine fluoride (AMF), sodium monofluorophosphate and sodium fluoride (NaF), which was used in the majority of studies. Only few investigations have focused on sodium monofluorophosphate [16–18], some of which

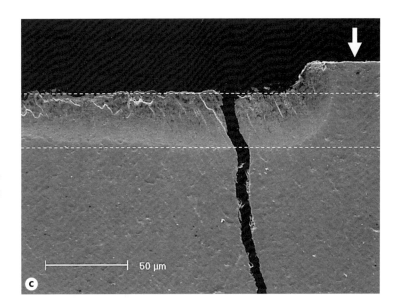

Fig. 1. c Cross-section of the same sample as in **b** (embedded in resin, cut and polished; gap within the sample is a drying artefact). The step between the untreated reference area (arrow) and the experimental area indicates bulk tissue loss. A broad structurally altered zone (dotted lines) is clearly visible, the less dense area of which indicates partial demineralisation. Within this zone, energy-dispersive X-ray spectroscopy analysis revealed that Sn was incorporated (approx. 6 wt%); underneath this zone, Sn was below the detection limit.

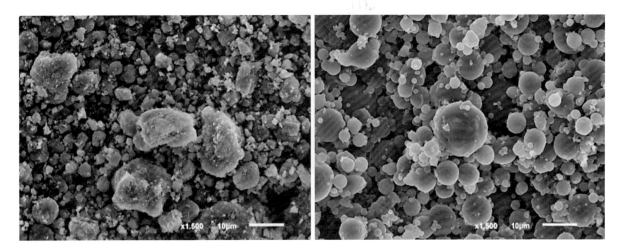

Fig. 2. Abrasives extracted from toothpaste slurries. Left: silica, right: polyethylene.

were in vitro studies without enzymic degradation of the compound. So far it seems as if there is no information about AMF toothpastes.

As mentioned above, monovalent fluoride compounds seem to have only limited anti-erosion effects and therefore highly concentrated formulations have mainly been investigated. In toothpaste experiments, formulations under study are mostly applied as slurries with a fluoride concentration ranging between 250 and 500 ppm depending on the F concentration in the toothpaste and the dilution factor. In vitro effects of slurry applications provided in the range of only between 18 and 39% protection of enamel loss [19–22], while no effect was observed in dentine [23]. In vitro erosion/abrasion experiments demonstrated effects ranging between none and 26–47% protection in enamel [18, 20–22] and between no effect and 23% protection in dentine [23, 24].

Whether or not brushing hampers the protective effect of F toothpastes is unclear. One study demonstrated similar protective effects after slurry application versus slurry application + brushing [20], one found a better protection with brushing [22] and another came to the conclusion that slurry application alone was more effective than when combined with brushing [21]. For dentine, there was no difference between the two application forms [24].

Few in situ studies investigating F toothpastes have been published, and the majority used an extra-oral erosion as well as brushing regime so that the only difference compared to the in vitro studies is that samples were harboured in the oral cavity instead of in a Ca/P solution or in artificial saliva. This means that the samples are covered with a natural pellicle and that between interventions the interaction of dental hard tissues with the surrounding fluid in terms of mineral exchange is mimicked in a more natural way than for simple (super-)saturated mineral solutions. From these studies it appears that the in situ effects are somewhat less promising. Two studies revealed no effect [17, 25], one study 7% protection [26] and two studies 21% protection [27, 28].

In view of these limited effects, highly concentrated NaF toothpastes seem worth consideration. Four studies were identified that investigated a 5,000 ppm F as NaF toothpaste, but these studies revealed conflicting results. An in vitro approach demonstrated a twice as good protection as a 1,100-ppm NaF toothpaste – both compared to placebo [20], which was corroborated by an in situ study revealing a 55% reduction of enamel loss compared to a 1,450-ppm formulation [29]. Another study did not find a significant effect compared to placebo [25], and in dentine, the 5,000-ppm formulation was not superior to a 1,100-ppm formulation [30].

Another approach is to add further active ingredients. Compounds in question are organic agents (e.g. mucin or various enzymes) or Ca and/or phosphate (e.g. sodium trimetaphosphate, or nano-hydroxyapatite). Sodium trimetaphosphate seems to distinctly enhance the effects of a low (500 ppm) concentrated NaF toothpaste [20], but hydroxyapatite in combination with fluoride (1,450 ppm) was not shown to be superior to conventional NaF toothpastes [21]. When combined with fluoride, nano-hydroxyapatite reduced the amount of available fluoride dramatically [21], which makes its caries preventive effect questionable. Nano-hydroxyapatite as such tested in a fluoride-free formulation had no significant effect [21]. Supplementing NaF toothpaste with a combination of various enzymes and mucin showed some effects over NaF alone [31].

Toothpastes with Polyvalent Metal Cations
Regarding the promising effects of polyvalent metal cations mentioned above it seems worthwhile to also consider toothpastes as carriers for such active ingredients. Indeed, when applied as slurries, a reduction of enamel loss between 55 and 67% has been demonstrated [19, 21]. When combined with brushing, effects are much more varying, ranging between no effect and 66% protection [21, 32–34]. From these experiments it seems as if the effects are inversely related to the severity of the acid challenge, obtaining the best protective effects under relatively mild experimental conditions. In an in situ trial, two different Sn-containing toothpastes reduced enamel loss between 26 and 37% [26]. Much less is known about effects in dentine. One in vitro experiment revealed reduction of wear in the order of 57–79% [32], whereas two others demonstrated a reduction of 17–25% [24, 34]. In contrast, an in situ study revealed an increase in tissue loss after brushing with a stannous fluoride (SnF_2) toothpaste compared to an NaF formulation, but the latter had a much lower RDA value [35].

The stannous ion is introduced in the formulation either as SnF_2 or as $SnCl_2$, which is often combined with different monovalent fluoride compounds such as NaF or AMF. Using $SnCl_2$ as a source for Sn allows for variable concentrations of Sn relative to F, but little is known about the relevance of such parameters. A study comparing various combinations of compounds and concentrations of Sn in marketed and experimental formulations did not find a significant difference from these formulation aspects [33]. Another study showed that an experimental formulation was much more effective than a marketed product with the same type and amount of active ingredients (1,100 ppm F as SnF_2 + 350 ppm F as NaF) [32], which again emphasises the importance of the overall formulation of a toothpaste.

Considering the variation in results from erosion/abrasion experiments compared to experiments with slurry application alone, the importance of abrasives becomes obvious (fig. 1). One plausible assumption is that abrasives not only scrub away partly demineralised tissue but may also hamper the retention and uptake of Sn. An additional important aspect is that Sn can be adsorbed to silica to various extents and that the amount of adsorbed Sn is inversely related to the available Sn in the slurry [33]. Furthermore, in an abrasive-free gel the amount of Sn detected after chemical extraction was the same as the amount of available Sn, whereas the latter was reduced up to 60% in toothpaste formulations containing silica [33]. It should be noted, however, that many types and grades of silica are currently available, which are aimed at optimizing stability of actives and providing effective cleaning.

Similar to formulations with monovalent fluoride compounds, attempts have been made to increase the efficacy by adding an organic compound. Chitosan, which is a cationic polysaccharide potentially capable of adsorbing to enamel, seems to be promising in this respect. In vitro as well as in situ studies have shown that this polymer increases the protecting effects in enamel [28,

33] and that an Sn formulation containing chitosan is much more effective than a corresponding NaF formulation [28]. In dentine, however, the order of protection was only 20–25% [24] compared to 67% in enamel [33]. Only one study investigated an experimental toothpaste with titanium tetrafluoride (TiF_4) revealing similar effects to Sn formulations [32].

Overall, protective effects of toothpastes have been demonstrated particularly for Sn formulations. It must, however, be taken into consideration that many of the erosion models used were relatively mild and that the obtained effect size seems to be smaller than for rinses or higher concentrated products. This makes toothpastes suitable for prevention, but in patients with more severe acid impacts and progressing lesions, additional measures should be considered.

Solutions and Rinses

Fluoride-containing solutions and rinses have a long tradition as vehicles for dental caries prevention [36]. Not surprisingly, research on the possible preventive effect of such solutions against erosive wear has therefore been extensive over the last decades. Although the bulk of studies have examined the preventive effects of fluoride solutions on erosion only in enamel, the clinically relevant combination of erosion and abrasion has also been addressed. In dentine, the presence of an organic matrix affects the mechanism for the effect of fluoride solutions [13], and studies examining the effects of fluoride solutions in both enamel and dentine are therefore important. So far there are no published clinical studies on the effects of fluoride solutions in preventing erosion or erosion/abrasion.

Effect on Erosion Only
Early studies on the effect of NaF solutions on dental erosion showed promising results [37, 38], but more recent studies demonstrated that low

concentrations of neutral NaF are not effective against enamel erosion [38, 39] and that the acidification of NaF greatly improved the protective effect [40–42]. NaF solution reduced enamel erosion by 18–19% and dentine erosion by 23% in situ [43, 44], and increasing the NaF concentration increased the protective effect [43, 12] (table 1). The combination of NaF toothpaste and mouth rinse had a significant effect on rehardening incipient enamel erosion lesions in situ, and increased their resistance to a second erosive challenge [4]. Only few studies have tested AMF alone and results are inconclusive. A single application of 1% AMF solution was shown to be effective in reducing enamel loss due to erosion by HCl in vitro [45], but 6 daily exposures to 250 ppm AMF did not prevent enamel erosion progression [41]. As described later in this section, AMF has been included in solutions containing both NaF and $SnCl_2$.

Polyvalent metal fluorides such as TiF_4 and SnF_2 (fig. 3) [46] have been extensively tested for their anti-erosive effects. Already several decades ago TiF_4 was considered to be a useful fluoride agent owing to its excellent complexing ability, protein-binding properties and resulting fast reaction with tooth substance, suggesting the possibility of a shorter application time [47, 48].

Many in vitro studies have reported a protective effect of TiF_4 against erosion, both due to endogenous acids [11, 42, 49–51] and to dietary acids such as citric acid or soft drinks [40, 52–55]. TiF_4 is more effective at the higher concentrations that are suitable for professional applications [46, 50] than at concentrations/pH suitable for home use products [42, 56]. TiF_4 and TiF_4-containing solutions had marked efficacy in enamel under mild erosive conditions in vitro, but the effect was lost under more severe erosive conditions [53].

TiF_4 solution was shown to protect against enamel erosion due to HCl significantly better in situ [46] (table 1) than in vitro [49]. In dentine, TiF_4 and acidified NaF solutions provided a similar level of protection in vitro [40, 56]. Highly concentrated TiF_4 solution reduced enamel surface softening due to repeated soft drink exposures [57] but did not protect against erosive wear in enamel [57, 58] and dentine [59], most likely due to a strong etching effect at this concentration.

Stannous fluoride has received increasing attention as a promising anti-erosive agent. In vitro studies have demonstrated the protective effect of SnF_2 solutions against enamel erosion, either alone [41, 45, 50, 60, 61], combined with other fluoride solutions such as AMF and NaF [41, 62, 63], or as part of a more intensive regime [64]. SnF_2 solution alone, or as part of an intensive fluoridation regime involving toothpaste, mouth rinse and gel containing SnF_2 combined with AMF and NaF, is shown to be significantly more protective against enamel erosion in situ [9, 46] (table 1) than in vitro [50, 64], and is more effective in enamel than in dentine in situ [9].

The efficacy of SnF_2 has been demonstrated in vitro for concentrated preparations under relatively mild erosive conditions [45, 50, 54] and for solutions with lower fluoride concentrations under more severe challenges [12, 41, 65–67] (table 1). Although no controlled long-term clinical erosion studies have yet been reported, a single application of SnF_2 did not protect the enamel 24 h later using an in vivo experimental model [68].

More recently, Sn-containing fluoride solutions rather than SnF_2 per se have been studied. The presence of the Sn ion is shown to contribute to the anti-erosive effect [41, 65], and the efficacy of solutions containing Sn and F is demonstrated to improve with increasing Sn to F ratio [62, 69, 70]. Experimental mouth rinses containing AMF, NaF and $SnCl_2$ have been shown to reduce enamel tissue loss by 78% and 67% in vitro and in situ, respectively [43, 71]. These solutions are more effective in enamel than dentine [12, 43], reducing enamel erosion by 78–82% and dentine erosion by 40–53% [67, 71]. In dentine, the protective effect of Sn- and F-containing solutions is shown to vary

Table 1. Compilation of results from in situ studies investigating fluoride solutions in prevention of erosion or erosion-abrasion

	Exposure days, n	Erosion/ abrasion protocol	Fluoridation protocol	Fluoride compound	Control	Quantification method	Order tissue loss	Effect size
Fluoride solutions in prevention of erosion								
Hove et al. [46], 2008	9	HCl, 2×2 min/day	1×2 min every 3rd day	NaF, SnF_2, TiF_4 (all 9,500 ppm F, all native pH)	erosion only	white light interferometry	0.5–21 μm	enamel SnF_2: 91% TiF_4: 100%
Schlueter et al. [12], 2009	9	citric acid, 6×5 min/day	1×30 s/day	$AmF/NaF/SnCl_2$ (1,900 ppm Sn), NaF (both 1,000 ppm F, pH 4.5)	placebo	profilometry	enamel: 9–34 μm dentine: 24–48 μm	enamel/dentine NaF: 28%/29% $AmF/NaF/SnCl_2$: 73%/50%
Ganss et al. [43], 2010	7	citric acid, 6×5 min/day	1×30 s/day	$AmF/NaF/SnCl_2$ (800 ppm Sn^{2+}), NaF (both 500 ppm, pH 4.5)	placebo	profilometry	enamel: 9–28 μm dentine: 23–44 μm	enamel/dentine NaF: 19%/23% $AmF/NaF/SnCl_2$: 67%/47%
Wiegand et al. [72], 2010	3	Sprite, 2×30 s/day	pretreatment 1×60 s/day	AmF (pH 4.5), TiF_4, HfF_4, ZrF_4 (pH 1.7–2.1) (all 9,500 ppm F)	no fluoride	profilometry	enamel: 0.4–1.0 μm dentine: 0.6–2.3 μm	enamel/dentine AmF: 50%/48% TiF_4: 50%/60% HfF_4: 44%/61% ZrF_4: 38%/68%
Schlueter et al. [67], 2011	7	citric acid, 6×5 min/day	1×30 s/day	Sn + F (250 ppm F, 409 ppm Sn^{2+}, pH 4.2), $AmF/NaF/SnCl_2$ (1,000 ppm F, 1,900 ppm Sn, pH 4.5)	placebo	profilometry	enamel: 10–55 μm dentine: 26–48 μm	enamel/dentine Sn + F: 55%/32% $AmF/NaF/SnCl_2$: 82%/45%
Mathews et al. [44], 2012	28	citric acid, 2-hour preformed erosive lesions	2×1 min/day	NaF: 225 and 450 ppm F NaF + fTCP: 225 ppm F	water	transverse microradio-graphy	ΔZ 240–350 vol% μm	enamel NaF (225 ppm): 18% NaF (450 ppm): 29% NaF + fTCP: 28%
Levy et al. [81], 2013	5	erosion: Cola, 4×90 s/day	4×90 s/day	NaF (pH 5), TiF_4 (pH 1), both 15,500 ppm F	erosion only	profilometry	enamel: 1.3–2.2 μm	enamel NaF: 28% TiF_4: 33%
Fluoride solutions in prevention of erosion-abrasion								
Wiegand et al. [72], 2010	3	erosion: Sprite, 2×30 s/day abrasion: brushing 2×30 s/day	pretreatment 1×60 s/day	AmF (pH 4.59), TiF_4, HfF_4, ZrF_4 (pH 1.7–2.1) (all 9,500 ppm F)	erosion only	profilometry	enamel: 0.8–1.3 μm dentine: 2.4–4.1 μm	enamel/dentine AmF: 30%/32% TiF_4: 38%/31% HfF_4: 17%/31% ZrF_4: 38%/17%
Stenhagen et al. [80], 2013	9	erosion: HCl, 2×2 min/day abrasion: brushing 1×30 s/day	1×2 min/day	NaF, SnF_2, TiF_4 950 ppm F (all native pH)	erosion only	white light interferometry	enamel: 1.8–32.2 μm	enamel NaF: 18% SnF_2: 94% TiF_4: 90%
Levy et al. [81], 2013	5	erosion: Cola, 4×90 s/day abrasion: brushing 2×10 s/day	4×90 s/day	NaF (pH 5), TiF_4 (pH 1), both 15,500 ppm F	erosion only	profilometry	enamel: 1.3–2.2 μm	enamel NaF: 27% TiF_4: 32%

Only experiments quantifying tissue/mineral loss in human or bovine dental hard tissues are shown. Effect size (reduction of tissue loss compared to control) is given for significant results only.

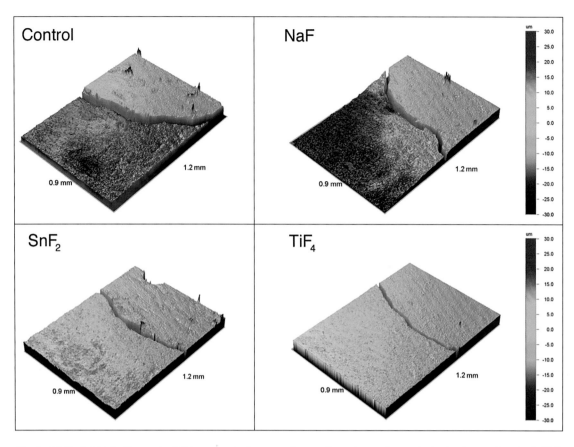

Fig. 3. White light interferometer 3D topography images of enamel specimens from a 9-day in situ erosion study [46]. Specimens were treated for 2 min every third day (in total 3 times) with different fluoride solutions: 2.1% NaF, 3.9% SnF_2, 1.5% TiF_4 (all 0.5 M F). Control specimens received no fluoride treatment. In order to simulate acidic challenge due to gastric reflux episodes specimens were subjected to 0.01 M HCl for 2 min twice daily. The figure shows different images obtained by subtracting the baseline image of the specimen from the image of the specimen obtained after the experiment. Compared to the control, TiF_4 completely prevented erosion, SnF_2 reduced erosion by 91% and NaF had no significant protective effect.

depending on whether the organic matrix is left intact or continuously removed. With an intact matrix SnF_2 reduced dentine tissue loss by 89%, AMF and NaF by about 60% and the combination AMF/SnF_2 by 74% [65]. Erosion inhibition was shown to be dependent on the incorporation of Sn into the demineralized organic portion of the dentine and underlying mineralized areas [13]. When the dentine matrix was continuously removed, SnF_2 reduced dentine tissue loss by 78%, AMF and NaF by 12–34% and AMF/SnF_2 by 67% [65], and

a surface accumulation of Sn was thought to be responsible for the effect [13]. Other polyvalent cations such as hafnium, zirconium, copper, and zinc have also been examined but they do not appear to have a better anti-erosion effect than conventional fluorides [53, 72] (table 1).

Effect on Erosion/Abrasion
Erosion seldom occurs alone and acid-softened enamel will succumb more easily to other surface challenges such as toothbrush abrasion [see

chapter by Wiegand and Schlueter, this vol., pp. 215–219]. Studies examining the effect of low-concentration fluoride solutions on toothbrush abrasion of softened enamel have not shown promising results [73, 74]. The concentration of the fluoride solution is an important factor as shown by the fact that application of a 2,000-ppm NaF solution prior to brushing of eroded dentine resulted in a significantly higher wear resistance than a 250-ppm NaF solution [75]. However, in a simulated in vitro regurgitation model, even highly concentrated NaF and SnF_2 solutions could not prevent erosion-abrasion in enamel [76], as was the case for concentrated acidified NaF and native TiF_4 solutions as treatment against a dietary acid [77, 78]. It was suggested that the low pH of the TiF_4 solution was responsible for the lack of protective effect in the latter studies. However, absence of a natural pellicle may also have played a role.

As is often the case with research, other studies have shown promising results of various fluoride solutions, such as for AMF in reducing abrasion of eroded enamel in vitro [79] and for AMF and various tetrafluorides in reducing enamel and dentine loss in situ [72]. In the latter study, the protective effect of the fluorides against erosion-abrasion was not significantly less than the effect against erosion only, and was similar in enamel and dentine [73]. Recently two in situ studies have shown encouraging results. Low concentrations of native SnF_2 and TiF_4 solutions suitable for mouth rinsing were reported to almost completely inhibit erosive/abrasive wear in situ when applied daily [80] (table 1). Highly concentrated TiF_4 and acidified NaF solutions also reduced erosive and erosive/abrasive wear in enamel, but to a lesser extent [81] (table 1). Although different study protocols were used in these latter studies, the results confirm that both pH and concentration play an important role in the protective effect of fluoride solutions against erosion-abrasion.

Fluoride Varnishes and Gels

The use of fluoride varnish was suggested for the prevention of erosion as early as 1994 [7]. In this study, a NaF varnish was applied to the teeth and then removed prior to the erosive challenge. Some effects were observed, but the idea did not gain widespread acceptance at the time.

Later on, one research group investigated three types of varnish: NaF varnish, $NaF-CaF_2$ varnish (either 5%/5% or 6%/6% combinations) and an experimental TiF_4 varnish, both on enamel and dentine in vitro. In a severe erosion challenge (60 cumulative min per day in a cycling set-up) no significant effect on enamel wear was observed [82], whereas in a milder regime (6 cumulative min per day) enamel wear was reduced compared to a placebo varnish by all varnishes [83]. These results were confirmed in another study using an intermediate challenge protocol (30 cumulative min per day), where a reduction of surface softening could be observed for the NaF varnish compared to a non-treatment control [84]. In a model simulating intrinsic erosion, a small protective effect of $NaF-CaF_2$ varnish was shown [76]. Very little effect on dentine wear (mild regime) could be observed for varnishes [59]. When expanding the model with toothbrushing abrasion, all three varnishes showed protective effects compared to a placebo varnish [78].

In all studies mentioned above the varnish was removed before the erosive challenge, after between 6 and 24 h of application time, thus considering only the fluoride effect and not a possible coating effect. With the advent of polyvalent metal fluoride formulations such as TiF_4, which was shown to leave a surface layer on the treated enamel [10], interest grew in the use of surface coatings in erosive wear prevention. Bonding material was suggested and tested in vitro and in vivo with some success [85, 86]. Using this mode of action a clear fluoride varnish was tested both in vitro and in situ, where the varnish was left on the enamel surface. In vitro the varnish was able to almost

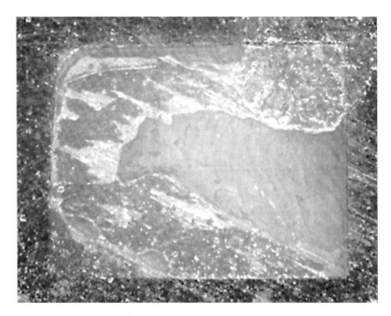

Fig. 4. Enamel sample embedded in polymethyl methacrylate and treated with fluoride varnish, after 10 days of erosion + brushing cycling [88]. It can be observed that the varnish has been partially abraded.

completely prevent surface loss after up to 70 min of cumulative erosive challenge [87]. In situ the varnish also almost completely prevented erosive wear compared to an untreated control for 15 days (cumulative challenge 15 min per day). However, when toothbrush abrasion was added to the model, the varnish was partially removed (fig. 4) and the effect reduced to about 50% [88].

Although fluoride varnish may be considered to be effective, the rationale for its application must be questioned. As a professional application, it is likely to be less cost-effective than home care products, and a minimal treatment effect duration of about 3 months should be established. None of the in vitro studies lasted for more than 7 days, and the in situ study lasted for 15 days, after which time the loss of varnish coverage was substantial [88] (fig. 4). As attrition was not even modelled in this study, one may assume that clinical loss on chewing surfaces will be even quicker.

Fluoride can also be applied in gel form. Traditionally, this has been a professional treatment option using high concentrations, usually 1.25% fluoride. However, a home application gel of this type is also available. Overall, fluoride gel application

was observed to be effective in reducing erosion and erosive wear [52, 89]. Acidic formulations such as APF gels and an AMF/NaF gel may have a stronger effect than pH-neutral NaF gels [89]. The preventive effect of TiF_4 appears to be much reduced by the application in gel form [87], which may be related to the higher pH of such formulations [90]. SnF_2 in gel form was highly effective (about 70% reduction) in preventing erosive wear [33].

A professional application gel has the same drawbacks as varnishes, as it may not be applied frequently enough to be clinically effective. An intensive fluoridation protocol including a gel application every other day, using an acidic AMF/NaF gel with 1.25% fluoride (for home use), was shown to be effective in situ but complaints of mucosal soreness occurred, indicating that the treatment was too aggressive for the oral soft tissues [9].

Conclusion

It may be concluded from the above that fluoride applications are very likely to be of use in the preventive treatment of erosive wear. Traditional formulations with monovalent fluorides in low-to-medium concentration and at neutral pH, such as most available fluoride toothpastes and mouth rinses, are probably not or only minimally effective, whereas high-concentration, acidic formulations provide a higher level of benefit. Most promising are the polyvalent fluoride formulations, with the best evidence for effectiveness available for Sn/F. However, the evidence base for clinical effectiveness is still quite small. Furthermore, effects appear to be reduced when models are used that mimic the clinical situation more closely, and also when the erosive challenge is more severe.

References

1 Buzalaf MA, Pessan JP, Honório HM, ten Cate JM: Mechanisms of action of fluoride for caries control. Monogr Oral Sci 2011;22:97–114.

2 Magalhães AC, Wiegand A, Rios D, Buzalaf MA, Lussi A: Fluoride in dental erosion. Monogr Oral Sci 2011;22:158–170.

3 Wegehaupt FJ, Tauböck TT, Stillhard A, Schmidlin PR, Attin T: Influence of extra- and intra-oral application of CPP-ACP and fluoride on re-hardening of eroded enamel. Acta Odontol Scand 2012;70:177–183.

4 Maggio B, Guibert RG, Mason SC, Karwal R, Rees GD, Kelly S, et al: Evaluation of mouth rinse and dentifrice regimens in an in situ erosion remineralisation model. J Dent 2010;38(suppl 3):S37–S44.

5 Holmen L, Thylstrup A, Artun J: Surface changes during the arrest of active enamel carious lesions in vivo. A scanning electron microscope study. Acta Odontol Scand 1987;45:383–390.

6 Lussi A, Megert B, Eggenberger D, Jaeggi T: Impact of different toothpastes on the prevention of erosion. Caries Res 2008;42:62–67.

7 Sorvari R, Meurman JH, Alakuijala P, Frank RM: Effect of fluoride varnish and solution on enamel erosion in vitro. Caries Res 1994;28:227–232.

8 Saxegaard E, Lagerlöf F, Rølla G: Dissolution of calcium fluoride in human saliva. Acta Odontol Scand 1988;46:355–359.

9 Ganss C, Klimek J, Brune V, Schurmann A: Effects of two fluoridation measures on erosion progression in human enamel and dentine in situ. Caries Res 2004;38:561–566.

10 Büyükyilmaz T, Tangugsorn V, Ogaard B, Arends J, Ruben J, Rølla G: The effect of titanium tetrafluoride (TiF$_4$) application around orthodontic brackets. Am J Orthod Dentofacial Orthop 1994;105:293–296.

11 Büyükyilmaz T, Øgaard B, Rølla G: The resistance of titanium tetrafluoride-treated human enamel to strong hydrochloric acid. Eur J Oral Sci 1997;105:473–477.

12 Schlueter N, Klimek J, Ganss C: Efficacy of an experimental tin-F-containing solution in erosive tissue loss in enamel and dentine in situ. Caries Res 2009;43:415–421.

13 Ganss C, Hardt M, Lussi A, Cocks AK, Klimek J, Schlueter N: Mechanism of action of tin-containing fluoride solutions as anti-erosive agents in dentine – an in vitro tin-uptake, tissue loss, and scanning electron microscopy study. Eur J Oral Sci 2010;118:376–384.

14 Walsh T, Worthington HV, Glenny AM, Applebe P, Marinho VC, Shi X: Fluoride toothpastes of different concentrations for preventing dental caries in children and adolescents. Cochrane Database Syst Rev 2010;1:CD007868.

15 Ganss C, Klimek J, Lussi A: Accuracy and consistency of the visual diagnosis of exposed dentine on worn occlusal/incisal surfaces. Caries Res 2006;40:208–212.

16 De Menezes M, Turssi CP, Hara AT, Messias DC, Serra MC: Abrasion of eroded root dentine brushed with different toothpastes. Clin Oral Investig 2004;8:151–155.

17 Turssi CP, Faraoni JJ, Rodrigues AL Jr, Serra MC: An in situ investigation into the abrasion of eroded dental hard tissues by a whitening dentifrice. Caries Res 2004;38:473–477.

18 Turssi CP, Messias DC, De Menezes M, Hara AT, Serra MC: Role of dentifrices on abrasion of enamel exposed to an acidic drink. Am J Dent 2005;18:251–255.

19 Hooper SM, Newcombe RG, Faller R, Eversole S, Addy M, West NX: The protective effects of toothpaste against erosion by orange juice: studies in situ and in vitro. J Dent 2007;35:476–481.

20 Moretto MJ, Magalhães AC, Sassaki KT, Delbem AC, Martinhon CC: Effect of different fluoride concentrations of experimental dentifrices on enamel erosion and abrasion. Caries Res 2010;44:135–140.

21 Ganss C, Lussi A, Grunau O, Klimek J, Schlueter N: Conventional and anti-erosion fluoride toothpastes: effect on enamel erosion and erosion-abrasion. Caries Res 2011;45:581–589.

22 Rochel ID, Souza JG, Silva TC, Pereira AF, Rios D, Buzalaf MA, Magalhães AC: Effect of experimental xylitol and fluoride-containing dentifrices on enamel erosion with or without abrasion in vitro. J Oral Sci 2011;53:163–168.

23 Ponduri S, Macdonald E, Addy M: A study in vitro of the combined effects of soft drinks and tooth brushing with fluoride toothpaste on the wear of dentine. Int J Dent Hyg 2005;3:7–12.

24 Ganss C, Klimek J, Schlueter N: Erosion/abrasion preventing potential of NaF and F/Sn/chitosan toothpastes in dentine and impact of the organic matrix. Caries Res 2014;48:163–169.

25 Rios D, Magalhães AC, Polo RO, Wiegand A, Attin T, Buzalaf MA: The efficacy of a highly concentrated fluoride dentifrice on bovine enamel subjected to erosion and abrasion. J Am Dent Assoc 2008;139:1652–1656.

26 Huysmans MC, Jager DH, Ruben JL, Unk DE, Klijn CP, Vieira AM: Reduction of erosive wear in situ by stannous fluoride-containing toothpaste. Caries Res 2011;45:518–523.

27 Magalhães AC, Rios D, Delbem AC, Buzalaf MA, Machado MA: Influence of fluoride dentifrice on brushing abrasion of eroded human enamel: an in situ/ex vivo study. Caries Res 2007;41:77–79.

28 Schlueter N, Klimek J, Ganss C: Randomised in situ study on the efficacy of a tin/chitosan toothpaste on erosive/abrasive induced enamel loss. Caries Res 2013;47:574–581.

29 Ren YF, Liu X, Fadel N, Malmstrom H, Barnes V, Xu T: Preventive effects of dentifrice containing 5,000 ppm fluoride against dental erosion in situ. J Dent 2011;39:672–678.

30 Magalhães AC, Rios D, Moino AL, Wiegand A, Attin T, Buzalaf MA: Effect of different concentrations of fluoride in dentifrices on dentin erosion subjected or not to abrasion in situ/ex vivo. Caries Res 2008;42:112–116.

31 Jager DH, Vissink A, Timmer CJ, Bronkhorst E, Vieira AM, Huysmans MC: Reduction of erosion by protein-containing toothpastes. Caries Res 2012;47:135–140.

32 Comar LP, Gomes MF, Ito N, Salomao PA, Grizzo LT, Magalhães AC: Effect of NaF, SnF_2, and TiF_4 toothpastes on bovine enamel and dentin erosion-abrasion in vitro. Int Dent J 2012;2012:134350.

33 Ganss C, von Hinckeldey J, Tolle A, Schulze K, Klimek J, Schlueter N: Efficacy of the stannous ion and a biopolymer in toothpastes on enamel erosion/abrasion. J Dent 2012;40:1036–1043.

34 Hara AT, Lippert F, Zero DT: Interplay between experimental dental pellicles and stannous-containing toothpaste on dental erosion-abrasion. Caries Res 2013;47:325–329.

35 West NX, Hooper SM, O´Sullivan D, Hughes N, North M, Macdonald EL, Davies M, Claydon NC: In situ randomised trial investigating abrasive effects of two desensitising toothpastes on dentine with acidic challenge prior to brushing. J Dent 2012;40:77–85.

36 Newbrun E: Evolution of professionally applied topical fluoride therapies. Compend Contin Educ Dent 1999; 20(1 suppl):5–9.

37 Graubart J, Gedalia I, Pisanti S: Effects of fluoride pretreatment in vitro on human teeth exposed to citrus juice. J Dent Res 1972;51:1677.

38 Lennon AM, Pfeffer M, Buchalla W, Becker K, Lennon S, Attin T: Effect of a casein/calcium phosphate-containing tooth cream and fluoride on enamel erosion in vitro. Caries Res 2006;40:154–157.

39 Pai N, McIntyre J, Tadic N, Laparidis C: Comparative uptake of fluoride ion into enamel from various topical fluorides in vitro. Aust Dent J 2007;52:41–46.

40 Schlueter N, Ganss C, Mueller U, Klimek J: Effect of titanium tetrafluoride and sodium fluoride on erosion progression in enamel and dentine in vitro. Caries Res 2007;41:141–145.

41 Ganss C, Schlueter N, Hardt M, Schattenberg P, Klimek J: Effect of fluoride compounds on enamel erosion in vitro: a comparison of amine, sodium and stannous fluoride. Caries Res 2008;42:2–7.

42 Wiegand A, Waldheim E, Sener B, Magalhães AC, Attin T: Comparison of the effects of TiF_4 and NaF solutions at pH 1.2 and 3.5 on enamel erosion in vitro. Caries Res 2009;43:269–277.

43 Ganss C, Neutard L, von HJ, Klimek J, Schlueter N: Efficacy of a tin/fluoride rinse: a randomized in situ trial on erosion. J Dent Res 2010;89:1214–1218.

44 Mathews MS, Amaechi BT, Ramalingam K, Ccahuana-Vasquez RA, Chedjieu IP, Mackey AC, et al: In situ remineralisation of eroded enamel lesions by NaF rinses. Arch Oral Biol 2012;57:525–530.

45 Wiegand A, Bichsel D, Magalhães AC, Becker K, Attin T: Effect of sodium, amine and stannous fluoride at the same concentration and different pH on in vitro erosion. J Dent 2009;37:591–595.

46 Hove LH, Holme B, Young A, Tveit AB: The protective effect of TiF_4, SnF_2 and NaF against erosion-like lesions in situ. Caries Res 2008;42:68–72.

47 Shrestha BM, Mundorff SA, Bibby BG: Enamel dissolution. I. Effects of various agents and titanium tetrafluoride. J Dent Res 1972;51:1561–1566.

48 Mundorff SA, Little MF, Bibby BG: Enamel dissolution. II. Action of titanium tetrafluoride. J Dent Res 1972;51:1567–1571.

49 Hove L, Holme B, Øgaard B, Willumsen T, Tveit AB: The protective effect of TiF_4, SnF_2 and NaF on erosion of enamel by hydrochloric acid in vitro measured by white light interferometry. Caries Res 2006;40:440–443.

50 Hove LH, Holme B, Young A, Tveit AB: The erosion-inhibiting effect of TiF_4, SnF_2, and NaF solutions on pellicle-covered enamel in vitro. Acta Odontol Scand 2007;65:259–264.

51 Hove LH, Holme B, Stenhagen KR, Tveit AB: Protective effect of TiF_4 solutions with different concentrations and pH on development of erosion-like lesions. Caries Res 2011;45:64–68.

52 van Rijkom H, Ruben JL, Vieira A, Huysmans MC, Truin GJ, Mulder J: Erosion-inhibiting effect of sodium fluoride and titanium tetrafluoride treatment in vitro. Eur J Oral Sci 2003;111:253–257.

53 Schlueter N, Duran A, Klimek J, Ganss C: Investigation of the effect of various fluoride compounds and preparations thereof on erosive tissue loss in enamel in vitro. Caries Res 2009;43:10–16.

54 Yu H, Attin T, Wiegand A, Buchalla W: Effects of various fluoride solutions on enamel erosion in vitro. Caries Res 2010; 44:390–401.

55 Vieira AM, Ruben JL, Bronkhorst EM, Huysmans MC: In vitro reduction of dental erosion by low-concentration TiF_4 solutions. Caries Res 2011;45:142–147.

56 Wiegand A, Magalhães AC, Sener B, Waldheim E, Attin T: TiF_4 and NaF at pH 1.2 but not at pH 3.5 are able to reduce dentin erosion. Arch Oral Biol 2009;54:790–795.

57 Magalhães AC, Rios D, Honorio HM, Jorge AM Jr, Delbem AC, Buzalaf MA: Effect of 4% titanium tetrafluoride solution on dental erosion by a soft drink: an in situ/ex vivo study. Arch Oral Biol 2008;53:399–404.

58 Magalhães AC, Rios D, Honorio HM, Delbem AC, Buzalaf MA: Effect of 4% titanium tetrafluoride solution on the erosion of permanent and deciduous human enamel: an in situ/ex vivo study. J Appl Oral Sci 2009;17:56–60.

59 Magalhães AC, Levy FM, Rios D, Buzalaf MA: Effect of a single application of TiF_4 and NaF varnishes and solutions on dentin erosion in vitro. J Dent 2010;38:153–157.

60 Willumsen T, Øgaard B, Hansen BF, Rølla G: Effects from pretreatment of stannous fluoride versus sodium fluoride on enamel exposed to 0.1 M or 0.01 M hydrochloric acid. Acta Odontol Scand 2004;62:278–281.

61 Hjortsjö C, Jonski G, Young A, Saxegaard E: Effect of acidic fluoride treatments on early enamel erosion lesions – a comparison of calcium and profilometric analyses. Arch Oral Biol 2010;55:229–234.

62 Schlueter N, Hardt M, Lussi A, Engelmann F, Klimek J, Ganss C: Tin-containing fluoride solutions as anti-erosive agents in enamel: an in vitro tin-uptake, tissue-loss, and scanning electron micrograph study. Eur J Oral Sci 2009;117:427–434.

63 Rakhmatullina E, Beyeler B, Lussi A: Inhibition of enamel erosion by stannous and fluoride containing rinsing solutions. Schweiz Monatsschr Zahnmed 2013;123:192–198.

64 Ganss C, Klimek J, Schaffer U, Spall T: Effectiveness of two fluoridation measures on erosion progression in human enamel and dentine in vitro. Caries Res 2001;35:325–330.

65 Ganss C, Lussi A, Sommer N, Klimek J, Schlueter N: Efficacy of fluoride compounds and stannous chloride as erosion inhibitors in dentine. Caries Res 2010;44:248–252.

66 Yu H, Wegehaupt FJ, Zaruba M, Becker K, Roos M, Attin T, et al: Erosion-inhibiting potential of a stannous chloride-containing fluoride solution under acid flow conditions in vitro. Arch Oral Biol 2010;55:702–705.

67 Schlueter N, Klimek J, Ganss C: Efficacy of tin-containing solutions on erosive mineral loss in enamel and dentine in situ. Clin Oral Investig 2011;15:361–367.

68 Hjortsjö C, Jonski G, Thrane PS, Saxegaard E, Young A: Effect of stannous fluoride and dilute hydrofluoric acid on early enamel erosion over time in vivo. Caries Res 2009;43:449–454.

69 Schlueter N, Klimek J, Ganss C: In vitro efficacy of experimental tin- and fluoride-containing mouth rinses as anti-erosive agents in enamel. J Dent 2009; 37:944–948.

70 Schlueter N, Klimek J, Ganss C: Effect of stannous and fluoride concentration in a mouth rinse on erosive tissue loss in enamel in vitro. Arch Oral Biol 2009;54:432–436.

71 Schlueter N, Neutard L, von Hinckeldey J, Klimek J, Ganss C: Tin and fluoride as anti-erosive agents in enamel and dentine in vitro. Acta Odontol Scand 2010; 68:180–184.

72 Wiegand A, Hiestand B, Sener B, Magalhães AC, Roos M, Attin T: Effect of TiF$_4$, ZrF$_4$, HfF$_4$ and AMF on erosion and erosion/abrasion of enamel and dentin in situ. Arch Oral Biol 2010;55: 223–228.

73 Kelly MP, Smith BG: The effect of remineralizing solutions on tooth wear in vitro. J Dent 1988;16:147–149.

74 Lussi A, Jaeggi T, Gerber C, Megert B: Effect of amine/sodium fluoride rinsing on toothbrush abrasion of softened enamel in situ. Caries Res 2004;38:567–571.

75 Attin T, Zirkel C, Hellwig E: Brushing abrasion of eroded dentin after application of sodium fluoride solutions. Caries Res 1998;32:344–350.

76 Austin RS, Stenhagen KS, Hove LH, Dunne S, Moazzez R, Bartlett DW, et al: A qualitative and quantitative investigation into the effect of fluoride formulations on enamel erosion and erosion-abrasion in vitro. J Dent 2011;39: 648–655.

77 Levy FM, Magalhães AC, Gomes MF, Comar LP, Rios D, Buzalaf MA: The erosion and abrasion-inhibiting effect of TiF$_4$ and NaF varnishes and solutions on enamel in vitro. Int J Paediatr Dent 2012;22:11–16.

78 Magalhães AC, Levy FM, Rizzante FA, Rios D, Buzalaf MA: Effect of NaF and TiF$_4$ varnish and solution on bovine dentin erosion plus abrasion in vitro. Acta Odontol Scand 2012;70:160–164.

79 Vieira A, Lugtenborg M, Ruben JL, Huysmans MC: Brushing abrasion of eroded bovine enamel pretreated with topical fluorides. Caries Res 2006;40: 224–230.

80 Stenhagen KR, Hove LH, Holme B, Tveit AB: The effect of daily fluoride mouth rinsing on enamel erosive/abrasive wear in situ. Caries Res 2013;47:2–8.

81 Levy FM, Rios D, Buzalaf MA, Magalhães AC: Efficacy of TiF$_4$ and NaF varnish and solution: a randomized in situ study on enamel erosive-abrasive wear. Clin Oral Investig, Epub ahead of print.

82 Magalhães AC, Stancari FH, Rios D, Buzalaf MAR: Effect of an experimental 4% titanium tetrafluoride varnish on dental erosion by a soft drink. J Dent 2007;35: 858–861.

83 Magalhães AC, Kato MT, Rios D, Wiegand A, Attin T, Buzalaf MAR: The effect of an experimental 4% TiF$_4$ varnish compared to NaF varnishes and 4% TiF$_4$ solution on dental erosion in vitro. Caries Res 2008;42:269–274.

84 Murakami C, Bönecker M, Corrêa MSNP, Mendes FM, Rodrigues CRMD: Effect of fluoride varnish and gel on dental erosion in primary and permanent teeth. Arch Oral Biol 2009;54:997–1001.

85 Sundaram G, Wilson R, Watson TF, Bartlett D: Clinical measurement of palatal tooth wear following coating by a resin sealing system. Oper Dent 2007;32: 539–543.

86 Bartlett D, Sundaram G, Moazzez R: Trial of protective effect if fissure sealants, in vivo, on the palatal surfaces of anterior teeth, in patients suffering from erosion. J Dent 2011;39:26–29.

87 Vieira A, Ruben JL, Huysmans MC: Effect of titanium tetrafluoride, amine fluoride and fluoride varnish on enamel erosion in vitro. Caries Res 2005;39: 371–379.

88 Vieira A, Jager DHJ, Ruben JL, Huysmans MC: Inhibition of erosive wear by fluoride varnish. Caries Res 2007;41: 61–67.

89 Attin T, Deifuss H, Hellwig E: Influence of acidified fluoride gel on abrasion resistance of eroded enamel. Caries Res 1999;33:135–139.

90 Rölla G, Jonski G, Saxegaard E: On inhibition of dental erosion. Acta Odontol Scand 2013;71:1508–1512.

Prof. M.-C. Huysmans, PhD
College of Dental Sciences, Radboud University Medical Center
Radboud University Nijmegen, PO Box 9101
NL–6500 HB Nijmegen (The Netherlands)
E-Mail marie-charlotte.huysmans@radboudumc.nl

Lussi A, Ganss C (eds): Erosive Tooth Wear. Monogr Oral Sci. Basel, Karger, 2014, vol 25, pp 244–252
DOI: 10.1159/000360557

Alternatives to Fluoride in the Prevention and Treatment of Dental Erosion

Marília Afonso Rabelo Buzalaf[a] · Ana Carolina Magalhães[a] · Annette Wiegand[b]

[a]Department of Biological Sciences, Bauru Dental School, University of São Paulo, Bauru, Brazil; [b]Department of Preventive Dentistry, Periodontology and Cariology, University of Göttingen, Göttingen, Germany

Abstract

In recent years, different agents have been discussed as potential alternatives to fluoride in the prevention of dental erosion. These agents are intended to form acid-resistant layers on the surface, to induce repair of eroded lesions by mineral precipitation or to prevent the enzymatic degradation of demineralised collagen. The application of adhesives and/or fissure sealants is considered to be an effective alternative to fluoride, but requires professional application and, depending on the product used, a re-sealing of the surface every several months. Studies testing film-forming products, such as polymers, have suggested the potential effectiveness of some of these approaches, such as chitosan, although further studies are needed to confirm the effectiveness of this approach. Other studies have demonstrated that products designed to deliver calcium and/or phosphate have not been successful at providing a significant anti-erosive effect. In advanced erosive lesions, the demineralised collagenous dentine matrix can be degraded by host enzymes such as matrix metalloproteinases (MMPs). As well as fluorides, epigallocatechin gallate and chlorhexidine have been identified as effective MMP inhibitors, with the potential to reduce the progression of dentine erosion. While fluoride compounds have been shown to have an anti-erosive potential, particularly those containing tin, alternative approaches that provide even greater protective capacity still need to be developed and proven to be effective.

© 2014 S. Karger AG, Basel

A possible alternative to the use of fluoride for the control of dental erosion is to establish the following: (1) an acid-protective layer on the tooth surface, such as through the use of sealants or polymers, (2) enhanced mechanisms of mineral precipitation and/or (3) the preservation of the organic matrix of dentine. The acid-resistant layers can be composed of different ions or molecules attached to the salivary pellicle or directly to the tooth surface. The second mechanism of protection is based on mineral precipitation that might be induced by the use of different sources of calcium phosphate such as casein phosphopeptide-amorphous calcium phosphate (CPP-ACP) and hydroxyapatite particles or non-fluoride polyvalent metal compounds.

It is also important to consider that the preservation of the exposed organic layer (in the case of dentine) is essential for the promotion of mineral precipitation. However, the organic layer can be degraded by collagenases such as matrix metalloproteinases (MMPs) and cysteine cathepsins (CCs), impairing the mineral repair and enabling the progression of tooth loss. Therefore, the use of protease inhibitors could be the third alternative strategy to control dentine erosion.

This chapter provides an overview of current strategies with respect to alternatives to fluoride and critically discusses their mechanism of action and anti-erosive potential in comparison to the established prevention provided by fluoride.

Acid-Protective Layers

Adhesive/Sealant Application

The prevention of dental erosion by the use of toothpastes, gels and rinses primarily depends on the compliance of the patients, while the professional application of adhesives and sealants presents a more patient-independent approach.

Depending on the filler content and the abrasion stability of the resin coatings, adhesives and fissure sealants were shown to prevent enamel and dentine erosion for limited periods of time [1, 2]. A series of laboratory, in situ and clinical studies [3–6] focused on the effect of resin coatings on dentine erosion.

As the resin coating of fissure sealants is significantly thicker than the coating of a bonding agent, surface sealants provided a longer duration of protection against erosive wear. Clinically, the coating of exposed dentine on palatal surfaces of eroded anterior teeth with a bonding agent (baseline thickness of coating: 150 µm) lasted for 3 months [5], while a fissure sealant (baseline thickness: 290 µm) had worn off after 6–9 months [6]. Interestingly, sealed teeth presented a higher wear than untreated controls after 12 months of intra-oral stress. It has been noted that remnants of the sealants break off together with some of the underlying dental substrate, so that the surface requires re-sealing on a frequent basis to achieve a preventive effect [7].

Only one study compared the protective effect of a resin coating with the repeated use of a 225-ppm fluoride solution in an in vitro erosion/abrasion model. The fluoride solution was able to reduce dentine wear, but was significantly less effective than the resin coating [4].

Mouth Rinses and Toothpastes Containing Polymers as Active Ingredients

The anti-erosive potential of film-forming polymers has not been extensively investigated. Most studies analysed whether the erosive potential of acids or soft drinks can be reduced by modification with polymers such as ovalbumin, casein, pectin or alginate [8, 9; see chapter by Barbour and Lussi, this vol., pp. 143–154]. Only few studies have tested the effect of specific polymers as active ingredients in toothpastes or mouth rinses on the development of erosive lesions.

Among these, chitosan-containing toothpastes were of interest, as chitosan was shown to physically adsorb on saliva-coated hydroxyapatite by forming a surface layer [10], probably resulting in a more hydrophobic surface [11]. The chitosan coating was shown to be quite resistant against citric acid erosion (pH 2.8, 50 min), but erosion of the underlying hydroxyapatite could not be prevented completely [10]. Both the concentration and exposure time of the biopolymer to enamel seemed to influence the demineralisation-inhibiting effect [12].

Brushing with a commercial chitosan-containing toothpaste without fluoride was shown to prevent enamel erosion [13] in vitro to the same extent as conventional sodium fluoride-containing toothpastes. The addition of chitosan enhanced the preventive effect of a tin-containing fluoridated toothpaste in vitro [14] and in situ [15]. However, there is no information about the protective effect of chitosan added to sodium fluoride-containing toothpastes.

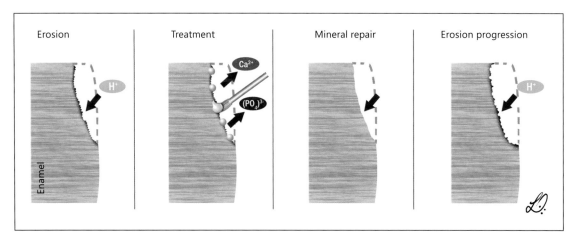

Fig. 1. Eroded enamel (erosion) treated with calcium/phosphate-based product (treatment), showing some superficial mineral repair; however, this was unable to make it more resistant to further acid challenge (erosion progression).

Besides the formation of multilayers on the surface, complex interactions between the positively charged biopolymer and the negatively charged dental hard tissue and pellicle, as well as the toothpaste abrasives, are considered to be relevant, but further studies are necessary to analyse the mode of action between chitosan and other ingredients of toothpastes [15].

Experimentally, the film-forming and anti-erosive properties of various polymers such as fluoropolymers [16], latex-deposited poly(alkyl methacrylate)s [17] or a polymer system containing carboxymethyl cellulose, xanthan gum and copovidone [18] have been tested. Under some test conditions, polymer-coated substrates have been shown to be somewhat protective against acid dissolution; however, when compared to aqueous sodium fluoride treatments (300 or 663 ppm fluoride), these polymer coatings were found to be less effective [16, 17].

Mechanisms of Mineral Repair/Precipitation

Remineralising agents such as CPP-ACP, hydroxyapatite with or without fluoride, Zn-carbonate hydroxyapatite or calcium sodium phosphosilicate have been tested for the control of dental erosion. Their mechanism of action is mainly based on delivering calcium or/and phosphate to the tooth, which might be incorporated into the apatite lattice to some extent (fig. 1).

However, a true remineralisation phenomenon does not occur in the case of dental erosion due to its histology [see chapter by Ganss et al., this vol., pp. 99–107]. Therefore, remineralising agents are generally limited to provide mineral precipitation (partial mineral deposition) onto the eroded surfaces rather than true remineralisation.

CPP-ACP has been added to acidic drinks [19, 20] as well as to chewing gums [21]. However, CPP-ACP has been generally tested as mousse or paste applied between the erosive challenges. It has shown no effect [22] to a slight decrease in tooth loss (about 30–35%) compared to control/ placebo in vitro [23, 24]. CPP-ACP application also induced some increase in hardness recovery (CPP-ACP: 25–46% and CPP-ACP + F: 62.2%) in situ [25, 26]. Interestingly, when CPP-ACP was applied for the control of combined erosion and abrasion, its protective effect was improved (63–79% reduction of tooth loss) compared to control. Based on this, the authors speculated that the protection might be due to both remineralising and lubricant effects [27, 28].

Only few studies compared the effect of CPP-ACP paste with fluoride (in the form of gel or solution), showing that CPP-ACP was as effective as a fluoride mouth rinse (250 ppm F) on the hardness recovery of eroded enamel [26], but less effective compared to fluoride gel (22,500 ppm F) on the enamel wear [29]. Based on a limited number of available studies, CPP-ACP appears to be less effective than fluoride in the control of dental erosion.

Other examples of such remineralising agents are pure and nano-sized hydroxyapatite (with or without F) and Zn-carbonate hydroxyapatite, which might be expected to induce some mineral precipitation on eroded enamel and dentine, as previously showed using surface-scanning methods [30, 31]. However, the incorporation of hydroxyapatite into toothpaste has not been demonstrated to increase the enamel resistance against erosion and erosion-abrasion compared to conventional toothpastes [13]. Nano-sized hydroxyapatite only showed minor protection when added to sports drinks [32].

Besinis et al. [33] has shown that sol-gel hydroxyapatite (combined with sodium hexametaphosphate and acetone as vehicle) and silica nanoparticles could infiltrate into collagen from demineralised dentine, providing a suitable scaffold for the dentine repair.

Similar results were also found for calcium sodium phosphosilicate. Despite being deposited on enamel and onto dentine surfaces [34], it had no preventive or repairing effect on erosion [22], or at least not superior to that provided by conventional fluoride toothpastes [35].

Sodium trimetaphosphate (TMP) is another source of phosphate that has been added to toothpastes and mouth rinses. A toothpaste containing 550 ppm F and 3% TMP had a greater protective effect (33.5% reduction) compared to conventional toothpaste (1,100 ppm F) in reducing enamel erosive-abrasive wear in vitro [36]. The addition of TMP (0.2, 0.4 and 0.6%) to a solution containing 100 ppm F also resulted in less erosion (35% reduction in enamel wear) than a solution containing 225 ppm F in vitro [37]. TMP associated with fluoride seems to have some promising effect as an anti-erosive agent compared to fluoride alone. TMP seems to act more as a surface-active agent that binds apatite and inhibits demineralisation rather than as a remineralising agent. However, its mechanism of action and the clinical relevance of the protective effect need to be tested in vivo before any concusion can be drawn regarding potential effectiveness.

Based on a review of the literature, there is no evidence that products delivering calcium or/and phosphate to the tooth significantly contribute to reduce enamel or dentine solubility under erosive challenges or to promote higher mineral precipitation compared to conventional fluoride products [13].

Besides calcium and phosphate, non-fluoride polyvalent metal compounds, particularly Sn and Ti compounds, are potentially effective against erosive demineralisation, presumably due to their ability to establish relatively acid-resistant surface precipitates. An early experiment [38] investigated the effects of Sn (as $SnCl_2$), on etched enamel. A 0.2% $SnCl_2$ solution was applied for 6×2 min and washed in between with running distilled water for 30 s after each treatment. Even after 6 days of storage in distilled water, SEM images clearly demonstrated a fine and continuous granular covering, which completely masked the etching pattern. The amount of Sn retained on the surface was 8.9 wt% (range 7.0–10.7) directly after application and 8.2 wt% (range 6.7–9.2) after 6 days of water storage. This indicates that, under neutral conditions, an Sn-rich precipitate of considerable stability was established. Though readily soluble in KOH [38], such precipitates seem to survive acid challenges [39]. $SnCl_2$ has been shown to be protective against demineralisation in both caries [40] and erosion models [39]. Similar to enamel,

SnCl$_2$ may also have a certain potential to help prevent dentine erosion [41].

Much less is known about the effects of the titanium ion, although there is one study indicating that TiCl$_3$ may also help inhibit enamel demineralisation [42].

Although some effects related to non-metal polyvalent compounds have been noted, these do not appear to be superior to the protection provided by conventional fluorides. In combination with fluoride, however, either as SnF$_2$, TiF$_4$ or mixed with monovalent fluoride compound (e.g. SnCl$_2$ + NaF), the polyvalent metals have demonstrated distinct protective effects for enamel and, to a lesser extent, for dentine. This will be addressed in the chapter by Huysmans et al. [this vol., pp. 230–243].

The Role of Protease Inhibitors

The rate of erosion progression over time is lower in dentine compared to enamel [43]. This is due to the presence of the demineralised organic matrix (DOM), constituted mainly of type I collagen, at the outer layers of the dentine [44]. The DOM acts as a barrier to ionic diffusion [44] and, because of its organic nature, cannot be degraded through the action of erosive acids. However, these acids make it susceptible to subsequent degradation by proteases [45], thereby allowing erosion to progress. Host-derived proteases, originating either from saliva or dentine, might be involved in the degradation of the DOM [46, 47]. To date, two main classes of proteases have been implicated in the demineralisation processes of dentine: MMPs and CCs. Among MMPs, isoforms 2, 3, 8 and 9 have already been identified in dentine [48–52]. Many isoforms of CCs are present in the dentin-pulp complex, with cathepsin B being the most abundant [53].

MMPs are secreted as inactive precursors (pro-forms) that are activated in low pH environments (around 4.5). However, despite being activated, they are not functionally active to degrade the DOM at acidic pH, which can occur upon pH neutralisation. In addition, latent MMPs can be activated by CCs that are functionally active at acidic pH [54]. Thus, the events essential for MMP and CC activation and functional activity typically occur in erosion processes [55], where the pH fall due to the acid influx is followed by the neutralisation action of salivary buffers. Since CCs can degrade collagen at acidic pH while MMPs are functional at neutral environments, and considering that CCs can activate MMPs [54], the interplay between these two classes of collagenolytic enzymes seems to govern the fate of the DOM after erosive demineralisation. The role of collagenolytic enzymes in the progression of erosive demineralisation is supported by clinical data showing higher activity of collagenase in saliva of bulimic patients with erosion compared to control patients [56]. In addition, evidence from in vitro studies suggests that the DOM is resistant to abrasion [57, 58]. With these concepts in mind, a recently proposed strategy to prevent dentine erosion involves the use of protease inhibitors with the aim of preserving the DOM (fig. 2), which has a protective role against further mineral loss [55, 59].

Among the vast array of inhibitors that act on collagenolytic enzymes, epigallocatechin gallate (EGCG) and chlorhexidine (CHX) have been evaluated in situ. These compounds were included in rinse solutions [60, 61] or gels for topical application [62]. Both CHX and EGCG are classical inhibitors of MMPs [63, 64] while CHX has recently been shown to also inhibit CCs [65]. Green tea rinse reduced dentine wear by around 30–40% compared to control (water rinse) [60]. In the subsequent study, a green tea extract (OM24™ containing 30% EGCG; Omnimedica, Zürich, Zurich Switzerland) was used to prepare the rinse solution (0.61% OM24). Another rinse solution containing 0.06% CHX was also tested, as well as a fluoride rinse (250 ppm F as SnF$_2$/AmF) that was included as control. The rinses with protease inhibitors (EGCG or CHX) or fluoride reduced the

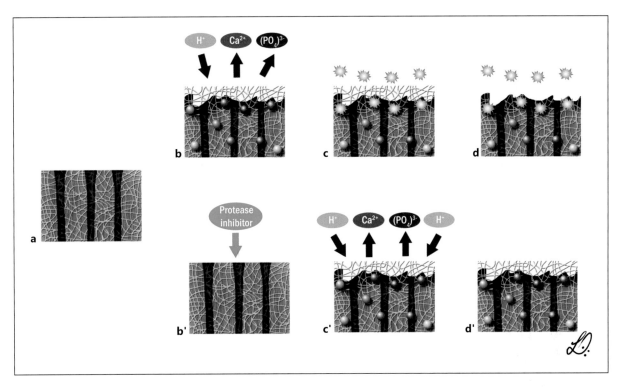

Fig. 2. Dentine (**a**) treated with protease inhibitor (**b'**), showing the preservation of the DOM (**c'**) and lower erosion progression (**d'**) compared to untreated dentine (**b–d**).

dentine wear significantly (around 30–40%) compared to the water rinse, but did not significantly differ from each other [61]. Although the rinses with protease inhibitors led to a significant reduction of dentine wear, the necessity of rinsing immediately after each erosive challenge is not practical for clinical application. Thus, as a further step, the protease inhibitors were included in gel formulations. Gels containing concentrations of EGCG or CHX that are known to inhibit MMPs (10 or 400 μM EGCG or 0.012% CHX) or NaF (control, 1.23%) were applied on the specimens for 1 min only once, before the first erosive challenge. The fluoride gel reduced dentine wear by more than 50% but did not significantly differ from placebo, while the gels containing protease inhibitors completely prevented dentine wear [62]. Thus, it appears that the protective effect is

higher when gels are used instead of rinse solutions. This might be due to the increased substantivity of the gels, which could allow enhanced penetration of the delivered agents into dentine. Additional studies are needed to evaluate how long the protective effect of the gels lasts and to assist in the development of protocols for clinical trials.

The results of these studies indicate that the use of compounds that are known for their ability to inhibit collagenolytic enzymes may be effective in the prevention of dentine erosion, which might be due to the preservation of the DOM itself or to its action on the de- and remineralisation processes. Preliminary evidence that the protective effect observed was due to the capacity of the compounds to inhibit collagen-degrading enzymes came from a recent in vitro proof-of-concept study. In this study, a superficial layer of

DOM was initially created on dentine by extensive demineralisation with citric acid (0.87 M, pH 2.3, 36 h). Demineralised dentine was then treated once for 1 min with gels containing EGCG (400 μM), CHX (0.012%), $FeSO_4$ (1 mM), NaF (1.23%) or no active compound (placebo). Following treatment, the DOM was degraded by collagenase from *Clostridium histolyticum* (5 days, 37°C). Collagen degradation was analysed by hydroxyproline assay and wear by profilometry. Both hydroxyproline concentration and dentine wear were significantly lower for dentine treated with protease inhibitors compared to fluoride or placebo [59]. Since hydroxyproline is one of the main amino acids present in collagen, which constitutes nearly 90% of the dentine organic matrix, this study provides evidence that the protease inhibitors are able to reduce the degradation of the DOM [see chapter by Shellis and Addy, this vol., pp. 32–45].

One interesting finding of the study by Kato et al. [59] was that the gel containing 1.23% NaF significantly reduced the DOM degradation. Due to this finding, it was hypothesised that besides its known action in erosive de- and remineralisation [66], fluoride could also inhibit MMPs. This hypothesis was confirmed using gelatin zymography that revealed decreased activities of pro- and active forms of salivary and purified human MMPs by incubation with NaF in a dose-response manner [67]. These findings might help to explain why the action of fluoride to prevent dentine erosion is dependent on the maintenance of the DOM [68] and provide new insights into the mechanism of action of fluoride for the prevention of erosion in dentine.

Despite the promising in vitro and in situ data showing the beneficial effect of protease inhibitors to prevent dentine erosion, clinical trials are required to confirm the relevance of this proposed preventive measure, as well as to establish protocols for its clinical use.

Conclusion

Based on this review of the literature, promising alternatives to the use of the fluoride ion include the deposition of protective barrier layers, whether through the use of sealants or polymers capable of depositing onto and protecting tooth surfaces against erosive acid attack. In addition, available data suggest that certain protease inhibitors, particularly when formulated as gels, may be of value in preserving the organic matrix of dentine, potentially reducing the progression of erosive wear. While there are clearly approaches that have demonstrated the potential to deliver effective preventive therapies against dental erosion (sealants, polymers, protease inhibitors), there is little data available to suggest that products containing calcium or phosphate are as effective as fluoride at preventing dental erosion. Additional studies, particularly in vivo studies, are needed to confirm the effectiveness of each of the potentially promising alternatives.

References

1 Wegehaupt FJ, Tauböck TT, Attin T: Durability of the anti-erosive effect of surface sealants under erosive abrasive conditions. Acta Odontol Scand 2013; 71:1188–1194.
2 Wegehaupt FJ, Tauböck TT, Sener B, Attin T: Long-term protective effect of surface sealants against erosive wear by intrinsic and extrinsic acids. J Dent 2012;40:416–422.

3 Sundaram G, Bartlett D, Watson T: Bonding to and protecting worn palatal surfaces of teeth with dentine bonding agents. J Oral Rehabil 2004;31:505–509.
4 Sundaram G, Wilson R, Watson TF, Bartlett DW: Effect of resin coating on dentine compared to repeated topical applications of fluoride mouthwash after an abrasion and erosion wear regime. J Dent 2007;35:814–818.

5 Sundaram G, Wilson R, Watson TF, Bartlett D: Clinical measurement of palatal tooth wear following coating by a resin sealing system. Oper Dent 2007;32: 539–543.
6 Bartlett D, Sundaram G, Moazzez R: Trial of protective effect of fissure sealants, in vivo, on the palatal surfaces of anterior teeth, in patients suffering from erosion. J Dent 2011;39:26–29.

7   Wegehaupt FJ, Tauböck TT, Attin T: How to re-seal previously sealed dentin. Am J Dent 2013;26:161–165.

8   Beyer M, Reichert J, Heurich E, Jandt KD, Sigusch BW: Pectin, alginate and gum arabic polymers reduce citric acid erosion effects on human enamel. Dent Mater 2010;26:831–839.

9   Barbour ME, Shellis RP, Parker DM, Allen GC, Addy M: An investigation of some food-approved polymers as agents to inhibit hydroxyapatite dissolution. Eur J Oral Sci 2005;113:457–461.

10 Lee IIS, Tsai S, Kuo CC, Bassani AW, Pepe-Mooney B, Miksa D, Masters J, Sullivan R, Composto RJ: Chitosan adsorption on hydroxyapatite and its role in preventing acid erosion. J Colloid Interface Sci 2012;385:235–243.

11 van der Mei HC, Engels E, de Vries J, Dijkstra RJ, Busscher HJ: Chitosan adsorption to salivary pellicles. Eur J Oral Sci 2007;115:303–307.

12 Arnaud TM, de Barros Neto B, Diniz FB: Chitosan effect on dental enamel de-remineralization: an in vitro evaluation. J Dent 2010;38:848–852.

13 Ganss C, Lussi A, Grunau O, Klimek J, Schlueter N: Conventional and anti-erosion fluoride toothpastes: effect on enamel erosion and erosion-abrasion. Caries Res 2011;45:581–589.

14 Ganss C, von Hinckeldey J, Tolle A, Schulze K, Klimek J, Schlueter N: Efficacy of the stannous ion and a biopolymer in toothpastes on enamel erosion/abrasion. J Dent 2012;40:1036–1043.

15 Schlueter N, Klimek J, Ganss C: Effect of chitosan additive to a Sn^{2+}-containing toothpaste on its anti-erosive/anti-abrasive efficacy a controlled randomised in situ trial. Clin Oral Investig 2014;18: 107–115.

16 Churchley D, Rees GD, Barbu E, Nevell TG, Tsibouklis J: Fluoropolymers as low-surface-energy tooth coatings for oral care. Int J Pharm 2008;352:44–49.

17 Nielsen BV, Nevell TG, Barbu E, Smith JR, Rees GD, Tsibouklis J: Multifunctional poly(alkyl methacrylate) films for dental care. Biomed Mater 2011;6: 015003.

18 Gracia LH, Brown A, Rees GD, Fowler CE: Studies on a novel combination polymer system: in vitro erosion prevention and promotion of fluoride uptake in human enamel. J Dent 2010; 38:S4–S11.

19 Ramalingam L, Messer LB, Reynolds E: Adding casein phosphopeptide-amorphous calcium phosphate to sports drinks to eliminate in vitro erosion. Pediatr Dent 2005;27:61–67.

20 Manton DJ, Cai F, Yuan Y, Walker GD, Cochrane NJ, Reynolds C, Brearley-Messer LJ, Reynolds EC: Effect of casein phosphopeptide-amorphous calcium phosphate added to acidic beverages on enamel erosion in vitro. Aust Dent J 2010;55:275–279.

21 Prestes L, Souza BM, Comar LP, Salomão PA, Rios D, Magalhães AC: In situ effect of chewing gum containing CPP-ACP on the mineral precipitation of eroded bovine enamel – a surface hardness analysis. J Dent 2013;41:747–751.

22 Wang X, Megert B, Hellwig E, Neuhaus KW, Lussi A: Preventing erosion with novel agents. J Dent 2011;39:163–170.

23 Rees J, Loyn T, Chadwick B: Pronamel and tooth mousse: an initial assessment of erosion prevention in vitro. J Dent 2007;35:355–357.

24 Piekarz C, Ranjitkar S, Hunt D, McIntyre J: An in vitro assessment of the role of Tooth Mousse in preventing wine erosion. Aust Dent J 2008;53:22–25.

25 Srinivasan N, Kavitha M, Loganathan SC: Comparison of the remineralization potential of CPP-ACP and CPP-ACP with 900 ppm fluoride on eroded human enamel: an in situ study. Arch Oral Biol 2010;55:541–544.

26 Wegehaupt FJ, Tauböck TT, Stillhard A, Schmidlin PR, Attin T: Influence of extra- and intra-oral application of CPP-ACP and fluoride on re-hardening of eroded enamel. Acta Odontol Scand 2012;70:177–183.

27 Ranjitkar S, Kaidonis JA, Richards LC, Townsend GC: The effect of CPP-ACP on enamel wear under severe erosive conditions. Arch Oral Biol 2009;54:527–532.

28 Ranjitkar S, Rodriguez JM, Kaidonis JA, Richards LC, Townsend GC, Bartlett DW: The effect of casein phosphopeptide-amorphous calcium phosphate on erosive enamel and dentine wear by toothbrush abrasion. J Dent 2009;37: 250–254.

29 Wegehaupt FJ, Attin T: The role of fluoride and casein phosphopeptide/amorphous calcium phosphate in the prevention of erosive/abrasive wear in an in vitro model using hydrochloric acid. Caries Res 2010;44:358–363.

30 Poggio C, Lombardini M, Colombo M, Bianchi S: Impact of two toothpastes on repairing enamel erosion produced by a soft drink: an AFM in vitro study. J Dent 2010;38:868–874.

31 Poggio C, Lombardini M, Vigorelli P, Colombo M, Chiesa M: The role of different toothpastes on preventing dentin erosion: An SEM and AFM study®. Scanning, 2013 Epub ahead of print.

32 Min JH, Kwon HK, Kim BI: The addition of nano-sized hydroxyapatite to a sports drink to inhibit dental erosion: in vitro study using bovine enamel. J Dent 2011;39:629–635.

33 Besinis A, van Noort R, Martin N: Infiltration of demineralized dentin with silica and hydroxyapatite nanoparticles. Dent Mater 2012;28:1012–1023.

34 Litkowski LJ, Hack GD, Sheaffer HB, Greenspan DC: Occlusion of dentin tubules by 45S5 Bioglass; in Sedel L, Rey C (eds): Bioceramics. Proceedings of the 10th International Symposium on Ceramics in Medicine. New York, Elsevier, 1997, vol 10, pp 411–444.

35 Turssi CP, Maeda FA, Messias DC, Neto FC, Serra MC, Galafassi D: Effect of potential remineralizing agents on acid softened enamel. Am J Dent 2011;24: 165–168.

36 Moretto MJ, Magalhães AC, Sassaki KT, Delbem AC, Martinhon CC: Effect of different fluoride concentrations of experimental dentifrices on enamel erosion and abrasion. Caries Res 2010;44: 135–140.

37 Manarelli MM, Vieira AE, Matheus AA, Sassaki KT, Delbem AC: Effect of mouth rinses with fluoride and trimetaphosphate on enamel erosion: an in vitro study. Caries Res 2011;45:506–509.

38 Ellingsen JE: Scanning electron microscope and electron microprobe study of reactions of stannous fluoride and stannous chloride with dental enamel. Scand J Dent Res 1985;94:299–305.

39 Ganss C, Schlueter N, Hardt M, Schattenberg P, Klimek J: Effect of fluoride compounds on enamel erosion in vitro-a comparison of amine, sodium and stannous fluoride. Caries Res 2008;42: 2–7.

40 Gray JA: Acid dissolution rate of sound and white-spot enamel treated with tin(II) and fluoride compounds. J Dent Res 1965;44:493–501.

41 Ganss C, Lussi A, Sommer N, Klimek J, Schlueter N: Efficacy of fluoride compounds and stannous chloride as erosion inhibitors in dentine. Caries Res 2010;44:172–176.

42 Shrestha BM, Mundorff SA, Bibby BG: Enamel dissolution. I. Effects of various agents and titanium tetrafluoride. J Dent Res 1972;51:1561–1566.

43 Ganss C, Klimek J, Schäffer U, Spall T: Effectiveness of two fluoridation measures on erosion progression in human enamel and dentine in vitro. Caries Res 2001;35:325–330.

44 Kleter GA, Damen JJ, Everts V, Niehof J, Ten Cate JM: The influence of the organic matrix on demineralization of bovine root dentin in vitro. J Dent Res 1994;73:1523–1529.

45 Klont B, ten Cate JM: Susceptibility of the collagenous matrix from bovine incisor roots to proteolysis after in vitro lesion formation. Caries Res 1991;25: 46–50.

46 Tjäderhane L, Larjava H, Sorsa T, Uitto VJ, Larmas M, Salo T: The activation and function of host matrix metalloproteinases in dentin matrix breakdown in caries lesions. J Dent Res 1998;77:1622–1629.

47 van Strijp AJ, Jansen DC, DeGroot J, ten Cate JM, Everts V: Host-derived proteinases and degradation of dentine collagen in situ. Caries Res 2003;37:58–65.

48 Martin-De Las Heras S, Valenzuela A, Overall CM: The matrix metalloproteinase gelatinase A in human dentine. Arch Oral Biol 2000;45:757–765.

49 Mazzoni A, Mannello F, Tay FR, Tonti GA, Papa S, Mazzotti G, Di Lenarda R, Pashley DH, Breschi L: Zymographic analysis and characterization of MMP-2 and -9 forms in human sound dentin. J Dent Res 2007;86:436–440.

50 Mazzoni A, Papa V, Nato F, Carrilho M, Tjäderhane L, Ruggeri A Jr, Gobbi P, Mazzotti G, Tay FR, Pashley DH, Breschi L: Immunohistochemical and biochemical assay of MMP-3 in human dentine. J Dent 2011;39:231–237.

51 Sulkala M, Tervahartiala T, Sorsa T, Larmas M, Salo T, Tjäderhane L: Matrix metalloproteinase-8 (MMP-8) is the major collagenase in human dentin. Arch Oral Biol 2007;52:121–127.

52 Kato MT, Hannas AR, Leite AL, Bolanho A, Zarella BL, Santos J, Carrilho M, Tjäderhane L, Buzalaf MA: Activity of matrix metalloproteinases in bovine versus human dentine. Caries Res 2011;45: 429–434.

53 Tersariol IL, Geraldeli S, Minciotti CL, Nascimento FD, Pääkkönen V, Martins MT, Carrilho MR, Pashley DH, Tay FR, Salo T, Tjäderhane L: Cysteine cathepsins in human dentin-pulp complex. J Endod 2010;36:475–481.

54 Nagase H: Activation mechanisms of matrix metalloproteinases. Biol Chem 1997;378:151–160.

55 Buzalaf MA, Kato MT, Hannas AR: The role of matrix metalloproteinases in dental erosion. Adv Dent Res 2012;24: 72–76.

56 Schlueter N, Ganss C, Pötschke S, Klimek J, Hannig C: Enzyme activities in the oral fluids of patients suffering from bulimia: a controlled clinical trial. Caries Res 2012;46:130–139.

57 Ganss C, Schlueter N, Hardt M, von Hinckeldey J, Klimek J: Effects of toothbrushing on eroded dentine. Eur J Oral Sci 2007;115:390–396.

58 Ganss C, Hardt M, Blazek D, Klimek J, Schlueter N: Effects of toothbrushing force on the mineral content and demineralized organic matrix of eroded dentine. Eur J Oral Sci 2009;117:255–260.

59 Kato MT, Leite AL, Hannas AR, Calabria MP, Magalhães AC, Pereira JC, Buzalaf MA: Impact of protease inhibitors on dentin matrix degradation by collagenase. J Dent Res 2012;91:1119–1123.

60 Kato MT, Magalhães AC, Rios D, Hannas AR, Attin T, Buzalaf MA: Protective effect of green tea on dentin erosion and abrasion. J Appl Oral Sci 2009;17:560–564.

61 Magalhães AC, Wiegand A, Rios D, Hannas A, Attin T, Buzalaf MA: Chlorhexidine and green tea extract reduce dentin erosion and abrasion in situ. J Dent 2009;37:994–998.

62 Kato MT, Leite AL, Hannas AR, Buzalaf MA: Gels containing MMP inhibitors prevent dental erosion in situ. J Dent Res 2010;89:468–472.

63 Gendron R, Grenier D, Sorsa T, Mayrand D: Inhibition of the activities of matrix metalloproteinases 2, 8, and 9 by chlorhexidine. Clin Diagn Lab Immunol 1999;6:437–439.

64 Demeule M, Brossard M, Page M, Gingras D, Beliveau R: Matrix metalloproteinase inhibition by green tea catechins. Biochim Biophys Acta 2000;1478:51–60.

65 Scaffa PM, Vidal CM, Barros N, Gesteira TF, Carmona AK, Breschi L, Pashley DH, Tjäderhane L, Tersariol IL, Nascimento FD, Carrilho MR: Chlorhexidine inhibits the activity of dental cysteine cathepsins. J Dent Res 2012;91:420–425.

66 Magalhães AC, Wiegand A, Rios D, Buzalaf MA, Lussi A: Fluoride in dental erosion. Monogr Oral Sci 2011;22:158–170.

67 Kato MT, Bolanho A, Zarella BL, Salo T, Tjäderhane L, Buzalaf MA: Sodium fluoride inhibits MMP-2 and MMP-9. J Dent Res 2014;93:74–77.

68 Ganss C, Klimek J, Starck C: Quantitative analysis of the impact of the organic matrix on the fluoride effect on erosion progression in human dentine using longitudinal microradiography. Arch Oral Biol 2004;49:931–935.

Prof. M.A.R. Buzalaf
Department of Biological Sciences, Bauru Dental School
University of São Paulo
Al. Octávio Pinheiro Brisolla, 9-75
Bauru, SP 17012-901 (Brazil)
E-Mail mbuzalaf@fob.usp.br

Lussi A, Ganss C (eds): Erosive Tooth Wear. Monogr Oral Sci. Basel, Karger, 2014, vol 25, pp 253–261
DOI: 10.1159/000360562

Restorative Therapy of Erosive Lesions

Anne Peutzfeldt · Thomas Jaeggi · Adrian Lussi

Department of Preventive, Restorative and Pediatric Dentistry, School of Dental Medicine, University of Bern, Bern, Switzerland

Abstract

When substance loss caused by erosive tooth wear reaches a certain degree, oral rehabilitation becomes necessary. Until some 20 years ago, the severely eroded dentition could only be rehabilitated by the provision of extensive crown and bridge work or removable overdentures. As a result of the improvements in resin composite restorative materials, and in adhesive techniques, it has become possible to rehabilitate eroded dentitions in a less invasive manner. However, even today advanced erosive destruction requires the placement of more extensive restorations such as overlays and crowns. It has to be kept in mind that the etiology of the erosive lesions needs to be determined in order to halt the disease, otherwise the erosive process will continue to destroy tooth substance. This overview presents aspects concerning the restorative materials as well as the treatment options available to rehabilitate patients with erosive tooth wear, from minimally invasive direct composite reconstructions to adhesively retained all-ceramic restorations. Restorative treatment is dependent on individual circumstances and the perceived needs and concerns of the patient. Long-term success is only possible when the cause is eliminated. In all situations, the restorative preparations have to follow the principles of minimally invasive treatment. © 2014 S. Karger AG, Basel

Early Diagnosis and Prevention

In order to plan adequate preventive and therapeutic measures, a thorough case history and diagnosis of each patient is mandatory. The teeth of all new patients and patients who are scheduled for a recall appointment (children as well as adults) should not only be examined for caries and periodontal diseases but also for noncarious tooth surface loss. Special consideration should be given to the following: dietary habits, drinking habits and sport activities, as well as gastric or esophageal problems. Furthermore, in patients judged to be at risk, the salivary flow rates and its buffering capacity should be measured. Patients with presumed reflux or vomiting problems require to be referred to a gastroenterologist or psychologist for further examination and therapy. If erosive tooth wear is diagnosed at an early stage it may be possible to protect the dentition against further damage. Local preventive measures may provide some protection against erosive challenge [1, 2]. For more information see chapter by Huysmans et al. [this vol., pp. 230–243].

Erosive Tooth Wear and Adhesion of Restorative Materials

Initially, erosive tooth wear is limited to enamel. At this stage of the erosive process, the teeth are not hypersensitive. Restorations may be inserted because of esthetic needs and/or to prevent further progression. Direct resin composite coverage or, in more advanced cases, ceramic veneers should be considered as the treatment of choice. This seals the enamel, re-establishes the tooth contour and minimizes further enamel loss by acid exposure. Both treatment options rely on effective adhesive bonding for clinical success. Reportedly, the structure of eroded enamel resembles that of enamel etched with phosphoric acid as a step in the adhesive procedure for the bonding of resin materials, i.e. a superficially softened layer with exposed enamel prisms [3, 4]. It appears that no information is available comparing bond strength to eroded enamel with the bond strength to normal, phosphoric acid-etched enamel, but it seems probable that there will be no difference [4].

In advanced cases, dentine becomes exposed, and there could be several reasons for treatment need, such as: (1) the structural integrity of the tooth is threatened, (2) the exposed dentine is hypersensitive, (3) the erosive defect is esthetically unacceptable to the patient or (4) pulpal exposure is likely to occur [5]. Most often the preferred treatment involves adhesive bonding. As a result of erosive processes dentine gradually becomes sclerotic, displaying a hypermineralized shiny surface along with tubular occlusion [6]. Although a few studies, using bovine dentine, have found no difference between resin bond strength to normal and sclerotic dentine [7, 8], most studies, using human dentine, have reported bond strength to sclerotic dentine to be lower than the bond strength to normal dentine [4, 9–13]. The decrease is thought to result from the tubular occlusion by mineral salts, preventing resin tag formation [6]. Two fundamentally different approaches have been investigated as to how to avoid impaired adhesion to sclerotic and/or erosively altered dentine: a chemical approach and a mechanical approach. Contradictory results exist as to the effect of the chemical approach. Whereas doubling the phosphoric acid etching time prior to application of a 2-step etch-and-rinse adhesive system increased the bond strength to sclerotic dentine [14], doubling the phosphoric acid or the primer etching time prior to application of a 2- or 3-step etch-and-rinse adhesive system or of a 1- or 2-step self-etching adhesive system had no effect on the bond strength to either normal or sclerotic dentine [15]. As regards the mechanical approach, a recent study found minimal roughening of eroded dentine with a diamond bur to be the pretreatment which caused the least drop in 1-year bond strengths compared to normal dentine [12]. Another recent study has reported pretreatment with an ER,Cr:YSGG laser to be just as effective or, depending on the adhesive system, even more effective than roughening with a diamond bur or pretreatment with an Er:YAG laser [16]. Thus, the published studies, although limited in number, indicate that adhesion to eroded dentine can be improved by a mechanical roughening pretreatment.

Numerous studies have shown tin-containing fluoride mouth rinses to be effective against erosive wear [17–20], the incorporated tin having a stabilizing effect on the eroded surface. It has been speculated that this positive effect is accompanied by a negative one. The incorporated tin might interfere with the adhesive applied during the following restorative procedure and thus impair the adhesion of the resin composite, reducing the longevity of the restoration. However, using an MDP-containing 2-step self-etching adhesive system (Clearfil SE Bond; Kuraray, Tokyo, Japan), bond strength to eroded dentine has been found not to decrease as a consequence of previous treatment with a tin-containing fluoride mouth rinse [13]. Indeed, bond strength increased. Subsequent studies investigated the effect on resin composite adhesion to enamel and dentine of including into the adhesive procedure a pretreatment with a 35% tin-chloride solution [21, 22]. Partial or total replacement of phosphoric acid etching with tin-chloride etching reduced bond strengths obtained with a 3-step etch-and-rinse adhesive (Optibond FL; Kerr, Orange, Calif., USA). In contrast, including an extra phosphoric acid or tin-chloride etching step prior to application of the self-etching primer increased bond strengths obtained with the MDP-containing 2-step self-etching adhesive system (Clearfil SE Bond) – etching with tin-chloride being more effective than etching with phosphoric acid. Consequently, it was concluded that the MDP-containing adhesive system seems to have a bond-promoting capacity to tin compounds incorporated in the enamel or dentine [21, 22]. However, further improvements, for example as regards concentration and stability of the tin-chloride solution, are needed before the tin-chloride treatment can be used in clinical practice.

Longevity of Restorative Materials under Acidic Conditions

The longevity of dental restorations depends on the durability of the material per se, the durability of the interface between tooth substance and restoration, and the extent of tooth destruction and its location and load, as well as on patient-related factors such as bruxism, dietary and tooth-cleaning habits. Although it would be preferable to eliminate the cause of the erosions and the erosive tooth wear before commencing restorative treatment, this approach is rarely feasible, implying that the restorations are bound to be exposed to erosive challenges.

A little more than a handful of studies have investigated and compared the behavior of various direct restorative materials under acidic and erosive conditions. Shabanian and Richards [23] measured, in vitro, the wear rates of a conventional glass-ionomer cement, a resin-modified glass-ionomer cement and a resin composite under different loads and varying pH. All three materials were more resistant to acid than enamel, with the resin composite demonstrating the highest resistance to acid. The acid and load resistance of the resin-modified glass-ionomer cement was less than that of the resin composite and higher than that of the conventional glass-ionomer cement. In a study of the interaction of restorative materials with acidic beverages, all materials evaluated were found to reduce the pH of the 0.9% NaCl solution (control) but to increase the pH of the acidic beverages [24]. Furthermore, the conventional glass-ionomer cement dissolved completely in apple and orange juice but survived in Coca-Cola despite a significant reduction in hardness after a 1-year immersion time. The resin-modified glass-ionomer cements and the compomers survived in apple and orange juice, but showed greater reductions in surface hardness in these beverages than in Coca-Cola. Fruit juices were thus shown to pose a greater erosive threat to the restorative materials than Coca-Cola, something that was claimed to be true also for enamel and dentine. The influence of different dietary solvents (0.02 M citric acid, 50% ethanol-water solution, heptane, distilled water as control) on the shear punch strength of a conventional glass-ionomer cement, a compomer and three types of resin composites has been determined in a study by Yap et al. [25]. The results showed lower strength for the nanofilled and the ormocer resin composites than for the minifilled resin composite, but higher strengths than those achieved for the compomer and the highly viscous, conventional glass-ionomer cement. Another investigation measured the effect of pH on the microhardness of a resin composite, a compomer and a so-called giomer. The results showed a material dependency: the compomer and the giomer were more affected by acids than was the resin composite [26]. Determining the effect of a prolonged erosive pH cycling procedure on microhardness and erosive wear of three restorative materials, Honorio et al. [27] found that the resin composite was much less sensitive to the erosive procedure than the resin-modified glass-ionomer cement, which performed better than the conventional glass-ionomer cement. In a study of the effect of erosion and/or toothbrush abrasion, the three resin composites tested presented higher durability under erosive and/or abrasive attacks than did the compomer and the conventional glass-ionomer cement evaluated. Human enamel presented higher substance loss than any of the restorative materials [28]. In their study of the susceptibility of five restorative materials to damage by common erosive acids, Wan Bakar and McIntyre [29] found in vitro restorations of resin composite or porcelain not to be affected at all by the erosive challenges, while restorations of the resin-modified glass ionomer cement were moderately damaged and the two conventional glass-ionomer cements were severely damaged. Besides confirming that resin composites have higher resistance to erosive attack than conventional glass-ionomer cement and compomer as well as reporting resin composite also to have higher resistance to topical fluoride application, Yu et al. [30] found the application of a high-concentrated AmF solution at native pH to increase the acid resistance of conventional glass-ionomer cement and compomer.

Only few studies have investigated the influence of dietary acids on ceramic materials. One study tested the effect of intermittent immersion in a carbonated beverage (Coca-Cola) on the wear of three ceramics and of human enamel specimens serving as antagonists. Exposure to Coca-Cola was found to accelerate enamel wear and to decrease the wear resistance of two of the ceramics [31]. Another study, simulating vomiting through 24 h using a simulated vomit solution (pH = 3.8), reported no effect on various surface roughness parameters for the three ceramic materials tested [32]. Finally, a very recent study investigated the effect of pH and time on the degra-

dation of glass ceramic veneers and a glaze material [33]. Whereas exposure to a basic pH buffer (pH = 10) led to substantial release of Si over time and to subsequent breakdown of the glass phase, exposure to an acidic pH (pH = 2) caused 'only' selective ionic leaching of the glass matrix.

To conclude, under acidic conditions all restorative materials show degradation over time (surface roughness, decrease of surface hardness, substance loss). However, it seems that ceramic materials and resin composites present much better durability than conventional glass-ionomer cements, resin-modified glass-ionomer cements and compomers, and that the latter materials should not be used in erosion patients.

Treatment Strategies

Initial restorative treatments should be conservative, using adhesive materials [34]. Modern therapeutic concepts determine that minimal amounts of healthy tooth substance should be sacrificed. Reconstructive restorative treatments should be adapted to the tooth and not vice versa. However, when teeth wear, the alveolar bone and the associated tissues adapt to some degree to the change with alveolar compensation [35]. Despite losing crown height, teeth maintain their occlusal contact and this may lead to problems for their reconstruction because there is not enough space for the restorative material. To prevent an invasive, full-mouth rehabilitation, it can be convenient to gain interocclusal space through orthodontic measures, especially if mainly groups of teeth (e.g. all teeth in the anterior region) are involved in the erosive tooth wear. The orthodontic treatment can be achieved with fixed or removable appliances such as the Dahl appliance [35]. Following orthodontic treatment, the eroded teeth can then be reconstructed [36]. Until some 20 years ago, the severely eroded dentition could only be rehabilitated by the provision of extensive crown and bridge work or, in more severe cases, by means of removable overdentures [37–39]. As a result of the improvements in resin composites and in adhesive techniques, it has become possible to rehabilitate eroded dentitions in a less invasive manner. The wear resistance of resin composites has gradually improved, and today direct resin composite restorations can provide excellent longevity, even in load-bearing situations [40–42]. Several case reports demonstrate the successful rehabilitation of (erosively) worn dentitions using adhesive techniques [43–46]. A very elegant method was described using direct resin composite build-up with the help of a vacuum-formed matrix template [47]. Good results were found after an average time in service of 5.5 years [48]. This method was later modified using the 'stamp' technique [49]. Tooth wear defects can be restored by copying the wax-up from the dental technician using silicone impressions. Both 'semi-direct' techniques facilitate the placement of large resin composite restorations and can be highly recommended.

Minimal Loss of Vertical Dimension: Sealant or Resin Composite

Treatment of erosive tooth wear should be performed at an early stage in order to prevent the development of functional and esthetic problems. The most minimally invasive measure is the sealing of the tooth surface. In one study [50], Seal and Protect (Dentsply DeTrey, Konstanz, Germany) and Optibond Solo (Kerr, Orange, Calif., USA) were each applied to extracted teeth and then subjected to an erosion/abrasion wear regime. It was concluded that both adhesive systems provided effective protection of the teeth. Another in vitro study examined the protective effect of adhesive systems on dentine after acid exposure and brushing abrasion in a cycling model. Twelve dentine samples were each pretreated with K-106 experimental varnish (Dentsply DeTrey), Prime & Bond 2.1 (Dentsply DeTrey), Syntac Classic with Heliobond (Vivadent, Schaan, Liechtenstein) or Gluma Desensitizer (Heraeus

Kulzer, Dormagen, Germany). Another twelve samples served as the untreated control group. Each test sample was subjected 120 times to the following procedure: 5 min of demineralization (Sprite Light), 1 h of storage in artificial saliva, and brushing abrasion (100 brush strokes) in an automatic brushing machine. Surface substance loss was measured by laser profilometry. It was concluded that adhesive systems can protect dentine from erosive tooth wear for a limited period of time [51]. In an in situ study, Azzopardi et al. [52] investigated the surface effects of erosion and abrasion on dentine with and without a protective layer (Seal and Protect or Optibond Solo). Dentine samples were attached to an appliance and worn 8 h per day for 20 consecutive days. Every day the samples were removed and immersed in citric acid for 24 min. The effects of the acid exposure and the mechanical influence of the soft tissues, especially the tongue, on tooth surface substance loss were measured using four assessment techniques. Results showed that the sealing materials remained in place despite the vigorous wear regime and therefore protected the tooth surface. The authors concluded that applying a dentine adhesive to exposed dentine in patients with erosive tooth wear is a practical measure which prevents further damage. This finding was later confirmed in vivo as a one-bottle sealant and a classic fissure sealant both showed good protection for up to 9 months [53, 54]. This is in corroboration with the in vitro study of Wegehaupt et al. [55], who found surface sealants to reduce erosive dentine mineral loss and to maintain the erosive-preventing efficacy during the entire erosive/abrasion cycling procedure applied, simulating 8 months in vivo. Thus, the sealing procedures have to be repeated periodically; fortunately, it has been shown that no additional pretreatment of previously sealed dentine is necessary to ensure stability of the new sealant [56]. The sealing of numerous lesions in one patient may also be time consuming because of the light-curing time needed to cure each sealant. Howev-

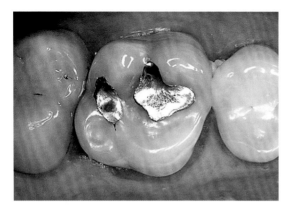 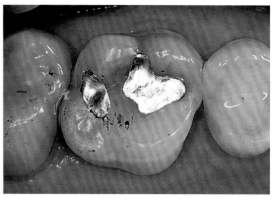

Fig. 1. Occlusal erosion with involvement of dentine. The margins of the amalgam restorations stand proud of the adjacent tooth surfaces.

Fig. 2. The groove-like defects of the molar were filled with resin composite after the cause (gastroesophageal reflux) had been treated. Control of the occlusion is important to prevent early contact on the groove restorations (same case as fig. 1); 2 years in situ.

er, a recent study found that reducing the light-curing time while keeping the energy density constant did not hamper the mechanical stability or the permeability of three different sealants [57]. This indicates that light-curing times may be shortened provided a high energy density light-curing unit is used.

Occlusal erosions typically appear as groove-like defects and restoration margins stand proud of the adjacent tooth surfaces. Following an acid attack the pH in these grooves is depressed for a prolonged period of time [unpubl. data], which will lead to further progression of the erosive process at this site. In such cases, minimally invasive resin composite restorations are able to protect the affected region (fig. 1, 2).

Distinct Loss of Vertical Dimension: Resin Composite or Ceramic

As long as there is only a loss of about 3–4 mm of interocclusal space, the teeth can be reconstructed directly or semi-directly with resin composites or with ceramics. Patients usually tolerate such an increase in the vertical dimension without any problem. Teeth are rebuilt with semi-direct methods or 'freehand' according to their original anatomy (fig. 3–5). The advantages of direct resin composite restorations are that they are adaptable to the defect and that repair is straightforward. The situation is more problematic if the occlusal and vestibular erosions merge; the original tooth shape becomes hardly recognizable and the loss of vertical dimension tends to be greater. In general, less invasive reconstruction procedures such as direct adhesive methods are preferable to indirect methods, but they are not always possible. For example, if the upper front teeth are severely eroded and need to be reconstructed, ceramic or resin composite veneers may be applied (fig. 6, 7). If the defects (on posterior teeth) show an extension over two or more tooth surfaces and the vertical tooth substance loss is massive, then reconstruction with full ceramic overlays is convenient. In patients with severe tooth surface loss on more than two surfaces per tooth and pronounced loss of vertical dimension, a complex reconstruction with indirect restorations (ceramic crowns, bridges) is often inevitable (fig. 6, 7). This measure should be restricted to very advanced erosion cases. However, such treatment is expensive. Therefore, it is important to combine active treatment with preventive measures and

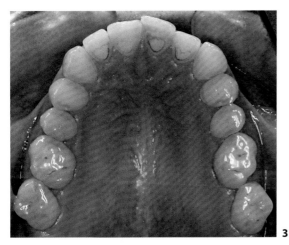
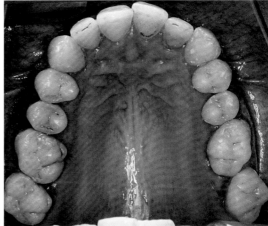

Fig. 3. Severe erosive tooth wear with involvement of dentine and loss of height.

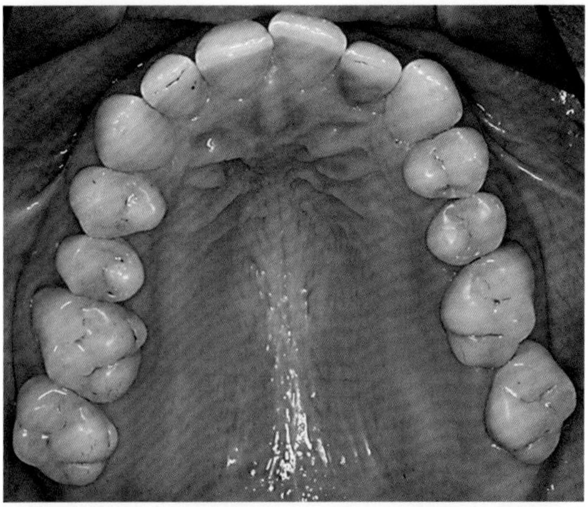

Fig. 4. The teeth were rebuilt freehandedly with direct resin composite restorations. Altogether, the vertical dimension was raised about 3 mm, which the patient tolerated without difficulty.

Fig. 5. The situation after 3 years in situ.

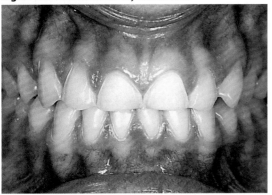

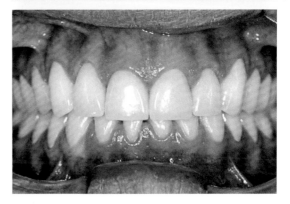

Fig. 6. Facial view of advanced dentinal erosive tooth wear. Also, the lower incisors have clearly eroded. The patient had a history of anorexia nervosa with unfavorable acidic nutrition.

Fig. 7. Completed restoration of the upper and lower arches with full ceramic crowns and veneers on the lower incisors. The vertical dimension had to be increased by 4 mm in the anterior region. This increase was accomplished and tested step-by-step by means of provisional crowns. The patient did not have any problems adapting to the new vertical dimension.

recall at regular intervals to ensure the long-term success.

To conclude, the restorative treatment should be adapted to the extent of tooth substance loss. It should be further kept in mind that erosive tooth wear is a multifactorial condition, and in many cases it is not possible to determine and eliminate all etiological parameters. In such cases, the long-term success of the rehabilitation may be compromised. Only in rare cases may restorations be inserted without treating the main causes (e.g. in patients with frequent vomiting, but who are already under psychological treatment).

Acknowledgements

The authors thank Drs. Matthias Strub and Anne Grüninger, Department of Preventive, Restorative and Pediatric Dentistry, University of Bern for providing some of the clinical pictures used in this chapter.

References

1 Amaechi BT, Higham SM: Dental erosion: possible approaches to prevention and control. J Dent 2005;33:243–252.

2 Vieira A, Ruben JL, Huysmans MC: Effect of titanium tetrafluoride, amine fluoride and fluoride varnish on enamel erosion in vitro. Caries Res 2005;39: 371–379.

3 Attin T, Koidl U, Buchalla W, Schaller HG, Kielbassa AM, Hellwig E: Correlation of microhardness and wear in differently eroded bovine dental enamel. Arch Oral Biol 1997;42:243–250.

4 Attin T, Wegehaupt FJ: Impact of erosive conditions on tooth-colored restorative materials. Dent Mater 2014;30: 43–49.

5 Lambrechts P, Van Meerbeek B, Perdigao J, Gladys S, Braem M, Vanherle G: Restorative therapy for erosive lesions. Eur J Oral Sci 1996;104:229–240.

6 Tay FR, Pashley DH: Resin bonding to cervical sclerotic dentin: a review. J Dent 2004;32:173–196.

7 Schmidlin PR, Siebenmann J, Kocher P, Seemann R, Attin T, Bindl A: Effects of de- and remineralization of dentin on bond strengths yielded by one-, three-, and four-step adhesives. J Adhes Dent 2008;10:119–126.

8 Cruz JB, Lenzi TL, Tedesco TK, Guglielmi Cde A, Raggio DP: Eroded dentin does not jeopardize the bond strength of adhesive restorative materials. Braz Oral Res 2012;26:306–312.

9 Perdigao J, Swift EJ, Denehy GE, Wefel JS, Donly KJ: In vitro bond strengths and SEM evaluation of dentin bonding systems to different dentin substrates. J Dent Res 1994;73:44–55.

10 Yoshiyama M, Sano H, Ebisu S, Tagami J, Ciucchi B, Carvalho RM, Johnson MH, Pashley DH: Regional strengths of bonding agents to cervical sclerotic root dentin. J Dent Res 1996;75;1404–1413.

11 Kwong SM, Cheung GS, Kei LH, Itthagarun A, Smales RJ, Tay FR, Pashley DH: Micro-tensile bond strengths to sclerotic dentin using a self-etching and a total-etching technique. Dent Mater 2002;18: 359–369.

12 Zimmerli B, De Munck J, Lussi A, Lambrechts P, Van Meerbeek B: Long-term bonding to eroded dentin requires superficial bur preparation. Clin Oral Investig 2012;16:1451–1461.

13 Flury S, Koch T, Peutzfeldt A, Lussi A, Ganss C: The effect of a tin-containing fluoride mouth rinse on the bond between resin composite and erosively demineralised dentin. Clin Oral Investig 2013;17:217–225.

14 Lopes GC, Vieira LC, Arauo E, Bruggmann T, Zucco J, Oliveira G: Effect of dentin age and acid etching time on dentin bonding. J Adhes Dent 2011;13: 139–145.

15 Oliviera GC, Oliviera GM, Ritter AV, Heymann HO, Swift EJ, Yamauchi M: Influence of tooth age and etching time on the microtensile bond strengths of adhesive systems to dentin. J Adhes Dent 2012;14:229–234.

16 Ramos TM, Ramos-Oliveira TM, de Freitas PM, Azambuja N, Esteves-Oliveira M, Gutknecht N, de Paula Eduardo C: Effects of Er:YAG and Er,Cr:YSGG laser irradiation on the adhesion to eroded dentin. Laser Med Sci, Epub ahead of print.

17 Ganss C, Schlueter N, Hardt M, Schattenberg P, Klimek J: Effect of fluoride compounds on enamel erosion in vitro: a comparison of amine, sodium and stannous fluoride. Caries Res 2008;42: 2–7.

18 Wiegand A, Bichsel D, Magalhaes AC, Becker K, Attin T: Effect of sodium, amine and stannous fluoride at the same concentration and different pH on in vitro erosion. J Dent 2009;37:591–595.

19 Ganss C, Lussi A, Sommer N, Klimek J, Schlueter N: Efficacy of fluoride compounds and stannous chloride as erosion inhibitors in dentine. Caries Res 2010;44:248–252.

20 Ganss C, Neutard L, von Hinckelday J, Klimek J, Schlueter N: Efficacy of a tin/fluoride rinse: a randomized in situ trial on erosion. J Dent Res 2010;89:1214–1218.

21 Schlueter N, Peutzfeldt A, Ganss C, Lussi A: Does tin pre-treatment enhance the bond strength of adhesive systems to enamel? J Dent 2013;41: 642–652.

22 Peutzfeldt A, Koch T, Ganss C, Flury S, Lussi A: Effect of tin-chloride pretreatment on bond strength of two adhesive systems to dentin. Clin Oral Investig 2014;18:535–543.

23 Shabanian M, Richards LC: In vitro wear rates of materials under different loads and varying pH. J Prosthet Dent 2002; 87:650–656.

24 Aliping-McKenzie M, Linden RWA, Nicholson JW: The effect of Coca-Cola and fruit juices on the surface hardness of glass-ionomers and 'compomers'. J Oral Rehabil 2004;31:1046–1052.

25 Yap AU, Lim LY, Yang TY, Ali A, Chung SM: Influence of dietary solvents on strength of nanofill and ormocer composites. Oper Dent 2005;30:129–133.

26 Mohamed-Tahir MA, Tan HY, Woo AA, Yap AU: Effects of pH on the microhardness of resin-based restorative materials. Oper Dent 2005;30:661–666.

27 Honorio HM, Rios D, Francisconi LF, Magalhaes AC, Machado MA, Buzalaf MA: Effect of prolonged erosive pH on different restorative materials. J Oral Rehabil 2008;35:947–953.

28 Hao Y, Wegehaupt FJ, Wiegand A, Roos M, Attin T, Buchalla W: Erosion and abrasion of tooth-colored restorative materials and human enamel. J Dent 2009;37:913–922.

29 Wan Bakar WZ, McIntyre J: Susceptibility of selected tooth-coloured dental materials to damage by common erosive acids. Aust Dent J 2008;53:226–234.

30 Yu H, Buchalla W, Cheng H, Wiegand A, Attin T: Topical fluoride application is able to reduce acid susceptibility of restorative materials. Dent Mater J 2012; 31:433–442.

31 Al-Hiyasat AS, Saunders WP, Sharkey SW, Smith GM: The effect of a carbonated beverage on the wear of human enamel and dental ceramics. J Prosthodont 1998;7:2–12.

32 Matsou E, Vouroutzis N, Kontonasaki E, Paraskevopoulos KM, Koidis P: Investigation of the influence of gastric acid on the surface roughness of ceramic materials of metal-ceramic restorations. An in vitro study. Int J Prosthodont 2001; 24:26–29.

33 Esquivel-Upshaw JF, Dieng FY, Clark AE, Neal D, Anusavice KJ: Surface degradation of dental ceramics as a function of environmental pH. J Dent Res 2013; 92:467–471.

34 Yip KH, Smales RJ, Kaidonis JA: The diagnosis and control of extrinsic acid erosion of tooth substance. Quintessence Int 2002;33:516–520.

35 Dahl BL, Krogstad O: The effect of partial bite raising splint on the occlusal face height. An X-ray cephalometric study in human adults. Acta Odontol Scand 1982;40:17–24.

36 Bartlett DW: The role of erosion in tooth wear: aetiology, prevention and management. Int Dent J 2005;4:277–284.

37 Hugo B: Orale Rehabilitation einer Erosionssituation. Schweiz Monatsschr Zahnmed 1991;101:1155–1162.

38 Ganddini MR, Al-Mardini M, Graser GN, Almong D: Maxillary and mandibular overlay removable partial dentures for the restoration of worn teeth. J Prosthet Dent 2004;91:210–214.

39 Kavoura V, Kourtis SG, Zoidis P, Andritsakis DP, Doukoudakis A: Full-mouth rehabilitation of a patient with bulimia nervosa: a case report. Quintessence Int 2005;36:501–510.

40 Hickel R, Manhart J: Longevity of restorations in posterior teeth and reasons for failure. J Adhes Dent 2001;3:45–64.

41 Opdam NJ, Bronkhorst EM, Roeters JM, Loomans BA: A retrospective clinical study on longevity of posterior composite and amalgam restorations. Dent Mater 2007;23:2–8.

42 Da Rosa Rodolpho PA, Donassollo TA, Cenci MS, Loguercio AD, Moraes RR, Bronkhorst EM, Opdam NJ, Demarco FF: 22-Year clinical evaluation of the performance of two posterior composites with different filler characteristics. Dent Mater 2011;27:955–963.

43 Hastings JH: Conservative restoration of function and aesthetics in a bulimic patient: a case report. Pract Periodontics Aesthet Dent 1996;8:729–736.

44 Tepper SA, Schmidlin PR: Technik der direkten Bisshöhenrekonstruktion mit Komposit und einer Schiene als Formhilfe. Schweiz Monatsschr Zahnmed 2005;115:35–42.

45 Aziz K, Ziebert AJ, Cobb D: Restoring erosion associated with gastroesophageal reflux using direct resins: case report. Oper Dent 2005;30:395–401.

46 Bartlett DW: Three patient reports illustrating the use of dentine adhesives to cement crowns to severely worn teeth. Int J Prosthodont 2005;18:214–218.

47 Schmidlin PR, Filli T, Imfeld C, Tepper S, Attin T: Three-year evaluation of posterior vertical bite reconstruction using direct resin composite: a case series. Oper Dent 2009;34:102–108.

48 Attin T, Filli T, Imfeld C, Schmidlin PR: Composite vertical bite reconstructions in eroded dentitions after 5.5 years: a case series. J Oral Rehabil 2012;39:73–79.

49 Perrin P, Zimmerli B, Jacky D, Lussi A, Helbling C, Ramseyer S: The stamp technique for direct composite restoration. Schweiz Monatsschr Zahnmed 2013;123:111–129.

50 Azzopardi A, Bartlett DW, Watson TF, Sherriff M: The measurement and prevention of erosion and abrasion. J Dent 2001;29:393–400.

51 Schneider F, Hellwig E, Attin T: Einfluss von Säurewirkung und Bürstabrasion auf den Dentinschutz durch Adhäsivsysteme. Dtsch Zahnarztl Z 2002;57:302–306.

52 Azzopardi A, Bartlett DW, Watson TF, Sherriff M: The surface effects of erosion and abrasion on dentine with and without a protective layer. Br Dent J 2004; 196:351–354.

53 Sundaram G, Wilson R, Watson TF, Bartlett D: Clinical measurement of palatal tooth wear following coating by a resin sealing system. Oper Dent 2007;32: 539–543.

54 Bartlett D, Sundaram G, Moazzaz R: Trial of protective effect of fissure sealants, in vivo, on the palatal surfaces of anterior teeth, in patients suffering from erosion. J Dent 2011;39:26–29.

55 Wegehaupt FJ, Tauböck TT, Attin T: Durability of the anti-erosive effect of surfaces sealants under erosive abrasive conditions. Acta Odontol Scand 2013; 71:1188–1194.

56 Wegehaupt FJ, Tauböck TT, Attin T: How to re-seal previously sealed dentine? Am J Dent 2013;26:161–165.

57 Wegehaupt FJ, Tauböck TT, Sener B, Attin T: Influence of light-curing mode on the erosion preventive effect of three different resin-based surface sealants. Int J Dent 2012;2012:874359.

Dr. A. Peutzfeldt, PhD
Department of Preventive, Restorative and Pediatric Dentistry
School of Dental Medicine, University of Bern
Freiburgstrasse 7
CH–3010 Bern (Switzerland)
E-Mail anne.peutzfeldt@zmk.unibe.ch

Lussi A, Ganss C (eds): Erosive Tooth Wear. Monogr Oral Sci. Basel, Karger, 2014, vol 25, pp 262–278
DOI: 10.1159/000360712

Erosive Tooth Wear in Children

Thiago S. Carvalho[a] · Adrian Lussi[a] · Thomas Jaeggi[a] ·
Dien L. Gambon[b]

[a]Department of Preventive, Restorative and Pediatric Dentistry, School of Dental Medicine, University of
Bern, Bern, Switzerland; [b]Department of Oral Biochemistry, Academic Centre for Dentistry Amsterdam
(ACTA), Amsterdam, The Netherlands

Abstract

Erosive tooth wear in children is a common condition. Besides the anatomical differences between deciduous and permanent teeth, additional histological differences may influence their susceptibility to dissolution. Considering laboratory studies alone, it is not clear whether deciduous teeth are more liable to erosive wear than permanent teeth. However, results from epidemiological studies imply that the primary dentition is less wear resistant than permanent teeth, possibly due to the overlapping of erosion with mechanical forces (like attrition or abrasion). Although low severity of tooth wear in children does not cause a significant impact on their quality of life, early erosive damage to their permanent teeth may compromise their dentition for their entire lifetime and require extensive restorative procedures. Therefore, early diagnosis of erosive wear and adequate preventive measures are important. Knowledge on the aetiological factors of erosive wear is a prerequisite for preventive strategies. Like in adults, extrinsic and intrinsic factors, or a combination of them, are possible reasons for erosive tooth wear in children and adolescents. Several factors directly related to erosive tooth wear in children are presently discussed, such as socio-economic aspects, gastroesophageal reflux or vomiting, and intake of some medicaments, as well as behavioural factors such as unusual eating and drinking habits. Additionally, frequent and excessive consumption of erosive foodstuffs and drinks are of importance.

Erosive tooth wear is a cumulative multifactorial process which begins following eruption of the teeth and can be considered, to a certain degree, a physiological condition. However, erosive damage to the permanent teeth occurring in early childhood may compromise the dentition for the child's entire lifetime and may require repeated expensive restoration [1]. Therefore, in order to provide children with complete dental care, it is important that dentists provide an early diagnosis of the tooth wear process, detect the main aetiological factor present in the patient and implement the required preventive measures.

Differences between Deciduous and Permanent Teeth

The most noticeable difference between deciduous and permanent teeth is related to their anatomy. Deciduous teeth are generally smaller than their permanent counterparts and have a significantly thinner enamel layer than permanent teeth [2, 3]. However, besides the anatomical differences between both kinds of teeth, there are additional histological differences that may influence their susceptibility towards dissolution and, consequently, the different patterns in erosive tooth wear.

It is well known that deciduous teeth have an outermost layer of aprismatic enamel, with a varying thickness of 15–30 μm [4–6]. The aprismatic layer is significantly thicker on buccal than lingual surfaces of anterior deciduous teeth, but no significant differences have been found between the surfaces in deciduous molars [7], though Horsted et al. [8] observed that the aprismatic layer is not common on the occlusal surfaces of the latter. Similarly, an aprismatic enamel layer has also been observed in permanent teeth, with a variable thickness of between 10 and 30 μm [9].

In relation to the enamel crystals, the arrangement of enamel prisms is reasonably similar in both deciduous and permanent teeth [10], reaching the surface of the tooth almost at a perpendicular angle in both dentitions [8]. Shellis [7] was able to trace the prisms in permanent teeth all the way to the surface, but the prisms in deciduous teeth were distinctly different – gently more curved, with slightly more pronounced Hunter-Schreger bands [11]. Furthermore, the prisms in deciduous teeth are smaller, with more complete boundaries, and are more widely spread than those in permanent teeth [11], which is suggestive of a more porous enamel in deciduous than in permanent teeth. The interprismatic fraction and prism-junction density are also greater in the enamel of deciduous teeth than in that of permanent teeth [7].

The organic content of enamel also varies according to the kind of teeth. It has been shown to range between 0.7 and 12% in deciduous teeth, which is a greater variation than that observed in permanent enamel, where organic content ranged between 0.4 and 0.8% [12]. In relation to the inorganic contents, a mineralization gradient from the surface to the amelo-dentinal junction is clearly observed in both dentitions, where a more mineralized layer of enamel is present nearer to the tooth surface and the mineralization decreases towards the amelo-dentinal junction. In general, deciduous enamel is considerably less mineralized than permanent enamel [13]. Moreover, Sønju Clasen and Ruyter [14] observed that deciduous enamel has greater total carbonate content than permanent enamel. The carbonate ion can occupy either the position of the hydroxyl (OH^-) groups (type A carbonated hydroxyapatite) or the phosphate (PO_4^{3-}) groups (type B carbonated hydroxyapatite) in the hydroxyapatite crystal. The authors observed that deciduous enamel contains more type A carbonated hydroxyapatite [14] compared to permanent enamel. Although the carbonate ion can cause distortion to the apatite crystal lattice in both positions, when it is in the position of type A it is assumed to be less tightly bound and to contribute to greater solubility of the enamel.

All these above-mentioned histological differences between deciduous and permanent enamel may be related to the fact that deciduous enamel has significantly lower surface microhardness [15–18] and elasticity [16] than permanent enamel. This, in turn, could render the deciduous teeth more susceptible to dissolution than permanent teeth.

Susceptibility of Deciduous and Permanent Teeth to Erosive Tooth Wear

Deciduous teeth have been shown to be more susceptible to in vitro caries-like acid dissolution than permanent teeth [7], and artificial caries lesions progressed 1.5 times faster in deciduous than in permanent enamel [19]. In relation to this, a number of comparative studies have also been carried out to verify whether deciduous and permanent teeth have different susceptibility to erosion. Amaechi et al. [20] examined the substance loss in both kinds of teeth after in vitro immersion in orange juice for different lengths of time (ranging from 6 to 12 h). They found a significantly greater mineral loss in deciduous teeth, which presented greater progression (1.5-fold) of erosive lesions into the enamel compared to permanent teeth. Another study by Johansson et al. [18] used enamel samples from deciduous and permanent teeth and observed that deciduous teeth were significantly softer than permanent teeth at baseline and also after immersion in citric acid (2%, pH 2.1, 37°C) for up to 30 min [18]. Moreover, in an in situ study, Hunter et al. [21] reported that deciduous enamel presented significantly greater tissue loss than permanent enamel, but no significant differences were found in their in vitro study with the same experimental set-up [22]. This led the authors to suggest that the increased susceptibility of deciduous enamel to erosion may be related, at least in part, to the presence of the salivary pellicle [21], but other studies concerning the presence of the salivary pellicle failed to find significant differences between deciduous and permanent enamel [17, 23].

Studies with relatively shorter demineralizing periods also showed no differences between the two kinds of teeth. Lippert et al. [16] used nanoindentation combined with atomic force microscopy to investigate the erosive effect of 4 different drinks on enamel (1 min immersion time for a total of 5 min) and concluded that deciduous enamel was not more susceptible to erosion than permanent enamel. Similarly, in another initial erosion study, 60 deciduous and 60 permanent human teeth were immersed in 12 different beverages and foodstuffs for 3 min, and no statistically significant differences were found in the decrease of surface microhardness between deciduous and permanent enamel [15]. In that case, it has been suggested that erosive wear in deciduous teeth appears rather over time and/or with the increasing presence of acid [21].

Deciduous enamel is significantly softer than permanent enamel [15–18]; therefore, it was reasonable to expect it to be more liable to abrasion and attrition. To analyse the effect of simultaneous erosion and abrasion in deciduous and permanent enamel, Correr et al. [24] carried out an in vitro experiment with an oral wear simulator. They observed that deciduous enamel presented more wear than permanent enamel. However, Attin et al. [25] studied the effect of erosion only or a combination of erosion and abrasion in enamel specimens and reported only negligible differences between deciduous and permanent human teeth in both treatments.

Although the aforementioned laboratory studies show conflicting results, epidemiological studies imply that deciduous teeth are less wear resistant than permanent teeth [26]. This suggests that many different factors may play a role on erosive tooth wear in vivo, which cannot be completely replicated in the laboratory.

Aetiology of Dental Erosion in Children

Identifying the main aetiological factor of tooth wear will allow the dentist to administer the required preventive measures for the patient. The aetiology of dental erosion in children does not differ greatly to that which has been previously discussed in this book, but in the present chapter we present an overview of erosive tooth wear with an emphasis on aspects related to the deciduous dentition.

General Factors Related to the Family and the Child

Taking a holistic approach to health, family-related factors like the family's household income and socio-economic status might contribute to different eating, drinking and (perhaps) oral hygiene habits in families, thus exerting some influence on the development of dental erosion in children. On the one hand, a higher socio-economic status can be related to higher educational levels of the parents, which could give them the discernment to provide their children with a healthier diet, lifestyle and better oral hygiene. On the other hand, a higher socio-economic status can also provide the family with the opportunity to acquire more sophisticated, yet erosive, substances such as soft drinks and bottle juices. In the systematic review by Kreulen et al. [26], out of the 29 selected studies reporting the prevalence of tooth wear in children and adolescents, 15 presented data on the effect of socio-economic status on erosive wear. From these, 6 studies showed that a higher socio-economic status was related to more tooth wear, whereas 7 studies reported the contrary, and 2 found no relationship between the two factors [26]. Consequently, it is still controversial whether, and to what extent, socio-economic factors can influence erosive wear in children.

The child's age is another important indicator of his/her oral health, as the prevalence of dental erosion has been shown to increase as children get older [27]. A linear association of extensive tooth wear to age has been observed in the deciduous teeth [26]. We know that when teeth erupt into the oral environment, they are susceptible to post-eruptive maturation and become more resistant to acid attacks. However, the longer the teeth are present in the mouth, the more likely they are to be exposed to the adverse effects of erosive substances and, consequently, the greater their chances of developing erosive wear.

In a similar manner to socio-economic status, the systematic review by Kreulen et al. [26] also presented data on the effect of a patient's gender on erosive tooth wear. They observed that 17 studies presented data on this issue; 8 of them observed an effect of gender on erosive tooth wear, while 9 studies showed that gender had no effect on erosion [26]. Interestingly, all of the 8 studies that presented data on the effect of gender showed that boys had significantly more erosive tooth wear than girls.

Patient-Related Factors Specific for the Child
Child's General Health
The child's general health will play a principal role in the development of dental erosion. Frequent intake of medications with an erosive potential can be a causative factor of dental erosion [1]. A recent study examined 154 Australian children aged 6–12 years and observed that 14% of them used a mouth rinse once or twice a week and 14% used one daily [28]. Although the authors did not specify the kinds of mouth rinses used by the children, they observed that the more frequent use of mouth rinse was associated with the presence of tooth wear [28]. The use of ascorbic acid (vitamin C) has also been implicated in childhood dental erosion. A recent meta-analysis on dietary factors showed that vitamin C is a risk factor for dental erosion, with an odds ratio of 1.16 [29]. As for the influence of medication for asthma on dental erosion, reports are still controversial [30–33]. Gurgel et al. [30] analysed a sample of 414 adolescents (aged 12–16 years) and reported that asthma was not associated with dental erosion. Similar results were also found by Dugmore and Rock [31] when they analysed a random sample of 1,753 children aged 12 years and re-examined more than 1,300 of them 2 years later. The presence of asthma was recorded on a self-completed questionnaire at the initial examination and the authors found that tooth erosion was present in 59% of children with asthma and in 60% of those who did not report suffering from the condition. Additionally, 88% of the drugs prescribed for the treatment of asthma for the participants in the study had a pH that does not harm the teeth [31]. Contrastingly, Shaw et al. [33] examined and recorded the level of tooth wear in a random sample of 418 children from 12 secondary schools and observed that the prevalence of dental erosion in children with asthma was higher. Al-Dlaigan et al. [32] compared three groups of adolescents aged 11–18 years: 20 with asthma requiring long-term medication, 20 referred with dental erosion and 20 age- and sex-matched chil-

dren in the control group. The authors concluded that the group of children with asthma had a higher prevalence of dental erosion compared to those in the control group. They also observed that the higher prevalence of erosion in children with asthma was associated with gastroesophageal reflux disease (GERD) [32]. This is noteworthy because children suffering from asthma also present a greater prevalence of GERD too [34], and the latter condition is probably more likely to cause dental erosion than the bronchodilators used by asthmatic children.

Gastroesophageal Reflux Disease and Eating Disorders

GERD and eating disorders are important factors related to erosive tooth wear. Eating disorders such as anorexia nervosa and bulimia are more frequently observed in adolescents and young adults than in children, but the study by Nicholls et al. [35], a national survey on eating disorders in Great Britain, found an overall incidence of eating disorders in 3 out of 100,000 children aged 6–12 years. Feeding problems are predominantly more common in children suffering from gastrointestinal problems [36], but it is estimated that 25% of normally developing children can also present this condition at some point [37]. GERD, on the other hand, is common in infants. In a longitudinal study, following a cohort of newborns in the course of 1 year, Osatakul et al. [38] found that the prevalence of GERD peaked at the age of 2 months (prevalence of 86.9%) and significantly decreased at the age of 4, 6 and 8 months, with prevalence values of 69.7, 45.5 and 22.8%, respectively. Also, the authors showed that after the age of 1 year the prevalence of children suffering from reflux was less than 8%. In a more recent nationwide cross-sectional study in France, Martigne et al. [39] estimated the prevalence of GERD to be 24.4% in infants aged between 0 and 23 months and 7.2% in children aged 2–11 years.

Regarding the association between GERD and erosive tooth wear in children, conflicting results are still found in the literature. A great variation in the prevalence of dental erosion in children suffering from GERD has been reported [40–42], which is possibly due to the small sample numbers in the studies. Aine et al. [41] examined 17 children (aged 1–16 years) with GERD and found that 87% of them presented dental erosion, whereas Dahshan et al. [42] examined 24 children (aged 2–18 years) with GERD and observed that 83.3% of them presented dental erosion. These numbers are considerably higher than those presented by O'Sullivan et al. [40], who found that, from a total of 53 children aged 2–16 years suffering from moderate-to-severe GERD, only 17% of them presented erosive tooth wear [40]. Conflicting results are also found in case-control studies. Ersin et al. [43] showed a significant difference in the number of affected teeth in children suffering from GERD in relation to the healthy control group. But in the study conducted by Linnett et al. [44], 52 children with GERD were matched with 52 control children made up of their healthy siblings and no significant differences were found in the prevalence of erosion between the two groups [44]. Similarly, Wild et al. [45] reported that children presenting GERD symptoms were not at greater risk of dental erosion than the asymptomatic children. This lack of difference is possibly due to a shorter history of GERD in young children or because reflux in older children is often limited to the oesophagus and, therefore, causes no erosive wear to the teeth. Remarkably, 2 systematic reviews on the subject also diverge on the issue; 1 study states that dental erosion related to GERD in children is of less importance than in adults [46], whereas the other states that children with GERD disease are found to be at increased risk of developing dental erosion [47]. In any case, frequent reported GERD has been associated with erosive tooth wear in young children (3-to 4-year-olds) [48]. Therefore, irrespective of the severity of the erosive wear on their patients, it is important for dentists to inquire about reflux symptoms. Additionally, low buffering capacity has been reported in adult patients suffering from GERD, but there are few studies on this topic relating to children [46]. In the study by Ersin et al. [43], the authors observed that both salivary flow rate and buffer capacity were similar in both healthy children and those suffering from GERD. Nonetheless, factors related to saliva should be further investigated in children, especially in relation to GERD.

Saliva and the Acquired Enamel Pellicle

Saliva is the main biological factor influencing dental erosion. In relation to the inorganic factors in the saliva, Järvinen et al. [49] showed that subjects with dental erosion had significantly lower salivary calcium and phosphorus concentrations than subjects without dental erosion [49]. However, when these factors were assessed in children during an epidemiological study, Wiegand et al. [50] found no differences in either calcium or phosphate concentration in saliva from children with and without erosive tooth wear. Differences in inorganic content between the saliva of adults and children have been previously shown by Anderson et al. [51], who analysed unstimulated and stimulated saliva from 15 children aged 6–12 years and 15 adults aged 19–44 years and found no difference in phosphate concentration but significantly lower calcium concentration in children's (0.31 ± 0.12 and 0.28 ± 0.05 mmol/l) than in adults' (0.53 ± 0.23 and 0.48 ± 0.19 mmol/l) unstimulated and stimulated saliva, respectively [51]. Though inorganic factors in saliva differ between adults and children, these factors might not play a crucial role in erosive wear in children, but organic factors present in saliva, such as proteins, will have some effect on the formation of the acquired enamel pellicle (AEP) and may have an impact on the susceptibility of children's dentition to erosion.

Analysing protein concentration in a group of 67 donors from different age groups, varying in age from 3 to 44 years, Cabras et al. [52] observed significantly lower protein concentrations in children aged 6–9 years than in older children and adults [52]. Similarly, Ben-Aryeh et al. [53] also analysed unstimulated whole saliva from 109 children and 25 adults and found a significant linear increase in salivary sodium, total protein concentration, amylase activity and salivary IgA with increasing age [53]. These differences in children's and adults' protein concentrations in whole saliva could lead to considerable differences between children's and adults' AEP, as well as different composition depending on whether the AEP is formed on deciduous or permanent teeth. Sønju Clasen et al. [54] collected AEP from deciduous and permanent teeth of 5 children with mixed dentition (aged 9–10 years). The AEP collected from the deciduous teeth presented a significantly greater quantity of serine and glycine but significantly less tyrosine than the AEP collected from the permanent teeth. The AEP from deciduous teeth was also thinner than the AEP from permanent teeth, corresponding to a thickness of about one third of the AEP formed on permanent teeth, and presented a slower protein adsorption process [54]. These differences were later confirmed by Zimmerman et al. [55], when they carried out a proteomic analysis of the AEP formed on deciduous enamel and showed that it consisted of only 42% of the proteins in common with AEP formed on permanent teeth. Given that AEP is formed by selective adsorption of proteins onto the enamel surface, differences between primary and permanent AEP could also be due to differences in enamel structure, surface properties and mineral content [55].

Behaviours and Drinking Habits

With regard to children's behaviours and drinking habits, these factors can significantly influence erosive wear [49, 56]. During eating/drinking, patients can adopt some specific behaviours that influence the onset and progression of dental erosion, especially those that increase the contact time between the tooth and the acidic substance. O'Sullivan and Curzon [57] carried out a case-control study with 3- to 16-year-old children presenting dental erosion in relation to matched control groups made up of children who were caries active or caries free. The authors found that 43% of the children in the erosion group had some kind of drinking habit, such as holding drinks in the mouth, sucking or swishing, whereas only 3 and 15% of the children in the caries-free and caries-active groups, respectively, presented such habits [57]. In relation to bottle-feeding, children who had used bottle-feeding for a longer time were shown to present fewer tooth surfaces affected by erosion [58], but other studies have shown the contrary. Ayers et al. [59] observed that a history of drinking from a feeding cup or bottle for longer than 6 months significantly increased cupping formations on deciduous upper first molars, and Luo et al. [60] reported that 3- to 5-year-old Chinese children were twice as likely to present dental erosion when they consumed fruit juice from a feeding bottle as a baby. In addition to how the erosive substance is consumed, the time of consumption also plays an important role in dental erosion. For example, the intake of fruit juice/syrup from a feeding bottle before bedtime also significantly increased the likelihood of tooth wear in children [60, 61], which could also be related to decreased salivary flow at night-time. However, the intake of sugary drinks before bedtime is also of great importance in relation to caries risk in children.

Nutritional Factors
Diet has been the most extensively studied aetiological factor in dental erosion. Lussi et al. [62] analysed the chemical properties (titratable acidity, buffer capacity, calcium, fluoride and phosphorus content, and degree of saturation) of 60 different dietary substances and medications and the variation in surface hardness of enamel after immersion for 2 and 4 min. In the multiple linear regression analysis, they showed that 52 and 61% of the variation in surface microhardness after immersion in the substances for 2 and 4 min, respectively, could be explained by pH, buffering capacity, calcium and fluoride concentrations in the substances [62]. The erosive potential of certain foods and drinks can be estimated using the values presented by Lussi and Hellwig [see table 3 in the chapter by Lussi and Hellwig, this vol., pp. 220–229], where the changes in enamel surface microhardness after 2 min incubation in different substances are presented.

In the meta-analysis regarding dietary factors, Li et al. [29] did not find an association between erosion and juice, sports drinks, milk or yoghurt, but vitamin C and soft drinks were significantly associated with erosion. In particular, soft drinks increased the risk of dental erosion with an odds ratio of 2.4 [29]. The excessive consumption of acidic (soft) drinks and foodstuffs has been described as the most important extrinsic factor for dental erosion [49, 63–65]. Data from the European Trade Association representing the non-alcoholic beverages industry show a continuous increase in the consumption of non-alcoholic beverages in Europe in the last years [66]. A study of 502 teenagers (aged 12–19 years) from the Netherlands showed a high level of soft drink intake among this age group, with a total of 85.2% of the participants reporting consumption of soft drinks [67]. The National Longitudinal Study of Children in Ireland recently published a research report stating that dietary behaviour in young children can be heavily influenced by the family environment, and showed that 40% of children as young as 3 years old – whose primary caregiver had a lower secondary qualification or less – consumed at least 1 portion of non-diet fizzy drinks, whereas this number decreased to 25% when the primary caregiver had a degree-level education background [68]. In the USA, soft drinks are the most prevalent sugar-sweetened beverage in adolescents and adults [69], and recent studies from national nutrition surveys have shown that at least 30% of children aged up to 5 years already consume soft drinks, with a significant increase in the amount of soft drinks consumed as the children get older [70]. Additionally, Lien et al. [71] concluded that adolescents reporting the most frequent consumption of soft drinks at age 14 still showed the most frequent consumption at age 21. Early studies have already shown the relationship between acidic substances and dental erosion in children. O'Sullivan and Curzon [57] described that children presenting erosive lesions had a greater daily consumption of carbonated drinks, fresh fruit juices and diluted cordial [57]. Additionally, if the frequency of soft drink consumption was greater than 3 times a day, the risk of presenting erosive lesions considerably increased [57]. In relation to diluted juice, Asher and Read [72] had already alerted to the fact that children could ingest such beverages in a far more concentrated form than that suggested by the manufacturer. Besides the mentioned drinks, baby drinks can also have an erosive potential. Although baby drinks seem innocuous, Hunter et al. [73] concluded that parents must be aware that commercially available baby drinks have an erosive potential, and some of the commercial products are as erosive as orange juice.

In the deciduous dentition, Gatou and Mamai-Homata [58] investigated tooth wear in 243 children aged 5–7 years and found that the consumption of soft drinks had a significant impact on tooth wear. Significant associations between tooth wear and dietary factors were also reported in younger children. Nayak et al. [74] assessed 1,002 children aged 5 years and found a 29% prevalence of dental erosion, which was significantly associated with acidic exposure from diet. In a pilot study including 202 children from Ireland (aged 5 years), an overall prevalence of dental erosion was found to be 47% and carbonated drinks and fruit squash were both significantly associated with more severe cases of dental erosion [75]. In China, a study with 1,949 children aged 3–5 years revealed a statistically significant correlation between dental erosion and intake of fruit drinks [60]. Similarly, in Brazil, Murakami et al. [48] reported that higher frequency of soft drink intake (twice a day or more than 3 times a day) presented significantly greater risk of erosive

tooth wear in a sample of 967 children aged 3–4 years. Although the above-mentioned studies observed the association between dietary factors and tooth wear on deciduous teeth, other reports have found no association between the two factors. In New Zealand, Ayers et al. [59] examined 190 children aged 5–8 years and found that the consumption of citrus fruits 2–3 times per week was associated with an increased frequency of dental cuppings. Nonetheless, in general, no association was found between tooth wear and frequency of consumption of low pH drinks. In a longitudinal study including 355 children (aged 4.5–5 years) selected from a birth cohort in the USA, no statistically significant association was found between tooth wear and soft drink or juice consumption [76]. Furthermore, besides having observed a 32% prevalence of dental erosion in 2- to 7-year-old German children, Wiegand et al. [50] found no significant association between dietary factors and erosion. Similarly, Rios et al. [77] found no significant association between tooth wear on deciduous teeth and consumption of citrus fruits or soft drinks in a convenience sample of 356 Brazilian children aged 6 years.

The above-mentioned studies show that, in the epidemiological setting, the influence of dietary factors on dental erosion in children is still equivocal. This is also reflected in the systematic review by Kreulen et al. [26], where 14 studies (out of the 29 selected) analysed the effect of diet on dental erosion, from which 6 studies reported a significant effect of diet on tooth wear in children and adolescents, and 8 studies showed the contrary [26]. However, numerous case reports and in vitro and in situ studies have confirmed the deleterious effects of different acidic substances on deciduous and permanent enamel and dentine. Such studies are relevant and should be taken into account within the clinical setting when analysing the causes of erosive tooth wear in patients.

Acidic candies are another important dietary factor. Children's affinity to sweets is notorious and the availability of candy increased dramatically in the last century, when the caries risk of sugar-containing candy became well known. However, there is a growing concern about sour sweets. In the last decades taste preference in children has changed for (extreme) sour candy and many new types and flavours of low pH candies were developed and marketed to children [78]. Solid and soft acidic candies contain organic acids, particularly citric, malic, and lactic acids, developing the characteristic fresh sour flavour. Davies et al. [79] showed that these organic acids have erosive potential for the hard dental tissues, inducing a drop in the salivary pH. In vitro, homogenized sour sweets dissolved in water lower the pH to a range of 2.3–3.1; by comparison with orange juice (pH 3.6) these sour candies were even more acidic [79]. Significant loss of enamel occurred after it was incubated for 1 h in sour sweet solution. Sucking this type of acidic candy, the salivary pH dropped to 4.5 [79, 80]. Testing lozenges in situ, Lussi et al. [81] concluded that the Knoop surface microhardness of human enamel reduced after sucking acidic candy. Brand et al. [82] determined the erosive potential of several commercially available lollipops showing different pH values. Fruit-flavoured and cola-flavoured lollipops had a very low pH (2.3–2.4), whereas yoghurt-containing and salty liquorice-flavoured lollipops had much higher pH values (3.8–4.7). In vivo, during consumption of fruit-flavoured and cola-flavoured lollipops the salivary pH dropped below pH 5.5. For strawberry yoghurt (containing calcium) and salty liquorice-flavoured lollipops the pH remained above pH 5.7. The salivary pH during consumption of the strawberry yoghurt and the liquorice-flavoured lollipops were both significantly different from all other lollipops tested (p < 0.05) [82]. Jensdottir et al. [83] also concluded that calcium-enriched candies reduced the erosive potential of acidic candies because the addition of calcium influenced the critical pH of hydroxyapatite dissolution [83, 84]. An in vivo study with fluid acidic candies, the so-called candy sprays (pH 1.9–2.2) which have to be sprayed directly on the tongue, showed a salivary pH decrease with values between pH 4.4 and 5.8 [85]. By repeated use of candy sprays and solid candies the teeth are exposed to acid for longer periods, which may exacerbate the erosive potential. During consumption, differences in the pH values of the oral saliva are related to different concentrations of citric acids [49, 86, 87].

The erosive potential of candy does not exclusively depend on pH – it is also strongly influenced by its titratable acidity. All studies on acidic candies showed a high titratable acidity, making them potentially erosive [79–83, 85, 88]. The greater the titratable acidity of the sour candy, the longer it will take for the saliva to neutralize the acids [63]. So the combination of low pH with a high buffer capacity can result in high levels of erosion. After introducing sour candies into the mouth the salivary flow is stimulated immediately, causing protective effects from the salivary buffer capacity and the acid clearance [63, 79, 80, 83]. Actively sucking during consumption obtains an even higher salivary flow rate [82]. Many in vivo results are based on the use of candy by healthy volunteers. However, lollipops, candies and candy sprays are frequently used by children and the volume of saliva in children is smaller than in adults [89, 90]. Therefore, in children the same candy in relation to lower salivary flow rates may result in even lower salivary pH values being more erosive. The volume of the sour candy in the mouth may also play a role in the loss of mineral. In situ, the mass of acidic lozenges was found to be significantly related to the level of dissolution of the enamel [81]. Many candies, like lollipops, seem to be designed to prolong acidic exposure to oral tissues during consumption [82]. In a study on 'jawbreakers' (several layers of candy around a chewing gum centre), of 302 children more than 50% estimated their time for consumption to be more than 15 min [88] – the longer the teeth are exposed to acids the longer the time for demineralization of the dental harder tissue to occur. However, after the layers of hard candy have been dissolved and the child starts chewing, the dentition is more prone to mechanical tooth wear due to attrition. It is well recognized that the interaction between erosion and attrition can have a synergetic effect on the risk of tooth wear [91, 92]. Bolan et al. [93] studied the effects of acid chewing gum and their erosive and abrasive potential and concluded that the acidic centre-filled chewing gum reduced the microhardness of primary and permanent enamel. Moreover, Paice et al. [94] showed that frequent chewers of acid-containing gums are susceptible to dentine erosion even in the presence of good salivary buffering. Since deciduous enamel is significantly softer than permanent enamel, in combination with the reduced dimension children are more at risk of developing dental erosion [18, 20–22]. When taking only 1 candy or spraying a single dose in the mouth of a child, the time of demineralization is limited. However, some labels suggest that children hold the candy in the mouth as long as possible, with a scoring chart measured by the number of seconds. Brand et al. [88] reported that some children compete with each other to keep the jawbreaker in the mouth as long as possible. The prolonged time in the mouth in combination with the very acidic pH of solid and fluid candies represent – besides tooth loss – irritation of soft tissues, lips, tongue and oral mucosa with blisters, burns and bleeding [79, 95]. There are warnings on labels to avoid spraying into the eyes. Nowadays 'tooth friendly' candies (non-cariogenic and non-erosive) form good alternatives to these acidic types recognizable by the 'Happy Tooth' logo on their label (fig. 1).

Diminishing the consumption frequency of acid-containing candy and the contact time with the dentition seems to be the best way to prevent dental erosion in relation to sour sweets.

Health promotion campaigns have encouraged the consumption of fruit and vegetables. Recently many fruit smoothies have entered the

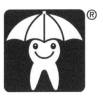

Fig. 1. Happy Tooth logo from Toothfriendly International.

market. All the smoothies investigated by Blacker and Chadwick [96] had baseline pH values of 5.0–5.3, though the smoothie on a yoghurt base had a baseline value of pH 5.7. Other smoothies tested by Ali and Tahmassebi [97] showed much lower pH values (3.7–3.9). Both studies concluded that smoothies have high titratable acidity. Although some of them had an erosive potential demonstrated with surface profilometry and microhardness testing [96, 97], different fruit varieties and fruit at different stages of ripening influence these outcomes. When children are consuming these drinks frequently, they may be heightening their risk of developing dental erosion [98].

Clinical and Histological Aspects of Dental Erosion in Children

Dental erosion in its early stages of development is difficult to diagnose, especially in primary teeth with the outermost layer of aprismatic enamel and the absence of perikymata. In children the most commonly reported areas are the palatal surfaces of the upper incisors and the occlusal surfaces of the molars. Air drying the surface of the teeth is essential for good examination. Initially, the early sign of vestibular erosion in primary teeth is the changing from the silky shining surface into a silky-glazed, sometimes even dull, appearance of enamel, progressing into concavities and surface loss and the involvement of dentine. In permanent incisors, the demineralization at first shows the loss of perikymata. Erosion on occlusal and incisal surfaces leads to rounded

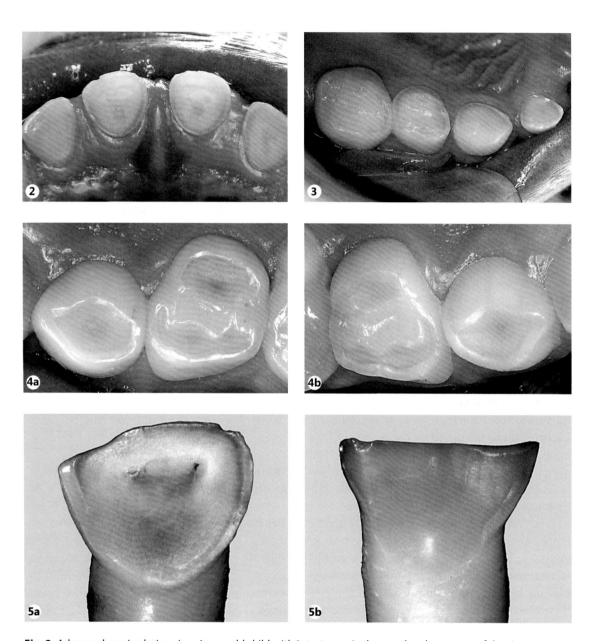

Fig. 2. Advanced erosive lesions in a 4-year-old child with intact marginal enamel and exposure of dentine.

Fig. 3. A 5-year-old child with altered morphology of the teeth. Tooth 51 was extracted because of exposure of the pulp (see fig. 5).

Fig. 4. a, b A 9-year-old child presenting severe erosive loss of tooth substance, considerable loss of anatomical features and extensive dentinal involvement.

Fig. 5. Tooth 51 from a 5-year-old child (same patient as fig. 3) presenting severe loss of tooth substance on the palatal (**a**) and labial (**b**) surfaces, with substantial alteration to the original morphology and pulp exposure.

cusps and grooves, and the overlapping edges of restorations rise above the level of adjacent tooth surfaces followed by indentations and the involvement of dentine (see fig. 2–6). In advanced stages, the original morphological features of the surface disappear with widespread dentine exposure (but intact marginal enamel) and ultimately even pulp exposure (fig. 5a, b).

Management of Dental Erosion in Children

Erosive tooth wear is a growing dental problem in society, but low severity of dental erosion in children does not cause a significant negative impact on their oral health-related quality of life [99]. This could be related to the fact that, in its initial stages, erosive lesions do not cause pain to the patient. Even though the early signs of dental erosion do not cause a considerable problem to the child, it ought to be of interest to the dental profession because it can compromise the dentition of the child for his/her entire lifetime [1]. For that reason, the early diagnosis of erosive wear lies entirely with the dentist, who should design an individual management programme for the patient in an attempt to reduce the progression of dental erosion.

For the management of dental erosion, it is important to focus mainly on its preventive aspects. For that, dentists should evaluate the different aetiological factors in a patient, identify the risk of the patient developing erosion and propose preventive measures to delay the advance of the condition [100]. The case history should contain information on the child as well as on the family. The socio-economic status of the family, i.e. household income and parental level of education, may not exert considerable influence on erosive tooth wear in children, but the background information on the child's family and environment can provide a bigger picture of the condition. Moreover, it is important to gather detailed information about the factors from the patient's side, such as the patient's general health, the presence of GERD, oral hygiene habits, salivary factors and deleterious eating and drinking habits. Also, detailed information about the factors from the aspect of nutrition should be investigated, with a comprehensive diet diary filled out by the parents/guardians [see chapter by Lussi and Hellwig, this vol., pp. 220–229]. This diary should be analysed by the dental professionals, who should be attentive to the presence and frequency of the intake of acidic substances in the patient's daily diet. These acidic substances should be avoided or their consumption decreased in frequency and quantity.

With regard to the factors from the patient's side, dental professionals should be watchful for children suffering from GERD. One sign of the presence of GERD may be in relation to food refusal. Children suffering from GERD can present more food refusal than children who do not suffer from reflux [36]. However, dental professionals must remain cognizant of the fact that if the child presents a more extreme case of food refusal, with a caloric intake lower than the daily requirement, closer observation and monitoring is necessary. In addition to the presence of GERD, it is also important to be aware of the patient's eating and drinking habits, in particular those that increase the time of contact between the erosive substance and the teeth. All such habits should be avoided, like sipping, swishing, holding drinks in the oral cavity before swallowing, chewing on drinks, or drinking acidic beverages before bedtime. Consumption should be decreased in frequency and quantity.

If a child presents erosive lesions in the deciduous dentition, it is important to bear in mind that this could be an indicating factor of erosive tooth wear in the permanent teeth. Ganss et al. [101] studied orthodontic study models from 265 children, which were initially made at a mean age of around 10 years and the final casts made 5 years later. The authors observed that children who initially presented erosive lesions in their

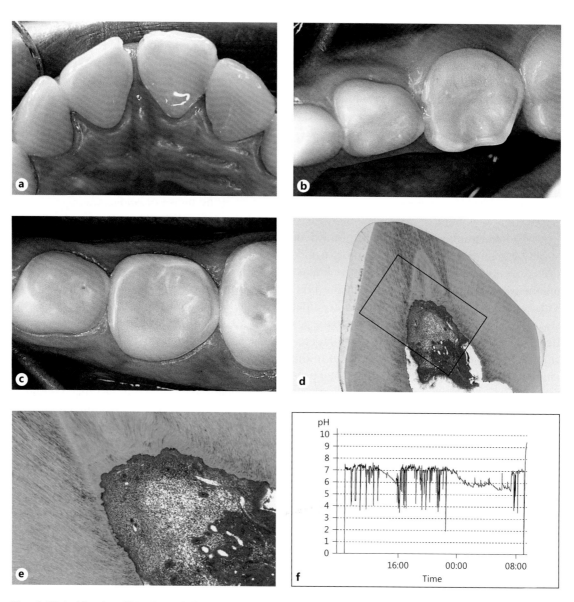

Fig. 6. Clinical (**a–c**) and histological (**d, e**) aspects of erosive tooth wear in an 8-year-old child later diagnosed with GERD (for the complete case report, see Lussi and Jaeggi [1]). **a** Erosive wear can be observed on the palatal surfaces of the upper permanent incisors. **b, c** Extensive erosive tooth wear with substantial loss of anatomical features and extensive dentinal involvement is also seen on the occlusal surfaces of the lower primary molars. **d, e** Histological section of the deciduous canine after exfoliation, showing denuded primary dentine due to tooth wear (**d**) and reactionary dentine with intact dentinal tubules (**e**), where the communication between the denuded surface of the dentinal tubules and the pulp explains the dentine hypersensitivity in this patient. **f** 24-hour pH measurements in the oesophagus after a 2-year period of medication, showing a reduction of the GERD and a pH <4 for only 3% of the measurement time.

deciduous teeth had a significantly greater risk (3.9-fold) of having erosive lesions in their permanent teeth [101]. Likewise, similar results were reported by Harding et al. [102], who assessed 123 children initially aged 5 years and re-examined them at a mean age of 12 years; they found that children who presented erosive tooth wear extending to dentine or pulp in the deciduous teeth at the age of 5 years were 5 times more likely to present erosive tooth wear on occlusal surfaces of first permanent molars at the age of 12 [102]. Considering these results, it may be suggested that tooth wear in deciduous teeth should not be considered solely as a short-term physiological process, which will be diminished with the eruption of the permanent dentition, but ought to be regarded as a predicting factor of wear in permanent teeth, and this should motivate dentists to implement early preventive measures still during childhood.

In order to determine whether the preventive measures were adequate and successful in delaying the rate of wear or if restorative interventions are necessary, it is important for dental professionals to assess the rate of progression of the tooth wear. In cases of significant areas of exposed dentine, dentine hypersensitivity, lack of functionality of the tooth or danger of pulp exposure due to proximity to the pulp [103, 104], minimally invasive restorative procedures are required. The first option in minimally invasive treatment is the sealing of the tooth surface. The use of sealants aims at ceasing any hypersensitivity and hampering erosion progression on the tooth, as it creates a physical barrier between the tooth and the erosive substance. A second choice of restorative procedure, essentially for cases of considerable substance loss, is restorative treatment with adhesive materials. A guide for clinical management has been proposed based on BEWE scores [see chapter by Ganss and Lussi, this vol., pp. 22–31]. The recommendations are based on the adult population, so some adaptations must be made in the case of erosive tooth wear in children. More specifically, with regard to young children with deciduous teeth, the time interval for repetition of the established criteria should be considerably decreased to between 6 and 12 months for routine maintenance, oral hygiene and dietary assessments in cases of no or low risk level. And in cases of medium and high risk of erosive tooth wear, the criteria should be repeated at 6-month intervals. Moreover, for older children and young adolescents, when the permanent teeth have been in the mouth for a relatively short period of time, not enough time will have gone by for clinically detectable erosive lesions to develop. Therefore, BEWE scores are bound to drop, and the cut-off values for the cumulative score of all sextants should be lowered for this age group (e.g. cumulative BEWE score of less than or equal to 2 for no risk level; between 3 and 6 for low risk level; between 7 and 10 for medium risk, and 11 or above for high risk level). This is important, considering that erosive lesions in deciduous teeth is a predicting factor for erosion in permanent teeth. Nonetheless, a meaningful longevity of any restorative procedure will only be guaranteed if the child and the parents rigorously comply with a long-term and effective preventive program [104, 105].

References

1 Lussi A, Jaeggi T: Dental erosion in children. Monogr Oral Sci 2006;20:140–151.
2 Grine FE: Enamel thickness of deciduous and permanent molars in modern Homo sapiens. Am J Phys Anthropol 2005;126:14–31.
3 Mahoney P: Testing functional and morphological interpretations of enamel thickness along the deciduous tooth row in human children. Am J Phys Anthropol 2013;151:518–525.
4 Kodaka T, Nakajima F, Higashi S: Structure of the so-called 'prismless' enamel in human deciduous teeth. Caries Res 1989;23:290–296.

5 Ripa LW, Gwinnett AJ, Buonocore MG: The 'prismless' outer layer of deciduous and permanent enamel. Arch Oral Biol 1966;11:41–48.

6 Ripa LW: The histology of the early carious lesion in primary teeth with special reference to a 'prismless' outer layer of primary enamel. J Dent Res 1966;45: 5–11.

7 Shellis RP: Relationship between human enamel structure and the formation of caries-like lesions in vitro. Arch Oral Biol 1984;29:975–981.

8 Horsted M, Fejerskov O, Larsen MJ, Thylstrup A: The structure of surface enamel with special reference to occlusal surfaces of primary and permanent teeth. Caries Res 1976;10:287–296.

9 Kodaka T, Kuroiwa M, Higashi S: Structural and distribution patterns of surface 'prismless' enamel in human permanent teeth. Caries Res 1991;25:7–20.

10 Radlanski RJ, Renz H, Willersinn U, Cordis CA, Duschner H: Outline and arrangement of enamel rods in human deciduous and permanent enamel. 3D reconstructions obtained from CLSM and SEM images based on serial ground sections. Eur J Oral Sci 2001;109:409–414.

11 Shellis RP: Variations in growth of the enamel crown in human teeth and a possible relationship between growth and enamel structure. Arch Oral Biol 1984;29:697–705.

12 Stack MV: Variation in the organic content of deciduous enamel and dentine. Biochem J 1953;54:xv.

13 Wilson PR, Beynon AD: Mineralization differences between human deciduous and permanent enamel measured by quantitative microradiography. Arch Oral Biol 1989;34:85–88.

14 Sønju Clasen AB, Ruyter IE: Quantitative determination of type A and type B carbonate in human deciduous and permanent enamel by means of Fourier transform infrared spectrometry. Adv Dent Res 1997;11:523–527.

15 Lussi A, Kohler N, Zero D, Schaffner M, Megert B: A comparison of the erosive potential of different beverages in primary and permanent teeth using an in vitro model. Eur J Oral Sci 2000;108: 110–114.

16 Lippert F, Parker DM, Jandt KD: Susceptibility of deciduous and permanent enamel to dietary acid-induced erosion studied with atomic force microscopy nanoindentation. Eur J Oral Sci 2004; 112:61–66.

17 Magalhães AC, Rios D, Honório HM, Delbem AC, Buzalaf MA: Effect of 4% titanium tetrafluoride solution on the erosion of permanent and deciduous human enamel: an in situ/ex vivo study. J Appl Oral Sci 2009;17:56–60.

18 Johansson AK, Sorvari R, Birkhed D, Meurman JH: Dental erosion in deciduous teeth – an in vivo and in vitro study. J Dent 2001;29:333–340.

19 Featherstone JD, Mellberg JR: Relative rates of progress of artificial carious lesions in bovine, ovine and human enamel. Caries Res 1981;15:109–114.

20 Amaechi BT, Higham SM, Edgar WM: Factors influencing the development of dental erosion in vitro: enamel type, temperature and exposure time. J Oral Rehabil 1999;26:624–630.

21 Hunter ML, West NX, Hughes JA, Newcombe RG, Addy M: Erosion of deciduous and permanent dental hard tissue in the oral environment. J Dent 2000;28: 257–263.

22 Hunter ML, West NX, Hughes JA, Newcombe RG, Addy M: Relative susceptibility of deciduous and permanent dental hard tissues to erosion by a low pH fruit drink in vitro. J Dent 2000;28:265–270.

23 Maupomé G, Aguilar-Avila M, Medrano-Ugalde H, Borges-Yáñez A: In vitro quantitative microhardness assessment of enamel with early salivary pellicles after exposure to an eroding cola drink. Caries Res 1999;33:140–147.

24 Correr GM, Alonso RC, Consani S, Puppin-Rontani RM, Ferracane JL: In vitro wear of primary and permanent enamel. Simultaneous erosion and abrasion. Am J Dent 2007;20:394–399.

25 Attin T, Wegehaupt F, Gries D, Wiegand A: The potential of deciduous and permanent bovine enamel as substitute for deciduous and permanent human enamel: erosion-abrasion experiments. J Dent 2007;35:773–777.

26 Kreulen CM, Van 't Spijker A, Rodriguez JM, Bronkhorst EM, Creugers NH, Bartlett DW: Systematic review of the prevalence of tooth wear in children and adolescents. Caries Res 2010;44:151–159.

27 Nunn JH, Gordon PH, Morris AJ, Pine CM, Walker A: Dental erosion – changing prevalence? A review of British national children's surveys. Int J Paediatr Dent 2003;13:98–105.

28 Fung A, Brearley Messer L: Tooth wear and associated risk factors in a sample of Australian primary school children. Aust Dent J 2013;58:235–245.

29 Li H, Zou Y, Ding G: Dietary factors associated with dental erosion: a meta-analysis. PLoS One 2012;7:e42626.

30 Gurgel CV, Rios D, de Oliveira TM, Tessarolli V, Carvalho FP, Machado MA: Risk factors for dental erosion in a group of 12- and 16-year-old Brazilian schoolchildren. Int J Paediatr Dent 2011; 21:50–57.

31 Dugmore CR, Rock WP: Asthma and tooth erosion. Is there an association? Int J Paediatr Dent 2003;13:417–424.

32 Al-Dlaigan YH, Shaw L, Smith AJ: Is there a relationship between asthma and dental erosion? A case control study. Int J Paediatr Dent 2002;12:189–200.

33 Shaw L, al-Dlaigan YH, Smith A: Childhood asthma and dental erosion. ASDC J Dent Child 2000;67:102–106.

34 Tolia V, Vandenplas Y: Systematic review: the extra-oesophageal symptoms of gastro-oesophageal reflux disease in children. Aliment Pharmacol Ther 2009; 29:258–272.

35 Nicholls DE, Lynn R, Viner RM: Childhood eating disorders: British national surveillance study. Br J Psychiatry 2011; 198:295–301.

36 Williams KE, Field DG, Seiverling L: Food refusal in children: a review of the literature. Res Dev Disabil 2010;31:625–633.

37 Arts-Rodas D, Benoit D: Feeding problems in infancy and early childhood: identification and management. Paediatr Child Health 1998;3:21–27.

38 Osatakul S, Sriplung H, Puetpaiboon A, Junjana CO, Chamnongpakdi S: Prevalence and natural course of gastroesophageal reflux symptoms: a 1-year cohort study in Thai infants. J Pediatr Gastroenterol Nutr 2002;34:63–67.

39 Martigne L, Delaage PH, Thomas-Delecourt F, Bonnelye G, Barthélémy P, Gottrand F: Prevalence and management of gastroesophageal reflux disease in children and adolescents: a nationwide cross-sectional observational study. Eur J Pediatr 2012;171:1767–1773.

40 O'Sullivan EA, Curzon ME, Roberts GJ, Milla PJ, Stringer MD: Gastroesophageal reflux in children and its relationship to erosion of primary and permanent teeth. Eur J Oral Sci 1998;106:765–769.

41 Aine L, Baer M, Mäki M: Dental erosions caused by gastroesophageal reflux disease in children. ASDC J Dent Child 1993;60:210–214.

42 Dahshan A, Patel H, Delaney J, Wuerth A, Thomas R, Tolia V: Gastroesophageal reflux disease and dental erosion in children. J Pediatr 2002;140:474–478.

43 Ersin N, Candan U, Aykut A, Onçağ O, Eronat C, Kose T: A clinical evaluation of resin-based composite and glass ionomer cement restorations placed in primary teeth using the ART approach: results at 24 months. J Am Dent Assoc 2006;137:1529–1536.

44 Linnett V, Seow WK, Connor F, Shepherd R: Oral health of children with gastro-esophageal reflux disease: a controlled study. Aust Dent J 2002;47:156–162.

45 Wild YK, Heyman MB, Vittinghoff E, et al: Gastroesophageal reflux is not associated with dental erosion in children. Gastroenterology 2011;141:1605–1611.

46 Firouzei MS, Khazaei S, Afghari P, et al: Gastroesophageal reflux disease and tooth erosion: SEPAHAN systematic review No 10. Dent Res J (Isfahan) 2011; 8:S9–S14.

47 Pace F, Pallotta S, Tonini M, Vakil N, Bianchi Porro G: Systematic review: gastro-oesophageal reflux disease and dental lesions. Aliment Pharmacol Ther 2008;27:1179–1186.

48 Murakami C, Oliveira LB, Sheiham A, Nahás Pires Corrêa MS, Haddad AE, Bönecker M: Risk indicators for erosive tooth wear in Brazilian preschool children. Caries Res 2011;45:121–129.

49 Järvinen VK, Rytömaa II, Heinonen OP: Risk factors in dental erosion. J Dent Res 1991;70:942–947.

50 Wiegand A, Müller J, Werner C, Attin T: Prevalence of erosive tooth wear and associated risk factors in 2- to 7-year-old German kindergarten children. Oral Dis 2006;12:117–124.

51 Anderson P, Hector MP, Rampersad MA: Critical pH in resting and stimulated whole saliva in groups of children and adults. Int J Paediatr Dent 2001;11:266–273.

52 Cabras T, Pisano E, Boi R, et al: Age-dependent modifications of the human salivary secretory protein complex. J Proteome Res 2009;8:4126–4134.

53 Ben-Aryeh H, Fisher M, Szargel R, Laufer D: Composition of whole unstimulated saliva of healthy children: changes with age. Arch Oral Biol 1990;35:929–931.

54 Sønju Clasen AB, Hannig M, Skjørland K, Sønju T: Analytical and ultrastructural studies of pellicle on primary teeth. Acta Odontol Scand 1997;55:339–343.

55 Zimmerman JN, Custodio W, Hatibovic-Kofman S, Lee YH, Xiao Y, Siqueira WL: Proteome and peptidome of human acquired enamel pellicle on deciduous teeth. Int J Mol Sci 2013;14:920–934.

56 Gambon DL, Brand HS, Nieuw Amerongen AV: Soft drink, software and softening of teeth – a case report of tooth wear in the mixed dentition due to a combination of dental erosion and attrition. Open Dent J 2010;4:198–200.

57 O'Sullivan EA, Curzon ME: A comparison of acidic dietary factors in children with and without dental erosion. ASDC J Dent Child 2000;67:186–192.

58 Gatou T, Mamai-Homata E: Tooth wear in the deciduous dentition of 5- to 7-year-old children: risk factors. Clin Oral Investig 2012;16:923–933.

59 Ayers KM, Drummond BK, Thomson WM, Kieser JA: Risk indicators for tooth wear in New Zealand school children. Int Dent J 2002;52:41–46.

60 Luo Y, Zeng XJ, Du MQ, Bedi R: The prevalence of dental erosion in preschool children in China. J Dent 2005; 33:115–121.

61 Al-Malik MI, Holt RD, Bedi R: The relationship between erosion, caries and rampant caries and dietary habits in preschool children in Saudi Arabia. Int J Paediatr Dent 2001;11:430–439.

62 Lussi A, Megert B, Shellis RP, Wang X: Analysis of the erosive effect of different dietary substances and medications. Br J Nutr 2012;107:252–262.

63 Lussi A, Jaeggi T, Zero D: The role of diet in the aetiology of dental erosion. Caries Res 2004;38(suppl 1):34–44.

64 Dugmore CR, Rock WP: A multifactorial analysis of factors associated with dental erosion. Br Dent J 2004;196:283–286, discussion 73.

65 Nahás Pires Corrêa MS, Nahás Pires Corrêa F, Nahás Pires Corrêa JP, Murakami C, Mendes FM: Prevalence and associated factors of dental erosion in children and adolescents of a private dental practice. Int J Paediatr Dent 2011; 21:451–458.

66 UNESDA: Statistics on the consumption of non-alcoholic beverages in Europe. http://www.unesda.org/industry.

67 Gambon DL, Brand HS, Boutkabout C, Levie D, Veerman EC: Patterns in consumption of potentially erosive beverages among adolescent school children in the Netherlands. Int Dent J 2011;61: 247–251.

68 Williams J, Murray A, McCrory C, McNally S: Growing up in Ireland. National Longitudinal Study of Children. Development from Birth to Three Years. Department of Children and Youth Affairs, 2013. http://www.growingup. ie/fileadmin/user_upload/documents/ Second_Infant_Cohort_Reports/ Development_from_Birth_to_Three_ Years.

69 Han E, Powell LM: Consumption patterns of sugar-sweetened beverages in the United States. J Acad Nutr Diet 2013;113:43–53.

70 Fulgoni VL, Quann EE: National trends in beverage consumption in children from birth to 5 years: analysis of NHANES across three decades. Nutr J 2012;11:92.

71 Lien N, Lytle LA, Klepp KI: Stability in consumption of fruit, vegetables, and sugary foods in a cohort from age 14 to age 21. Prev Med 2001;33:217–226.

72 Asher C, Read MJ: Early enamel erosion in children associated with the excessive consumption of citric acid. Br Dent J 1987;162:384–387.

73 Hunter L, Patel S, Rees J: The in vitro erosive potential of a range of baby drinks. Int J Paediatr Dent 2009;19:325–329.

74 Nayak SS, Ashokkumar BR, Ankola AV, Hebbal MI: Distribution and severity of erosion among 5-year-old children in a city in India. J Dent Child (Chic) 2010; 77:152–157.

75 Harding MA, Whelton H, O'Mullane DM, Cronin M: Dental erosion in 5-year-old Irish school children and associated factors: a pilot study. Community Dent Health 2003;20:165–170.

76 Warren JJ, Yonezu T, Bishara SE: Tooth wear patterns in the deciduous dentition. Am J Orthod Dentofacial Orthop 2002;122:614–618.

77 Rios D, Magalhães AC, Honório HM, Buzalaf MA, Lauris JR, Machado MA: The prevalence of deciduous tooth wear in six-year-old children and its relationship with potential explanatory factors. Oral Health Prev Dent 2007;5:167–171.

78 Gambon DL, Brand HS, Veerman EC: Dental erosion in the 21st century: what is happening to nutritional habits and lifestyle in our society? Br Dent J 2012; 213:55–57.

79 Davies R, Hunter L, Loyn T, Rees J: Sour sweets: a new type of erosive challenge? Br Dent J 2008;204:E3, discussion 84–85.

80 Jensdottir T, Nauntofte B, Buchwald C, Bardow A: Effects of sucking acidic candy on whole-mouth saliva composition. Caries Res 2005;39:468–474.

81 Lussi A, Portmann P, Burhop B: Erosion on abraded dental hard tissues by acid lozenges: an in situ study. Clin Oral Investig 1997;1:191–194.

82 Brand HS, Gambon DL, Paap A, Bulthuis MS, Veerman EC, Amerongen AV: The erosive potential of lollipops. Int Dent J 2009;59:358–362.

83 Jensdottir T, Nauntofte B, Buchwald C, Bardow A: Effects of calcium on the erosive potential of acidic candies in saliva. Caries Res 2007;41:68–73.

84 Ericsson Y: Enamel-apatite solubility: investigations into the calcium phosphate equilibrium between enamel and saliva and its relation to dental caries. Acta Odontol Scand 1949;8:1–139.

85 Gambon DL, Brand HS, Nieuw Amerongen AV: The erosive potential of candy sprays. Br Dent J 2009;206:E20, discussion 530–531.

86 Hunter ML, Patel R, Loyn T, Morgan MZ, Fairchild R, Rees JS: The effect of dilution on the in vitro erosive potential of a range of dilutable fruit drinks. Int J Paediatr Dent 2008;18:251–255.

87 Lussi A, Jaeggi T: Erosion – diagnosis and risk factors. Clin Oral Investig 2008; 12(suppl 1):S5–S13.

88 Brand HS, Gambon DL, Van Dop LF, Van Liere LE, Veerman EC: The erosive potential of jawbreakers, a type of hard candy. Int J Dent Hyg 2010;8:308–312.

89 Crossner CG: Salivary flow rate in children and adolescents. Swed Dent J 1984; 8:271–276.

90 Watanabe S, Dawes C: Salivary flow rates and salivary film thickness in five-year-old children. J Dent Res 1990;69: 1150–1153.

91 Litonjua LA, Andreana S, Bush PJ, Cohen RE: Tooth wear: attrition, erosion, and abrasion. Quintessence Int 2003;34: 435–446.

92 Addy M, Shellis RP: Interaction between attrition, abrasion and erosion in tooth wear. Monogr Oral Sci 2006;20:17–31.

93 Bolan M, Ferreira MC, Vieira RS: Erosive effects of acidic center-filled chewing gum on primary and permanent enamel. J Indian Soc Pedod Prev Dent 2008;26:149–152.

94 Paice EM, Vowles RW, West NX, Hooper SM: The erosive effects of saliva following chewing gum on enamel and dentine: an ex vivo study. Br Dent J 2011;210:E3.

95 Robyn RL, Robert JM, John DR: Pucker up: the effects of sour candy on your patients' oral health. A review of the dental erosion literature and pH values for popular candies. Northwest Dent 2008;87:20–21, 24–25, 28–29 passim.

96 Blacker SM, Chadwick RG: An in vitro investigation of the erosive potential of smoothies. Br Dent J 2013;214:E9.

97 Ali H, Tahmassebi JF: The effects of smoothies on enamel erosion: an in situ study. Int J Paediatr Dent, Epub ahead of print.

98 Brand HS: Summary of an in vitro investigation of the erosive potential of smoothies. Br Dent J 2013;214:172–173.

99 Vargas-Ferreira F, Piovesan C, Praetzel JR, Mendes FM, Allison PJ, Ardenghi TM: Tooth erosion with low severity does not impact child oral health-related quality of life. Caries Res 2010;44: 531–539.

100 Taji S, Seow WK: A literature review of dental erosion in children. Aust Dent J 2010;55:358–367, quiz 475.

101 Ganss C, Klimek J, Giese K: Dental erosion in children and adolescents – a cross-sectional and longitudinal investigation using study models. Community Dent Oral Epidemiol 2001;29: 264–271.

102 Harding MA, Whelton HP, Shirodaria SC, O'Mullane DM, Cronin MS: Is tooth wear in the primary dentition predictive of tooth wear in the permanent dentition? Report from a longitudinal study. Community Dent Health 2010;27:41–45.

103 Lambrechts P, Van Meerbeek B, Perdigão J, Gladys S, Braem M, Vanherle G: Restorative therapy for erosive lesions. Eur J Oral Sci 1996;104:229–240.

104 Harley K: Tooth wear in the child and the youth. Br Dent J 1999;186:492–496.

105 Schlueter N, Jaeggi T, Lussi A: Is dental erosion really a problem? Adv Dent Res 2012;24:68–71.

Dr. T.S. Carvalho, PhD
Department of Preventive, Restorative and Pediatric Dentistry
School of Dental Medicine, University of Bern
Freiburgstrasse 7
CH–3010 Bern (Switzerland)
E-Mail thiago.saads@zmk.unibe.ch

Author Index

Subject Index

Ion pair 166

Knoop hardness test, erosive tooth wear
    assessment 128, 129

Laser therapy, dentine hypersensitivity 117
Literature trends, erosive tooth wear 1, 2
Longitudinal microradiography, erosive tooth wear
    assessment 132, 133
Lussi index 50–52

Matrix metalloproteinases
    erosive tooth wear role 39
    inhibitors for remineralization promotion 248–250
Measuring light microscopy, erosive tooth wear
    assessment 125, 126, 137
Medications, erosive tooth wear epidemiology 84, 85,
    158–161
Microadiography, erosive tooth wear assessment 132,
    133, 137
Mouth rinse
    acid protection with polymers 245, 246
    erosion studies 156, 157
    fluoride mouth rinse
        erosion/abrasion studies 237–239
        erosion-only studies 235–238
    restorative therapy considerations 254, 255

Nanoindentation, erosive tooth wear assessment 135,
    138
Noncarious cervical lesions (NCCL) 39–41

Occupational risks, erosive tooth wear 85–94, 149–151
Optical coherence tomography, erosive tooth wear
    assessment 127, 128, 137
Optical reflection, erosive tooth wear assessment 126,
    127, 137
Oxalates 116

Pellicle
    acid diffusion 2, 3
    acid-protective properties 208, 209
    brushing effects 41, 42
    children 267
    composition 2, 206
    enhancement 212
    erosive tooth wear protection mechanisms 209–
        212
    formation 199, 206–208

pH
    beverages and foodstuffs 6, 165
    buffering capacity, undissociated acids, and
        chelation 144, 145
    erosive tooth wear studies 5–7, 14
    oral hygiene products 156–158
    restorative material longevity under acidic
        conditions 255, 256
Phosphate, food and beverage content 147
Potassium, dentine hypersensitivity management
    114
Pregnancy, erosive tooth wear epidemiology 193
Proteomics, pellicle 208
Proton-promoted dissolution 173

Quantitative light-induced fluorescence, erosive tooth
    wear assessment 134, 137

Reflux Disease Questionnaire 185
Relative dental abrasivity 34, 39
Restorative therapy, erosive tooth wear
    adhesion of restorative materials 254, 255
    longevity of restorative materials under acidic
        conditions 255, 256
    overview 256, 257
    prevention and early diagnosis importance 253
    resin composite or ceramic for deep loss
        258–260
    sealant or resin composite for minimal loss 257,
        258
Rumination, erosive tooth wear epidemiology 192,
    193

Saliva
    children 267
    erosive tooth wear protection 41, 42, 227
    flow rate 198
    hyposalivation erosion studies 158, 200, 201
    individual variation 201–203
    pellicle, *see* Pellicle
Saturated solution 164, 171
Scanning electron microscopy
    erosive tooth wear assessment 124, 125, 136, 137
    histology, *see* Dentine, Enamel
Sealants
    acid protection 245
    restorative therapy 257, 258
Secondary ion mass spectrometry, erosive tooth wear
    assessment 135, 136